The Miracle of Pain

The Miracle of Pain

David E. Smalley, M.D.

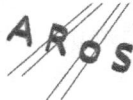

AROS

All Rays of Sunshine
Book Publishing

Riverside, California

Published by All Rays of Sunshine Book Publishing,
6185 Magnolia Avenue #264, Riverside, California 92506.
Phone 951-850-1472. Email: arosBooks@att.net. On the
web: https://themiracleofpain.com.

ISBN: 978-1-7322873-2-7 (paperback with full color cover)
Total of 384 pages with 19 grayscale illustrations and index
Paperback bulk orders (family, friends, companies): 3-5 books
(20% off), 6-47 books (35% off) and 48+ books (50% off)

ISBN: 978-1-7322873-1-0 (eBook)
ISBN: 978-1-7322873-0-3 (hardcover)

Cataloging—
HEA036000 Health & Fitness: Pain Management
HEA028000 Health & Fitness: Health Care Issues
SEL026000 Self Help: Substance Abuse and Addictions
Thema Subjects—VF: Family & health; VS: Self-help &
personal development; VXA: Mind, body, spirit: thought &
practice; MKAL: Pain & pain management

The author does not endorse any referenced medication, procedures, products, treatments or physicians in this book or on any website, such as https://www.orthoinfo.org, from the American Academy of Orthopedic Surgeons. The content is educational and should not be used as medical advice.

All who are seeking orthopedic (orthopaedic) advice should ask their orthopedic surgeon or should find one through the American Academy of Orthopaedic Surgeons "Find an Orthopaedist" link at their website: http://www.aaos.org.

The use of trademarks is for informational or editorial purposes only and are not endorsements for this book or for the trademark.

❦ Contents ❧

—— **Dedication** ——

To my wife and family, my patients and
the Lord God, the God of Abraham, Isaac and Jacob,
an unchanging, loving and eternal God of Miracles

৶৶

ᔓ **Illustrations, by Chapter** ᔒ

All images are by the author, including the full color cover.

Chapter 1

How My Interest in Pain Began

During my years of medical practice in the specialty of orthopedic surgery, I found tremendous satisfaction in helping patients one at a time, both with and without surgery. By listening to my patients in the office and dealing with their challenges, I was learning more about pain with each patient. Prescribing medications was easy. When the indications were right, performing surgery was gratifying. However, over the 30 years of my practice, I found increasing numbers of patients with pain who needed neither medication nor surgery.

Many patients needed to have someone listen to them. After listening, examining and telling patients what was wrong with them, I described the treatment options for them. Many wanted the details of what to do and what not to do. They may have already taken a lot of medication or had surgery. I saw many new patients who had failed treatments elsewhere and still had painful conditions. Some patients were addicted to medication, but they were still struggling with worsening pain. Some were seeing "alternative" health care practitioners and wanted better options. Some were struggling with overbearing restrictions of insurance or government health care systems and did not know what else to do.

Teaching patients the basic principles of what to do for healing and recovery from pain was fun. It became important because of the prevalent misinformation in our world. By applying what I learned from patients who did not need surgery, I was better able to help my patients who had surgery. They achieved better long-term pain relief. Patients were excited to learn basic things that they had never been told by their previous physicians or their family doctor.

It became apparent that I needed to teach patients more specifically what I was asking them to do. For example, I gave them the number of minutes for an activity or the number of repetitions for an exercise. More specifics at home, at work or during sports became essential to resolve pain for many patients. After finding the level of the patient's function, the specific things I gave the patient to do were an educated guess.

1

The patient could modify the specifics based on the principles I also taught them in our visits. I asked them to remember the principles and learn to apply them consistently.

Learning from our mistakes is good. To learn from the mistakes of others is better. It is, however, best if we trust and learn from our parents or other good sources before seeing the damage or pain that occurs with mistakes. Most of us do not ask for the challenges that we face with pain. Nevertheless, as we feel pain, we can learn from the waxing and waning that naturally occurs with it.

Without pain reminding us that we have done too much, we would wear out many parts of our body. Pain is a gift from our Creator for our benefit and to help us learn in many ways. Pain is always a warning sign. Pain is one of the first lessons we learn as a child. What happens if we do not feel pain? A hot stove may destroy an area of our skin. As adolescents, many of us learn that a bad sunburn is miserable. As adults, we learn to be more careful, respect our skin, get some sunlight and avoid sunburns.

I graduated from George Washington University Medical School in Washington, D.C. in 1976 with an M.D. degree. Afterwards, our young family with 2 children moved to Columbus, Ohio, where I trained at Ohio State University (OSU). I was a surgical intern the first year and then, a general surgery resident the next year. The surgical specialty training rotations in my second year were all exciting to me, but I found a passion for orthopedic surgery. All the mechanical aspects of it were interesting to me. The anatomy, drills, saws and screws were just a small part of what I enjoyed. For the next 3 years from 1978 to 1981, also at OSU, I served as an orthopedic surgery resident and loved it.

In 1981, I joined a small private practice with 3 other orthopedic surgeons in Riverside, California and stayed with the same partnership until I retired in 2010. During my years in orthopedic surgery, I wanted to help patients make better choices. In time, I was better at being more specific and more proficient at explaining principles. Then, it was easier for patients and their families to understand. Applying principles for their recovery from pain also became easier. Without principles, they were figuratively lost without a compass.

The application of principles for taking care of pain is more difficult than understanding them. It takes effort and practice to remember them, get good at them, be consistent with them and learn from pain as we go. Most principles are not complicated. A few of them are difficult to understand because of widespread fads and disinformation. This book illustrates the principles in diverse ways. Because varied experiences are ways we learn to apply principles, in time, the principles will start sounding familiar.

By not ignoring pain, we are able to learn from it. When we feel less pain or the pain goes away, we need to learn from what we are doing right. For some patients to make more consistent progress, teaching them what to do every 10 to 15 minutes was necessary. When I was injured, stiff or sore, I became a patient. Many experiences I had as a patient allowed me to experiment with and fine-tune my ideas. Later in my practice, principles about pain became more real for patients when I shared experiences as a father, a husband, a medical doctor and a Boy Scout leader.

When patients were trying to change habits, they needed to use some of the principles I was teaching them. Change is always difficult, but they had to if they wanted to improve. Bad habits and not taking care of or abusing our bodies comes in many forms. Smoking and obesity adversely affect the recovery of patients. Many asked for help.

Other less obvious habits can be just as limiting and destructive, such as risky behavior and fatigue with high activity levels. Often, both the patient and I did not know they had bad habits. Finding the bad habits was difficult. Another challenge was motivating them to stop habits they clung to. I could not force them to change. They had to want to change before it could begin to happen. Then, I had to give them tools or things to do that they needed to use instead.

A change in the habits of most patients happens over time, usually months and sometimes longer. I had to learn patience with them while they tried to change. They had to learn patience with themselves. They had to have patience with me as I tried to understand and help. Habits include addictions to many things. When a patient is willing, addictions are also possible to stop. For the healing and recovery of a patient from pain, I had to find and deal with any counterproductive habit, or there was no improvement.

Since 1998 when I began this book, I recognized it as an opportunity to help more people than one patient at a time. My purpose is to offer hope to those who are struggling with all types of musculoskeletal pain. By hearing true account stories and principles, we can improve our capacity to cope with pain and improve the likelihood of resolving pain. Though we often feel alone in our pain, everyone has experienced pain. It is a part of life with few exceptions.

Basic principles of movement, position changes, stretching, strength, adequate rest and hydration with fluids, especially water, will never change. We should never overlook these good tools. Like so many other good things, however, any valuable tool can be misunderstood or misused. Many people have tested and used both the old and new concepts I describe in this book, some for over 30 years.

In 1972, I remember being in a large classroom auditorium for a lecture. It was my first year of medical school in downtown Washington, D.C. A professor told us, "Once you have a back problem, you will always have a back problem." I wondered about the truth of that statement. Was there any scientific basis for his opinion? Though what the professor said is a common experience and belief, he did not cite any sources or give any reasons. It seemed to be a negative assessment for a very common problem.

I wondered if conquering back pain was possible. I decided then that I should try to prove or disprove that negative opinion. My hypothesis was, "When you have a back problem, you can get over it." Until then, I had never had any back pain. I had no idea how I was going to test the hypothesis. The scientific method is seeing a problem, studying it, forming a hypothesis, designing an experiment, conducting tests, looking at the results and finding truth and principles.

We retest the conclusions many times to confirm them and to fine-tune their use. Truth is exciting to discover and to use, whether the truth confirms or refutes the hypothesis. We can also use isolated experiences to study a phenomenon and suggest a hypothesis (anecdotal evidence). Strength in a research study conclusion comes from a sufficient number of tests and from honestly reporting what is found.

The opportunity to test my hypothesis came sooner than I thought. Near the end of my first year of medical school, I had finished building and staining a large bookcase, from the top of my desk to our apartment ceiling. Later while sitting at my desk, I noticed some mild low back pain when I arose from the chair. I felt it for a few months if I stood and bent forward at the waist. It was a low back strain (lumbar strain).

Because I wanted to see if I could get over the pain completely, I decided to avoid bending for a year. I was afraid to bend over until I discovered the first of many stretching modifications. The first one was spreading my feet apart while bending forward at the waist, which felt amazingly good! I stretched often and had no pain. Gradually, I resumed all extracurricular activities, including pickup basketball and slow pitch softball. Our church had a softball league that played on the CIA fields in McLean, Virginia near our apartment. That year, I coached and played on our softball team.

Since then, learning about pain continued when I had pain in other areas of the body. I looked at the pain as an opportunity and experimented with what to do and what not to do. Over a period of years, I gradually incorporated principles I learned into what I encouraged my patients to try if they did not improve with the usual approaches. After listening to their responses, we made slight to major adjustments in what they were doing.

Sometimes patients came back for a follow-up visit and told me what they thought I wanted to hear. I had to encourage them to tell me honestly what they felt and not what they thought I wanted to hear. When they did not improve or were worsening, hearing the truth was hard for me. But I had to hear it, so I could understand them, make changes and do some effective fine-tuning. If patients did not continue to improve, additional medical testing had to be considered.

At each office or hospital visit, I asked patients with pain if their pain was overall better or worse. I had to learn to spend time with them on that question. Glossing over the question and the answer was a disservice to them, and it would be misleading for me. Because a 0 to 10 pain scale did not give enough information, I learned to quantify pain in better ways. Variations of the pain and time periods with an absence of pain are only two of many examples. Pain characteristics are more important than a pain scale number.

As a patient, I learned that doing everything correctly is difficult even when we know what to do. As patients tried what I asked, the successes came sooner and more consistently if I could get them to learn along the way. If they were "no better," they often expressed frustration with their situation and with what I told them to do. It was a huge red warning flag when a patient returned for a second office visit and said, "I did everything you said." Did they really?

I could not remember or do everything I said. It was usually a lot. My medical notes gave me a summary of what I told them and had asked them to do. If I asked them what they had tried, they usually gave me a warped version of what I had asked them to do, especially if I asked for specifics. We had to change what the patient was doing or at least fine-tune it. When responding and encouraging change, I had to learn to be patient and specific with what I wanted them to do differently.

In my training program at OSU, I had seen a few times where getting angry helped motivate a patient to make better choices. But within a few years of medical practice, I learned that getting angry with a patient for making mistakes did no good at all. Instead, if I showed patience and explained the diagnosis again and what I wanted them to do and why, then I had a patient who was willing to try again. We were on the same side of the battle.

As I learned to patiently clarify and repeat things as often as the patient needed, they always appreciated it. Repeating instructions was never destructive. If a patient chose to disagree, despite explanations and encouragement, I simply explained the consequences and left it alone. I let them have their opinion. I believe it is true that, "Anger... builds nothing, but it can destroy everything."[1]

Another exciting principle I learned years ago was that many of the exercises and stretches I told patients to do were correct. But I was not communicating enough to patients how often to do them. I did not know. I was not a physical therapist. Because of reimbursement decreases from insurance carriers, physical therapists were beginning to spend less time with patients. To keep their business open, they had to be more efficient, especially with difficult patients. It took learning from my own trials with pain to find some details that were being lost, not used or were not known.

This book is for individuals who are having problems with musculoskeletal pain and for their family and friends. When a family member or a friend attends an appointment with the patient, they understand the doctor's diagnosis and recommendations better. Listen to the patient's complaints and the doctor's response. The family member or friend can help the patient remember. They cannot help the patient if the patient is not willing to learn from the pain. They should avoid enabling poor habits, risky behavior and other activities that contribute to the problem. To listen, learn and ask questions about how to apply the recommendations is important for a patient. With better understanding of the medical doctor's diagnosis and recommendations, they remember and do more of what they should do.

In this book, I offer insights for both common and unusual orthopedic diagnoses that are poorly understood. For example, common, chronic sprains and resulting severe, chronic pain are greatly under diagnosed and often poorly explained. Because the problems are under appreciated or ignored, over testing, poor healing, poor compliance and over

---

[1] Deseret News, "Early Hardships Shaped Candidates," Lawrence Douglas Wilder, Governor of Virginia 1990–1994, quoted by Jill Lawrence, Associated Press writer, December 1, 1991, www.deseretnews.com/article/196604/early-hardships-shaped-candidates.html?pg=all, accessed May 9, 2018.

use of medication are a natural and unavoidable result. Risks increase dramatically when pain or reinjury continues, whether it is in the arms, legs, back or neck.

Frequently, patients asked me if I could write anything down for them or if they could read something. A patient listening to understand and then asking questions about anything that does not make sense is better. They could also write notes during or after the appointment. For patients with memory, mental or emotional challenges, I often agreed to write down basic principles or tools for them.

All patients need a doctor who will listen. Then, patients need concise, direct answers for their specific problems and questions. I encouraged patients between visits to remember as much as they could and to put into practice what they learn from pain. That was reinforced by comparing notes and answering questions when a patient came back. We can then sort out what they can do next. Most patients cannot remember everything from the first visit, and the same is true for me if I am a patient. The medical record gives a summary of complaints, findings and recommendations.

To my back and neck pain patients, I gave 20-page booklets written by others that helped some. For pain with a recent onset, their principles were straightforward. They were less helpful for persisting pain. Pain that persists 3 months or more is the definition of chronic pain. The only part of the back booklet that I had a problem with was a recommended, preferred sleeping position on the side (lateral decubitus position). The sleeping position is good, but patients need to know that they should not stay there. If the position feels good, use it and come back to it often. The key is to change positions often.

The neck booklet, however, had some paragraphs I crossed out that suggested the use of above-the-head neck traction, chiropractic and acupuncture. There are better ways to deal with neck problems. They start with simple instructions of what to do and what not to do. The rest of the neck booklet information was okay. The booklet did not mention surgery, which is rarely an early answer.

Another orthopedic diagnosis with chronic pain is reflex sympathetic dystrophy (RSD). Most doctors and patients poorly understand it, and it is much more difficult to deal with than pain from a chronic sprain. RSD is a complex group of symptoms and findings with a common denominator of pain that is out of proportion to what we normally expect. It can be after an injury, a surgery or another trigger. Its name describes a specific mechanism of pain, which is dysfunction of the sympathetic nervous system.[2] It occurs in an area or a large region of the body, especially an arm or leg.

Reflex sympathetic dystrophy is a condition that strikes fear into most orthopedic surgeons. Dealing with it is problematic and time consuming. Many patients with it get worse and tend to be litigious. Some doctors have relabeled RSD since the mid-1990s as chronic regional pain syndrome (type 1 or type 2). But that diagnosis is a step backwards and is only a descriptive diagnosis. It gives patients no understanding of what is contributing to the pain and what to do about it. Another example of a descriptive diagnosis of little help is a diagnosis of "low back pain." Some doctors give it in place of the most likely real diagnosis of chronic low back sprain. Real diagnoses often take longer to explain, which should be a good thing.

Though RSD is always a challenge, I became more comfortable dealing with it over the last 20 years of my active practice. With patience on my part and effort by the patient, RSD can usually go in the right direction with less pain before the next office visit. Knowing what RSD is, what to do and what not to do is a huge help. But even with a doctor's one-on-one evaluation and specific caring treatment, it often remains a problem with severe pain and stiffness.

---

[2] The complex anatomy and physiology of the sympathetic nervous system includes nerve cells that extend from the spinal cord of the mid back, thoracolumbar levels T1 to L2, to just in front of and on either side of the spinal vertebrae as nodules, chains and nets. Additional nerve cells extend from there as tiny nerves that, among many other things, control muscle tone of blood vessels. For most blood vessels, increased sympathetic nerve activity constricts the blood vessel, but for others, such as in deep muscle, it dilates the blood vessel for greater blood flow. This generally gets many internal organs of the body ready for quick action, "fight or flight."

The Miracle of Pain

This book is a compilation of many true accounts with many different, difficult pain syndromes that I have learned from. They have helped me help others. I hope that these accounts will improve understanding of pain by patients and their families as the experiences have done for me. I also hope that the coping skills of patients will improve. They must, to lessen pain. With a little additional knowledge and practice, patients can begin to understand how much control over pain they have. I have carefully selected concepts to help as many people with ongoing musculoskeletal pain as possible.

Musculoskeletal pain can be directly from an injury such as a wrist sprain. It can also be from a problem in the muscles, joints or bones such as a bone tumor. These are examples of primary musculoskeletal pain. Other conditions in other structures of the body, such as a head injury, gall bladder attack, heart attack, infection or colon cancer, can result in pain indirectly affecting the muscles and joints. This indirect or referred pain is secondary musculoskeletal pain.

I have added limited medical terms in parentheses. For explanations of selected medical terms, I have used footnotes. To protect privacy, I have changed the names of my patients, ages, other details and the doctors or others associated with them. Any likeness of these names or details to persons is purely coincidental. The names of public persons are used with sources in footnotes where needed.

While reading this book or listening to others, as is always the case, bring any health concerns or serious issues to your licensed health care professional or personal physician. This book does not take the place of proper examination, testing, diagnosis, treatment recommendations and follow-up visits by an orthopedic surgeon or other appropriate, licensed medical specialists.

10

Chapter 2

"No Pain, No Gain?"

For me, learning about pain began well before I attended medical school. At the age of 5, I developed a severe autoimmune illness, Henoch-Schönlein purpura, resulting in pain and complications.[3] From French Hospital, the doctors transferred me by ambulance to Children's Hospital in Los Angeles, California. I was there for a total of 4 months and have vivid memories of part of it. I had pneumonia, headaches and groin pain. At one point, I remember having difficulty breathing in an oxygen tent in an Intensive Care Unit (ICU).

Other than having a lot of pain in my joints, abdomen and many other places, I do not remember much of the first few weeks. My parents and my pediatrician, the late Merl J. "Kit" Carson, M.D., were very concerned because I had the dreaded complication of kidney damage (glomerulonephritis). After enduring many episodes of pain, doctor consultations and a new treatment at the time with cortisone, I gradually began to feel better.

After being in a hospital bed for over 3 months, I could not get up out of bed to sit or stand. For 3 weeks, therapists lifted me into a hospital pool and encouraged me to move. Because I love water, I was in heaven and usually was the only one in the pool. As I tried to move, a therapist and flotation devices supported me. I could not do much at first, but with pool therapy, I learned how to walk again.

Back at home, I continued to recover mobility and strength over the next year. After the follow-up tests, doctors told us that there were no residuals of purpura, kidney damage or other problems. My parents felt that my recovery was a miracle. My dad told the story many times, and I am grateful he wrote about the details in his journal.

---

[3] Henoch-Schönlein purpura is an autoimmune illness that affects multiple body systems, including bleeding and pain, especially in the skin, joints, gastrointestinal tract, genitals and kidneys of young children, mostly males. Glomerulonephritis is a complication that can occur early or late. For a detailed medical definition, see Stedman's Medical Dictionary, Lippincott Williams & Wilkins, 28th Edition, 2005, at Drugs.com, www.drugs.com/dict/henoch-sch-ouml-nlein-purpura.html, accessed May 9, 2018.

The Miracle of Pain

Two years later, when I was 7 years old, I climbed high in a tree in our backyard. My concerned mother yelled at me, "Get down out of that tree or you might break something." I reluctantly scaled down out of the tree. A few minutes later, my brother was chasing me in the backyard. I slipped on wet grass and fell backwards onto a cement sidewalk, hitting my left elbow. Though there were no breaks in the skin, it swelled immediately. My father took me back to Children's Hospital in Los Angeles. I had broken my left elbow.

The doctor said that a piece of bone was turned around 180 degrees (displaced intra-articular closed distal humerus fracture). That night, he performed surgery, repairing the fracture with stainless steel pins (open reduction and internal pin fixation). My souvenir is a residual 5-inch scar on the outer side of the left elbow. About 2 months after the fracture repair, I remember the orthopedic surgeon, Dr. Peterson in Glendale California, taking out the two stainless steel pins in his office with a pair of pliers. He told me it would hurt for a few seconds. He was right, but it hurt a lot for a few seconds.

I still appreciate and respect the doctor's honesty. He told me ahead of time, what he was going to do. Years later, I tried to do the same for my patients. Some children and adults have phobias of doctors because a doctor, years before, did a procedure on them quickly without telling them or explaining it. For some, the trauma can be difficult to overcome. Patients appreciate doctors talking to them honestly. Patients want the doctor to explain what they need to do.

The recovery from my left elbow fracture and surgery was full and without deformity. At the start of third grade, the doctor allowed me to go outside for recess without restrictions. The next year, I played Little League baseball. My older brother and I were on the same team. I loved it because he was the catcher for our team, and I was one of the pitchers. Local newspapers listed the battery of Smalley-Smalley when I pitched. Before I was 40 years old, I only had one other broken bone. On the first day of a college wrestling class, a large class member landed directly on top of me and broke one of my ribs.

After I was 40 years old, I have had six other injuries with broken bones. I do not have soft or brittle bones, such as osteogenesis imperfecta, osteomalacia or osteoporosis. I am otherwise healthy, and the likely cause of my fractures is some mild risk taking. The first of the six injuries was when I fell while waterskiing at 40 miles per hour and sustained a couple of right rib fractures. While snowboarding, I sustained a left ankle fracture (nondisplaced medial malleolus).

The third injury included fractures of the tips of my right middle and ring fingers while getting up on a slalom waterski. Trying to stay up, I held on to the tow rope too long (distal phalanx tuft fractures). Then, left rib fractures occurred from a slide tackle while playing keep-away with a soccer ball in the backyard. I rolled on the grass, but my left elbow hit my chest. Because of the pain, I had to miss Thanksgiving dinner.

The fifth injury was from falling off a ladder while picking apricots. I held on to a large branch and fractured my left ring finger. The last injury was a right ankle fracture (medial and lateral malleoli). I slipped on decomposed granite, descending on the South Ridge Trail from 8,800-foot Tahquitz Peak in August 2010. The recovery from this last fracture was prolonged by right foot reflex sympathetic dystrophy (RSD) after a few days of a tight fiberglass cast and doing too much.

All six of these injuries included nondisplaced or minimally displaced fractures. They all healed without the need for surgery and without persisting problems. Accounts of what I learned from two of the six injuries are in later chapters of this book. All injury mechanisms were low-energy. However, I admit some risk taking with participation in fast and slow pitch softball, rock climbing, snow skiing, snowboarding, heliboarding, cliff and waterfall rappelling, canyoneering, waterskiing, wakeboarding, snorkeling, sea kayaking, wind surfing, hiking and mountain biking.

With good conditions and good instructors, I have had fun with many activities at appropriate skill levels. I like to learn new things if the level of risk is reasonably low. But I will not do dirt bikes, bungee jumping or sky diving. Wii Sports Resort sky diving is good enough for me. Gardening and pruning trees are also passions of mine that do not have a lot of risk, usually. Fortunately, I have not been in any automobile accidents.

I remember patients and families in my office asking, "Do fractures run in families or are they genetic?" Although we see exceptions, genetics is not likely playing a role when we notice what patients or their families are doing. Dirt bikes, motorcycles, horses, dune buggies and all-terrain vehicles (ATVs), especially when mixed with alcohol, are a frequent source of business for orthopedic surgeons.

Moderate to extreme risk taking is normal for some patients and some families. They knowingly make choices involving higher risks than the rest of us. Football, motocross and snow ski racing are common examples. There are many less common examples such as waterski racing and hang gliding. People engaged in all these activities do many things to minimize injury that they know is inevitable. Sometimes as badges of honor, however, they accept the injuries. The more injuries we have and the greater the severity, the more likely we will have permanent residual effects. Risk taking has nothing to do with genetics. It is a result of our choices.

I have found many fun things to do in this life, and I will pick things that for me have a reasonable risk. The risk is minimal if I choose wisely and have sufficient strength, training and experience. I stood again on top of Tahquitz Peak with my scouts in July 2015, happy and without pain. I also look forward to and hope for a longer period without pain or additional injuries. The longer we can go without injuries or pain after recovering, the better our flexibility, strength and endurance will likely be.

Fractures were not the only painful problems I had since I retired from orthopedic surgery private practice in January 2010. I had more opportunities to learn from:

    1. A black widow spider bite (envenomation) on the right elbow with severe pain in the right shoulder, right shoulder blade, entire right arm, right neck and right upper back with muscle weakness causing shoulder blade protrusion with full temporary nerve

damage (scapular winging from anterior serratus muscle weakness from long thoracic nerve loss).
2. Left inguinal hernia surgical repair (herniorrhaphy).
3. Neck strain with radiating pain to the left shoulder (left cervical radiculopathy).

Thankfully, I have resolved all the problems and pain that I have had so far. The neck and shoulder pain were the last major areas of my bones and joints that I had not yet dealt with. After dealing with sinus headaches years ago, I learned to deal with and resolve pain in many areas of my body.

In my orthopedic practice, I helped patients lessen or resolve their pain from a chronic low back sprain 90 percent of the time. This included the patients covered by Workers' Compensation. When patients know more about what is causing the pain, it is easier for them to make good choices. Seeing the success of many patients who had a large decrease in pain has been rewarding. Many had a complete resolution of musculoskeletal chronic pain from various sources.

In my experience, many painful conditions are not the fault of the one suffering. Pain may happen because of the choices of others, including friends and family. Because of their unfailing efforts to do the best they can with the challenges they face, I have profound respect for what patients and their loved ones try to do. If I listen to patients and their family members or friends, fortunately I do not have to walk in their shoes to learn from them and understand them.

In the late 1980s, I noticed that a few patients were slowing down their recovery with the mindset that they needed to, "just push through the pain." Since then, the frequency of patients I found with this stumbling block increased. When I asked them why they tried to push through pain, they quoted a common saying, "No pain, no gain, right?" The question after the saying meant that they were not sure about it. Others had assured them that the adage was right and to, "just ignore the pain." I grew to detest that saying. Soon, I began telling my patients that, "no pain, no gain," was wrong, and I felt justified. I did not like what was happening. The common saying was getting patients into trouble.

Then in October 1994, I remember listening to a Music and the Spoken Word radio broadcast that caught my attention. The narrator, Lloyd D. Newell said that, "no pain, no gain," was true! I have listened to the weekly broadcast by the Mormon Tabernacle Choir for years, and I respect it. On the air since 1929, Music and the Spoken Word is the world's oldest continuing weekly network broadcast.[4]

I know that we learn from pain, but I was incredulous and thought, "How could the saying be true if it gets my patients into trouble?" The narrator explained that, "no pain, no gain," was true because we grow from our experiences with pain. He said, "...the kind of pain that makes us grow, that carves for us real character, must be endured well." Then he concluded, "Even a cliché has captured the necessity of suffering... We all seem to accept the fact that out of pain may come growth, wisdom, and strength."[5]

That made sense, but how could, "no pain, no gain," be true if patients who embraced it were having problems? At that time, I recorded Music and the Spoken Word broadcasts, so I could listen to them as I drove to work. After listening to that broadcast again, I pondered what I had heard. A few patients continued to ask about the concept of, "no pain, no gain," as they struggled to improve. Most did not ask, yet many were suffering under the same misconception. They were trying to push through the pain or forget about it.

I began using a concept of, "not pushing through pain," more often with my patients. They frequently worry that others will view them as weak or label them as a "wimp" if they keep complaining of pain. When they fail to improve or get worse, they assume that there must be something terribly

---

[4] Mormon Tabernacle Choir, Music and the Spoken Word, www.musicandthespokenword.org/, accessed May 9, 2018. Mormon Tabernacle Choir and Music and the Spoken Word are trademarks of the Corporation of the President of The Church of Jesus Christ of Latter-day Saints or Intellectual Reserve, Inc., and are registered in the United States and other countries. This book is not endorsed by or affiliated with the Church or its leaders.
[5] Mormon Tabernacle Choir, Music and the Spoken Word, October 2, 1994, Text of Broadcast #3398 by Lloyd D. Newell, Bonneville Distribution, © By Intellectual Reserve, Inc.

wrong. It usually does not even cross their minds that they might be doing something wrong. After the pain continues for a while, out of frustration they feel that there must be something causing the pain that I can take care of by surgically cutting it out.

Weeks went by after that radio broadcast. Then one day, I was explaining to a patient what to do to get over back pain when the answer hit me. It was so obvious. I do not know why I did not see it before. We need to learn from pain in many ways. If we do not try, we will not learn. If we do try, we will make mistakes, but we can learn from our mistakes and from the pain. Hopefully, we will not keep making the same mistakes.

The old saying, "no pain, no gain," is true because we should learn from the pain. The saying is, however, grossly misused. Many have never realized its correct meaning. We cannot learn from pain or improve by ignoring or masking it. Learning from our mistakes is necessary for pain control. Pain of all kinds, physical, emotional and spiritual, responds in the same way. Paying attention to pain is troublesome and hard to want to do. It is work, but the knowledge it brings is worth it. Knowledge is better when we appreciate the gift of knowing what is wrong and what to do about it.

Because patients are getting older, sometimes they assume that they cannot heal. There may be a little truth to that because we tend to be more set in our ways. As we age, we tend to have difficulty learning new things. We are stiffer. We like our ruts! Learning or memorizing good things as we get older will tend to counteract that. A patient in his mid-thirties with elbow pain asked me, "I cannot heal because I am getting older, right?" I could not believe he said that. I was much older than he was at the time and told him, "If you cannot heal, then I am in real trouble." Age is important, but a much bigger influence on healing is what we do and what we do not do.

As I noticed patients understanding and applying the concept of learning from pain, the cliché, "no pain, no gain," became less of a hindrance. Some family members were skeptical when the patient returned home and tried to explain what I had said. When family members, however, came to appointments, they usually did not ask many questions because they were listening to the whole story. They heard the complaints of the patient as I heard them. And they heard my follow-up questions. Then at the end of the appointment, they heard my explanations of what was wrong, what to do and what not to do. It made sense to them. They knew what to expect and what the patient should do.

Many say, "no pain, no gain," to encourage a friend. But the saying is wrong when used to challenge the patient to get tough, ignore the pain or work through the pain. The only time pushing through pain works is when the patient merely needs to warm up. Even for that pain, there is a better way. Often, runners tell me that when they run, it hurts at first. If they continue and run through the pain, it goes away temporarily. That is better than getting worse. Nevertheless, if what they are doing is working, then why did they come to my office?

They came to my office because they needed direction for pain that kept coming back when the muscles, joints and other soft tissues cooled down. The pain vicious cycle continued to reappear. Warming up slowly enough so there is no pain is a better way to deal with it. Then, run much shorter intervals than usual, so it does not tighten up as much afterwards. That decreases the irritation of the muscles and other soft tissues. Then, stretch after the run for a cool-down that is like the warm-up, again without pain.

Both warm-ups and cool-downs can be deterrents for pain and can be done much more often than running. If a runner has already stopped running on their own, they can do warm-ups and cool-downs to stay away from the pain longer before trying to resume running. When recovering from an injury or when having pain with only warming up, "to just ignore the pain," is a mistake.

Before the 1990s, Medicare and private insurance coverage had no limits on how long patients could stay in the hospital. Getting some to go home was hard. They may have liked the pain medications or the hospital food. In those days, when patients were spending lengthy periods of time in bed for back pain, physicians had to encourage patients to get up and try to move. As they tried to get up and go, it hurt. So, they stopped completely. It became apparent that they spent too much time in bed.

The saying, "no pain, no gain," was often used to motivate patients to get up out of bed and get going. As they warmed up and loosened up, the pain lessened, and they felt better. In the 1970s and 1980s, physicians were hesitant to discharge patients who did not want to go home because the malpractice crisis was pervasive in California and elsewhere. There were no copayments or deductibles. Therefore, there was little patient responsibility. These were primary causes of increasing health care costs.

In the 1990s, states enacted laws that began allowing insurance companies to contract with doctors. It was an ill-advised effort to control health care costs. Cost control is always better when consumers or patients have enough choices and more responsibility. If doctors have more control, like any other business, they can keep the patient and their families happier. Private insurance companies, with their new-found power, soon developed copayments and deductibles for the new Preferred Provider Organization insurance products (PPOs). Because they curbed insurance abuse, they found more power and company profits.

It was years before Medicare began following their example with copays and deductibles. Later, when Medicare started retrospective reviews of hospitalizations and denials for days "not approved," suddenly persuading Medicare patients to go home was much easier. Within 5 years, inpatient treatment disappeared for out of control back pain that did not need surgery. After that, my orthopedic partners and I no longer needed to admit patients to the hospital for back pain control. Patients were taking better care of themselves at home because they had some financial responsibility. Others were using higher doses of prescription pain medications.

Accounts of three of the last few of my patients who were hospitalized for back pain are described in the next three chapters. I learned a lot from each one of them. As I think about them, each was uniquely different. One was male, and the other two were female. One was obese, and the other two were thin. One was athletic, and the other two were not. Two learned from their experiences and my encouragement. The other with a "high pain tolerance" did not learn.

Were there similarities? Yes, all were hospitalized by their internal medicine primary care physicians, and their pain was severe. When I first saw them, they could not lie down. All of them were afraid to lie down because it hurt worse. Each of them thought that if they did lie down, they would be giving up and would not be able to get up again. They could not rest or get comfortable even with all the medications their physicians could give them. All were being given more than the maximum recommended doses of intravenous (IV) narcotic pain medications (opiates or opioids) and muscle relaxants, but the medications were not helping the pain. They all told me that they could not tolerate the pain any longer.

For all three patients, their doctors asked me to do a consult for pain control, not for the option of surgery. Though the three consultation requests were odd, I was willing. I knew two of the individuals well and remember their names. One was a friend at church who had cancer. The other was a long-standing patient of mine though I had not heard from her for several years. I do not remember the name of the third patient. I refer to her as my "nightmarish referral." Her severe pain in the spine had the possibility of being cancer.

I have used each of their experiences many times for examples to help other patients. The lessons I learned were striking. Each of the three patients learned to deal with severe pain more appropriately and not ignore it. Their dreadfully ominous situations forced them to do so. These three patients had to learn how to not be afraid of the pain. They had to learn from the ups and downs of their pain over a period of months and at different pain levels.

As I helped them for several days, I felt fortunate for the privilege of learning with them. Each of them learned that ignoring their pain was impossible. Each had to learn to ignore unwanted advice from others. As they experienced the changes in their pain, they had to try to trust me and trust what their bodies were telling them. They had to trust that their bodies were still capable of improving. In that way, "no pain, no gain," was true. They had to learn from the pain.

Patients with a high pain tolerance will find some advantages, but they will have many disadvantages. Many are proud of their high pain tolerance and consider it a talent. I tend to believe that those patients do have a high pain tolerance. Regardless, pain is still a warning sign. "No pain, no gain," does not mean to work through the pain. It never did mean that. If we ignore or mask pain, there will always be negative consequences.

Occasionally, patients acknowledge that they have lost their high pain tolerance. It is not so much that they lose a talent. The talent becomes counterproductive. Their pain becomes bad enough that they cannot ignore it any longer. When those patients come to that realization, it takes them longer to recover because of the severity of their pain and the damage that has occurred. Their abnormal habit patterns are hard to break. Changing a patient's counterproductive habits is one of the more difficult tasks physicians have. It can be impossible, unless the patient is willing to learn. Fortunately, most patients who see a doctor want to learn.

Having an attitude of learning is vital to improve. We can learn from both the ups and the downs of pain. In that way, "no pain, no gain," is true. It means to not be afraid to try, and when you feel pain, learn from it. So, what can you say to those who say, "Just push through the pain!" and to those who think that you are a wimp? Tell them, a better way allows more consistent improvement. It is almost as quick and gives better early and long-term results.

Chapter 3

Will She Ever Learn?

I first met Alice Ramirez in the early 1980s. She had already had five back surgeries elsewhere. I remember thinking at the time, "I really do not want to add another back surgery to her list of surgeries." She had two abnormal curves of the middle and lower back (adult idiopathic combined thoracic and lumbar scoliosis). Dense, solid bone healing on the back side of the spine extended from the upper mid back to the pelvis except for one level that had not healed (posterior lumbar fusion nonunion or pseudarthrosis).

This unhealed joint level at L4-5 was one level above the lowest joint of the low back at L5-S1 (the lumbosacral junction). It continued to hurt after months of trying many good things. To help finish the bony healing at that one level, I recommended a revision surgery. I used bone graft from the patient and hardware fixation (posterior L4-5 fusion with local bone autograft and stainless steel rods and hooks). She did well and had less pain. Though the bone healing was not very robust, it healed.

One year later, Alice bruised her right leg and developed severe generalized pain in the right leg that was obvious reflex sympathetic dystrophy (RSD). The x-rays were normal. She had widespread stiffness from her right toes to her knee, a dusky discoloration over the same area and constant, burning, excruciating pain that required hospitalization. With rest, her pain improved only slightly and was still out of control. There was little if any swelling. We tried physical therapy in the hospital, but the relief was partial and temporary. It helped some for a few hours at a time.

I requested an injection of the sympathetic nerves in the right low back by an anesthesiologist with a local anesthetic and synthetic cortisone (lumbar sympathetic corticosteroid injection). This gave her excellent relief. She went home from the hospital, but the pain came back within a few weeks. After two more injections and shorter amounts of temporary relief with each one, it became clear that we needed to do something else.

I spoke to a general surgeon in our community about doing an open surgical removal of the sympathetic nerves. They are inside the abdomen and outside the spinal canal. We considered it a definitive procedure for ongoing problems with RSD of the lower extremity (right lumbar sympathectomy). General surgeons also use this procedure to help narrowing of the arteries (vascular occlusive disease). The procedure is familiar and well known to them. The general surgeon and patient were both willing to do it. With it, she received excellent relief of her pain.

Within a few months, the right leg burning pain, dusky skin and hypersensitivity gradually came back. Her office visits were long because she complained and talked. Then she complained some more. I tried to answer her questions, but the answers never satisfied her. She was dependent on a muscle relaxant, Robaxin (methocarbamol), and a narcotic pain pill, Vicodin (hydrocodone and acetaminophen). I did my best to get her off the medications, especially Vicodin. She was manipulative and good at it. She had noticeable difficulty doing what she said she would do. Her words seemed hollow because they did not appear to mean anything. She had a habit of complaining, and she had difficulty learning from what she was experiencing. Her pain gradually resolved.

For the next 10 years, her right leg pain was gone. After that, I hesitantly performed 2 more surgeries for recurrent back pain. First, I did a definitive single level bony fusion in front of the spine, using bone graft from the patient and hardware (anterior L4-5 fusion with stainless steel rods and screws, rib and iliac crest bone autograft). Then lastly 2 years later, again for recurrent back pain, I removed the rods I had used in the first surgery I had done for her. They were on the back side of the spine. During surgery, I was excited to find that the bone of her back had healed solidly. Even better, she had excellent pain relief after the surgery. Her good results continued. At her last follow-up visit a year later, I cautioned her because she was still having difficulty staying within her strength and endurance limits. Then, for a number of years I did not hear from her.

The Miracle of Pain

In the late 1990s, her internal medicine family doctor, Dr. Dennis Carr, asked me to see Alice at the hospital for an orthopedic consultation for back pain. He told me that she had fallen and broken her back. She was in so much pain that none of the medications were working. I worried that she had ruined the bony healing or broken the remaining hardware from prior surgeries. When I went to see her, she was writhing in pain, yelling in agony, but she was sitting upright cross-legged in bed. I cannot forget that picture in my mind. Something was wrong with that position. Though her fall was a few weeks before, she could not lie down without increasing the already intense pain. A pain management anesthesiology specialist had already tried injections and had increased her intravenous narcotic medications to dangerous levels. She was getting morphine with no benefit.

Since the patient told them that she would not accept another surgery, Dr. Carr and the anesthesiologist were, in fact, asking me, an orthopedic surgeon, to help with pain management. That was ironic because that has been what orthopedic surgeons had been doing quite well for years, both with and without surgery. But even at that time, an increasing number of physicians, including orthopedic surgeons and neurosurgeons, were sending patients to pain management physician specialists. I went to check on the x-rays.

Her x-ray findings were impressive. She had a slightly displaced fracture in the upper part of the low back and through her spinal bony fusion. The fracture opened like a book from front to back at a new level (a Chance fracture through the L2 vertebral body anteriorly and through the posterior spinal column bone fusion at L2). This was several levels above the surgeries I had done at the L4-5 level. Her healed bone from my surgeries was still solid. The old hardware at L4-5 in front of the spine was also still solid. Both the bone fusion healing and the hardware from my surgeries had withstood the challenge of a new injury. Her nerve and spinal cord functions were normal. The only realistic options she had now were bone fusion surgery at the new level (L2), external custom spinal bracing or extended bedrest.

Even before I gave her the treatment options, Alice told me that she did not want to accept surgery. She agreed to try a custom back brace. When the custom brace was fitted 2 days later, she could not tolerate it. The pain increased as soon as she put it on. At first, that did not make sense to me because the brace fit well and was supportive. It took the stress off the spine fracture. I then reasoned that the increased pain from the brace meant that her muscles were very irritable. Additional pressure on her muscles increased the pain-spasm vicious cycle. There were no other reasonable explanations. I told her that she could stop using the brace.

Because she still did not accept surgery, the patient had no other options. I listened to her and understood her hesitation. Then I did something that was bold. It was not only bold then, it still is now. I told Alice that she had to learn to lie down, and we would have to taper off her intravenous narcotics, muscle relaxants and pain pills. She looked at me incredulously and asked, "How can you do that?" I asked her if she wanted to try since we had no other good options. She hesitated but agreed. The first step was to stop the intravenous morphine. It turned out that this was the easiest step. The medication was not working anyway. I simply wrote an order for the nurses to discontinue it. After that, I heard nothing else about it, from Alice or the nurses.

The next step was the most difficult. I had to teach her how to lie down again. I had to coax her into trying it a little at a time. When muscles get bad enough, they can only recover in horizontal positions. She had been getting worse while she was staying upright, but it hurt her to lie down. Her muscles would never recover if she did not try to help them relax. Accepting what she needed to do was tough for her. Gradually, as she tried to lie down a few minutes at a time, her muscles began to relax.

Without surgery or a brace, I knew that extended, total bedrest would eventually help her fracture heal. Within a few days, she could stay in bed. But to keep the muscles out of painful spasm, she had to learn to squirm and to move more frequently. She had limited options for medications. The patient had already been complaining of difficulty breathing. Continuing narcotics would have been dangerous and would not have helped. Skin patches with numbing medication were not yet available (transdermal anesthetics). The numbing medications may have helped temporarily but would have led her into the same problematic vicious cycle of doing too much.

A few weeks after her discharge from the hospital, Alice came back to the office on a stretcher. She was lying down constantly and doing better with it. Her fracture was not healing yet but was still in good position on x-rays. She announced to me that she was getting married. Her fiancé attended her appointments, and initially he was supportive. But, by the second appointment he attended, he asked about questionable treatments that have little or no benefit.

Marriage dynamics with a spouse are complicated, but chronic conditions are known to add significant stresses to any relationship. A spouse can be supportive, especially if they attend some appointments and try to understand. They can give encouragement and help remember the diagnosis. They can help remember recommendations, particularly if they are complicated. The patient must take ownership of their choices. If a patient does not, they will wear out the spouse before the spouse cures them. The patient must be responsible for their own choices, especially with a chronic condition.

For Alice, the pressure and stresses from her spouse were not helpful. His encouragement was in the opposite direction from the instructions I was giving her and from what she knew was right. I encouraged her to finish tapering off her pain medications completely and to be up only a few minutes at a time. As she was gradually getting up more, she began going back to her old habits. She was doing too much, ignoring the pain and using more medication to cover it up. I wanted her to try the custom back brace again a few weeks after leaving the hospital, but she refused.

Alice did not finish tapering off her medications and had an increasing number of pain pill prescriptions from her primary care physician. She returned soon to my office with new complaints of pain in the front of her shins. Initially, I thought that she had shin splints until I saw the impressive x-rays. She had stress fractures above the ankles in both legs (bilateral distal tibia metaphysis fatigue fractures). They occurred because of the choices the patient was making. She was weight bearing more than the bones were ready for at that time. I have seen a lot of fractures, but I had never seen that before. Alice had done it again. She had worked herself into another limiting corner.

I put her in bilateral short leg fiberglass casts and reinstituted bedrest. She healed the leg fractures in 2 months, and the L2 spine fracture healed completely in 6 months. I had anticipated a much longer time. When the leg casts came off, keeping her off her feet was difficult. She did not even try to understand what to do and what not to do, unless I listened to her first. She had the same habits as before, doing too much, too fast. Doing surgery, writing a prescription and putting a cast on is enjoyable because, when needed, they give relief to patients immediately. I have found, however, an increasing number of patients with bad habits that hold them back from healing. If I do not pay attention to those habit patterns, improvement cannot happen, and the condition of the patient can continue to deteriorate.

Alice also had multiple old rib fractures of various ages. Some of them had not healed (nonunions). It surprised me that they did not continue to hurt. Most orthopedic surgeons have seen some chronic nonunions that do not hurt. About 10 percent of them do not hurt. Alice also had pelvis fracture nonunions. Fortunately for her, most of them did not hurt. The connective tissue healing of the bone nonunions in her pelvis was strong enough to support her level of activity without pain (fibrous union). I am still not sure why, but I have a strong suspicion that abusing all of them at the same time was biomechanically impossible.

Treating Alice helped me to understand why pressure from a brace or a support can increase pain. Problems wearing a brace can also happen if there is muscle spasm in the spine. That much intense, chronic muscle irritability or spasm is uncommon in patients. These observations made bracing trials understandable for me, when considering spinal fusion surgery for other patients. If an off-the-shelf neoprene back brace feels good and if x-ray or other findings justify it, the likelihood of success with a custom brace or invasive surgery is better. If the neoprene brace or support does not feel good, a custom brace or surgery will not help at least at that time. After more time and proper care, we can repeat the trial. Within a few weeks or months, the negative results of a bracing trial can change to a positive benefit for the spine.

I treated Alice on and off for 20 of my 30 years of orthopedic practice. I hope that others will also learn from her experiences. I learned much more than the benefits of a bracing trial. I saw the benefits of surgery with the right indications and timing. In some situations, I saw the necessity and benefits of holding back on surgery. I witnessed the frustrating consequences of non-compliance by a patient. I found the immense healing capacity of the human body when we put it in the right circumstances.

She occasionally told me that she had a high tolerance for pain. Because of the multitude of her complaints as I treated her, I did not believe her initially. After a few years of dealing with her, however, I felt that she did have a high pain tolerance. Most likely, it contributed to many of the problems she developed. Will she ever learn to conquer the bad habits that contributed to her recurrent trouble? I can only hope.

As everyone else must, she lived with the consequences of her choices. I am glad that I learned to have patience with her and how to be firm but kind. I will always be grateful for what I learned with her help.

Chapter 4

A Nightmarish Referral

Near the end of a long day in the office in about 1993, I was chatting with my secretary. She told me that a doctor in Moreno Valley, California called and asked if I wanted to accept the transfer of his hospitalized patient who had back pain. She said that the patient was in so much pain that the doctor thought the patient had spine cancer. She said that she had already asked two of my partners who also did spine surgery. They had no interest in taking the referral. They did not want to do cancer surgery and preferred doing arthritis spine cases that were easy and more profitable (degenerative disc disease).

For me, challenging and unusual cases kept things interesting. At that time in my practice, the profit margins were good enough that I did not have to worry about them as much as I did later. I could not have taken that same referral 10 years later in my practice because of very thin profit margins in our group practice. Increasing economic realities forced me to be more efficient and selective like my partners or close my doors.

I spoke with the doctor in Moreno Valley. He wanted to know if I could accept a female patient who was having severe back pain. He thought she had a "tumor" of the spine in the mid back at one level, the seventh thoracic vertebral body. I had become comfortable dealing with patients with severe spinal pain, and each one seemed to be an interesting puzzle to sort out. Severe pain can be many other things besides tumors. I had treated tumors of the spine before, and the case sounded interesting. My training in spine and tumor surgery had been well-rounded. I agreed to evaluate the patient and figure out what she needed. If it turned out to be more complicated than I was comfortable with, I knew other spine surgeons who would accept complicated cases at regional university hospitals (tertiary care institutions).

The patient arrived after a 20-minute ambulance ride from the other hospital. That afternoon, I went to see her as soon as I finished with my office patients. This unfortunate patient was visibly in pain. She was writhing in agony and could not get comfortable. I asked her where she hurt. She said that she hurt all over. While at the other hospital, she had received massive amounts of intravenous narcotic pain medication. For the transfer to our hospital, she had received an additional amount of pain medication and was still not obtaining any relief.

After introducing myself and asking a few basic questions, I went to find the patient's imaging studies that came from the other hospital. Within a few minutes, I found her x-rays in the nursing unit. The findings were not very impressive. She had a stable, mid back, partially healed, spinal column 50 percent compression fracture at the seventh thoracic vertebral body (T7).

The findings were consistent with the location of her worst pain, but the findings were not consistent with the intensity of her pain. In other words, her symptoms were much more impressive than her findings. She had no history of a fall, injury or automobile accident. Because compression fractures can sometimes be as a result of cancer, I ordered a nuclear medicine bone scan, which uses a radioactive tracer isotope, Technetium-99m.

The bone scan results would be ready the next day. While waiting, I tried to help her make the best of the situation. I reassured her that the x-rays showed no signs of a tumor and encouraged her to continue to change positions often. I also gave her pain medication with an intramuscular injection. That gave her longer relief more consistently. The muscle spasms appeared to be her biggest problem. What the bone scan might reveal was still worrisome for both of us.

The next afternoon, I went over the bone scan films with the radiologist. There was only a single lesion at the seventh thoracic vertebral body, which was consistent with her x-rays. That meant she had no other lesions or obvious tumor. Both the radiologist and I felt that a tumor was much less likely now based on the x-rays and bone scan. I went back to the patient's room to give her the good news. Worry and anxiety about the possibility of having a tumor still consumed her. It was because of the pain she was having and what her previous doctor had told her. Even with the good news, reassuring her was nearly impossible.

In answer to her questions, I had to acknowledge that an underlying cancer could still be contributing to the spinal fracture. Her pain was still excruciating though she admitted that the pain was a little better than the day before. She was not writhing in pain as much as she had been. The laboratory studies of her blood and urine were normal. I also requested an internal medicine consultation. That would help me make sure that there was no evidence of cancer anywhere else. It would also lessen the risk of missing something that we needed to worry about.

My diagnosis for her was osteoporosis with severe thoracic and lumbar muscle spasm and acute muscle strain along with the stable, partially healed, T7 vertebral body compression fracture. It was based on her symptoms, physical exam findings, x-rays, bone scan and a CT scan (computerized tomography). Normal healing time from the onset should have been 2 months. The patient's pain had already persisted for 3 months. We needed more time and more improvement of her symptoms to finalize and confirm the diagnosis.

She kept her time upright shorter as I had encouraged her to do. I also asked her to stretch more gently and deliberately. Over the next few days, gradually her pain continued to improve. It was reassuring to her and to me as well. She had to focus on which movements helped and which ones did not. It took about 6 days for her to get the pain under enough control, so she could go home with pain pills. She could not tolerate much movement without creating more pain. That compromised how much the physical therapist could do. During her time in the hospital, she needed much more reassurance and guidance than the average patient to control the muscle spasms and pain.

Once she was steadily heading in the right direction, there were other needed modifications of her behavior. What she was doing for movement and position needed fine-tuning. Teaching her how to move and turn without increasing the pain came in 3 parts. The first was to teach her to slow down. The next two parts were to teach her to move in small amounts and to move more often. That sounds easy, but recognizing habit patterns is hard. Then, getting a patient to change bad habit patterns is the most challenging thing we must do.

I have had no significant training in behavior modification, addiction or habits. Nevertheless, without a change in her behavior, she could not improve. I had to help her replace counterproductive habits with habits that were helpful for healing the problem that was causing her pain. I have a distinct advantage of knowing how the anatomy and physiology of the body functions. I also know how to place it in circumstances that will help it heal.

The patient wanted what I wanted. I knew it, and she knew it. She began to trust and gradually gained confidence in her ability to heal. The changes that she made were subtle, but without them, her body could not have healed. She learned to slow her movements down. She learned to be consistent with the changes that were helping and allow her muscles to warm up. She learned to remember her back, pay attention to it often and respect it. She needed to remember that her back was not yet normal even when it was feeling better.

When she was out of the hospital and was finishing the recovery at home, more fine-tuning was necessary to allow the pain to finish going away and stay away. Follow-up visits are very helpful for that and are the best way to continue towards a full recovery. If patients do not come back, the progress they make often stalls out. They eventually rationalize that they, "will probably not get better anyway." Or they may say, "I just have a bad back." Patients are often comfortable with a certain frequency of recurrent pain. When recovering, full function is ideal, but patients choose to settle at many different levels of function. If they want a full recovery, their level of function needs to be less than what it takes to cause recurrent pain.

This patient stayed motivated to continue her recovery. She wanted to return to work and resolve the pain. There was no Workers' Compensation claim. As she improved, she had to remind herself to keep from being impatient and doing too much. I encouraged her to, "let it stay good." She had to be without pain for 2 to 3 weeks before advancing up to the next level of function. The advances in function had to be gradual enough to continue without pain. To be able to make it back to work, she had to be able to sit. However, sitting too long caused recurrent pain. After only 15 minutes of sitting, her back tightened up and hurt. Then, it took several hours to get the muscles to relax again. With encouragement, she learned to keep her sitting time short. To get up and go lie down in the middle of doing something is frustrating.

Her pain and stiffness continued to lessen. If she sat for less than 5 to 10 minutes, she did not have pain. She noticed that some chairs would help the pain and others would cause pain. Some chairs were okay to sit in for a brief period. Some were not comfortable the moment she sat down. For all normal chairs tested by a patient, the least amount of sitting time without pain is sitting endurance. Therefore, the patient's sitting endurance at that time was zero. After teaching her that each chair allowed different amounts of sitting time, she kept track of it. To improve her sitting endurance or to be able to sit longer in any chair, she needed to practice keeping the time short enough that she did not have any setbacks.

That seems to be a huge, burdensome task, but without the effort and consistency what will happen? Setbacks happen easily. There are many ways to aggravate pain. A patient must learn how to stay away from all aggravating sources of pain. Even if this patient only set herself back once a day or once a week, how far will she get with that? The effort to improve is worth it because the payoff is big. The payoff is longer and longer periods without pain. The periods of time without pain can also increase in frequency. They rarely increase steadily. Ups and downs always occur. What counts is the direction of the trend. Of course, learning from what we feel helps the direction of the trend remain positive.

Increasing endurance for many things, including sitting, can occur over a period of months. Eventually we all reach a limit of our endurance for sitting. Pushing our limits for sitting eventually gets all of us into trouble of some kind. That is true whether we have a problem with our back or not. There are three main reasons for this. First, sitting for lengthy periods allows muscles to become tighter than they should be. Tight muscles put more pressure on the spinal discs and bony spinal column. Second, when muscles eventually fatigue in an upright sitting position, we have less muscle support for the spine. That also puts more pressure on the discs and bone of the spine. Third, when the spinal muscles are not strong enough to do what we ask them to do, it also puts more pressure on the discs and bones of the spine, just like prolonged sitting.[6]

Normally during the day, the soft-tissue center of the disc loses water content (desiccation). Because we have many discs, we lose a little height, and at the end of the day we are a little shorter. At night, the body restores the water content of the discs (rehydration). If we stay up too late at night, especially if we stay up all night, the discs struggle to regain their normal water content. Have you ever stayed up all night and noticed how you feel the next day? We do not feel well, and it often takes a few days to recover. When more pressure on the discs occurs from tight muscles that do not relax overnight, the discs will not as easily regain their normal water content. When we squirm and change positions while lying down at night, it helps the muscles to relax and the discs to recover more effectively.

As discs degenerate, they also lose water content, and they also lose the ability to recover water content at night. In some of our discs, we accumulate degenerative change as we age. But fatigue, overuse and injury may take a greater toll. Age plays a role, but I see 80-year-old patients with normal looking discs on an MRI scan (magnetic resonance imaging). Usually the lowest two discs in the low back take the most abuse (lumbar L4-5 and lumbosacral L5-S1).

---

[6] Spinal discs are fibrocartilaginous joints shaped like a jelly doughnut and filled with a gelatinous soft tissue (nucleus pulposus). Each disc is located between two cylindrical bones at each level of the spine (vertebral bodies). The spinal canal and spinal cord are immediately behind the vertebral bodies and discs. They are covered and protected on the back side by more bone (vertebral laminae).

34

When the discs are functioning properly as joints, they protect the spinal muscles and bones of the neck and back. Similarly, when the muscles are functioning properly, they protect the bones and joints. When the bones are normal, they protect the joints and muscles. When a patient's muscles fatigue, prolonged upright activity overloads their bones if their bones are weak or brittle (osteoporosis). Overloading cause pain, and patients are at risk for collapse of the bones of the spinal column (vertebral body compression fracture).

Like sitting endurance, the duration of other activity can be monitored to resolve pain in patients with osteoporosis. Standing or walking are simple, good examples. Setbacks are common if patients do not monitor activity duration. Endurance for standing in a line at the bank or at a grocery store is one of many steps while recovering from pain. These steps are not easy to resume without making mistakes.

To stand in a line for 15 minutes and leave your place in line without accomplishing what you were standing there for is hard. I learned that from an experience at the California Department of Motor Vehicles. I had to come back later to finish my driver license renewal when I was recovering from one of my injuries. Each activity has a unique endurance level measured in minutes. Each activity also has a certain endurance level for the total amount of it each day without setting ourselves back. This total endurance per day is also often measured in minutes.

The referral patient with the T7 spinal compression fracture, muscle strain, spasm and osteoporosis resolved her pain. She returned to work successfully after several months and caught up to where she should have been. She could sit long enough to do her work, and she continued to improve. The best part was that she stayed pain free and knew how to keep it that way.

Chapter 5

Our Lives are Fragile and Precious

In about 1988, a good friend at church, Lucius Wood, was in the hospital with cancer throughout his entire spine and other places as well (metastatic cancer). He was a retired business executive. His oncologist and internist had prescribed heavy doses of intravenous narcotic pain medication with some risk to his breathing (respiratory arrest). His pain was still out of control, and it was frustrating for him. Because nothing was helping, he and his family asked his doctors for my help. His physicians agreed. They knew that I did spine surgery. Because the cancer involved the entire spine, they also knew I could not do anything for him with surgery. He only had a few months to live.

Before seeing the patient, I went to look at his x-rays. Unexpectedly, they were normal except for mild generalized thinning of the bone (osteoporosis). There were no fractures or weak spots. Then, I looked at his bone scan and MRI scan. In contrast to the x-rays, the scans were strikingly abnormal. Widespread malignant spine cancer extended from the upper back all the way to the lower back. Though the bones were weak (mechanically insufficient), there was no pressure on the spinal cord, collapse of the bones or narrowing of the spinal canal (spinal stenosis). There was, indeed, nothing I could do with surgery.

Next, I went to see the patient in his room at the oncology nursing unit. In the early afternoon, I remember walking into the darkened room with the thick window drapes drawn tightly closed. There was an oppressive atmosphere of gloom. With light shining in from the opened door, I could see him propped up in a chair on the far side of the room near the windows. He was afraid to move, but he was grimacing and groaning with severe pain. I asked him if he wanted to lie down. He whispered to me, "I am afraid if I lie down, I will die." I knew he could be right.

I also knew that if I could not talk him into lying down, his pain would not let up. His muscles would not recover enough to support him comfortably in upright positions. I

36

explained to him what he had, including the extent of the cancer. I also explained that although he would eventually die, he was not going to die right now, and he could be more comfortable by lying down. He then explained, "It hurts more to lie down." I acknowledged to him that more pain is not good. I encouraged him to squirm as he was lying there and change positions more often.

I also encouraged him by telling him that I would order a spinal brace after his pain was doing better. When it felt okay, he could start sitting up a little at a time. With that encouragement, he did try to lie down. I ordered the custom back brace (thoracolumbosacral orthosis). The brace fit well the next day, and it felt good to him when he was up. Within a few days he was able to go home. Seeing him in church a few weeks later surprised me. Propped up in a wheelchair, he was doing okay in his brace. He came to church a few more weeks. Within a few months, he died from the cancer, but during that time he was much more comfortable than he was in the hospital.

Lucius learned that lying down to help muscles relax, so they can recover, is okay. In addition, the muscles need encouragement to relax with little movements such as squirming, position changes and gentle stretching. When muscles are tight or fatigued, stretching too far or too fast is easy but damaging. In the right situations, bracing or surgery can be very helpful. Muscles can often recover better than we give them credit for.

My own physical challenges have helped me understand Lucius and many others. Life is fragile, and none of us know when our time on earth is over. While serving as a scoutmaster on a Saturday in December 2009, I went on a 15-mile bike ride with our 11, 12 and 13-year-old Boy Scouts and other adult leaders. We rode the paved, off-street Trabuco Creek Bikeway in the hills of Orange County, California. To complete the 15 miles that we wanted to accomplish that day, we continued down the Trabuco Creek dirt hiking trail for about 2 miles. We turned around after stopping for snacks and biked back uphill, 7.5 miles to our campsite.

The Miracle of Pain

After cleaning our campsite and a 90-minute drive home, I helped our scouts unload the equipment and all the bikes from the scout trailer. After I put away my camping gear, I hung two bikes in the garage. I was tired, but otherwise I felt great. My wife made a wonderful dinner. After helping in the kitchen, I sat down to watch a digital video recorder to catch up on things I had missed during the week.

After an hour, I felt a painful catch in the front of my left hip (flexor muscle spasm). The pain went away when I squirmed, but I still felt it every time I stretched. I felt it even with little stretches. I felt other pain in the side muscles of my left hip (left hip abductor muscles) below the brim of the pelvis (iliac bone). When I stood, I felt pain in the left groin with weight bearing on the left side. The pain was worse when I tried to walk or hop. I worried that maybe arthritis had worn out the hip joint.

After another hour of trying to get comfortable, it was more uncomfortable. The muscles were stiff. I still could not bear any weight on my left leg without pain. I tried lying down, stretching easier and waiting. Even with that, the pain was getting worse. I did not have crutches at home to help me get upstairs. When I tried to limp, the pain was too intense to even go a few steps. Staying on the couch downstairs was too uncomfortable, so I crawled on my hands and knees up the stairs to get to bed.

While crawling, it hurt if I stayed in one position too long. I had to stop crawling after 5 feet to squirm, rest and change position. The left hip hurt to be upright on my knees. It might have been funny if the pain had not been so severe. My wife was asleep, so I did not want to wake her. I did not get much rest that night. All night long, I had to toss and turn slowly and carefully. Early the next day, I could not get up out of bed well enough to go to church. To get to the bathroom, I had to crawl. It was still painful if I moved too quickly.

As I was resting, I started to get a different pain on the back of the head on the left side and in the left neck. It went down to the left mid back, but the worst pain was in the back of the head. It did not quit. Because of nasal congestion and left ear popping, I knew I was still dehydrated from the bike ride the day before. Getting to the bathroom was difficult with the spasm of the left hip muscles, so I did not want to drink too much water. I drank slowly and frequently. With more rest, position changes and stretching, the left hip pain was better. I went to work Monday, and the hip pain was completely gone by Tuesday. With plenty of water hydration, the rest of the pain resolved in 3 more days (mastoid sinusitis). I recovered fully without decongestants or antibiotics.

In retrospect, it is surprising how many years it took me to discover the relationship of mild chronic dehydration to headaches, allergy symptoms and sinusitis. In the fall of 1973, I was in my second year of medical school at George Washington University in Washington, D.C. That summer, our school had moved from the old downtown medical school building at 1335 H Street, NW, where it had been since 1868. We moved to Ross Hall at 2300 Eye Street, NW. In the new, spacious auditorium, I remember asking a professor a question about the triggers for sneezing. He did not have an answer. I had suffered bouts of sneezing for years, especially if I was outside and looked towards the sun. I suspected that the sneezing was from allergies, but I had no other symptoms that I had recognized.

The amount of knowledge in the medical sciences is imposing. Yet all physicians admit a multitude of things we do not know. Some of us hang on to superstitions for years. Withholding water had been engrained in football at all levels for many years in the United States. There was fear of getting stomach cramps and limited playing time. While I was a surgery resident at Ohio State University from 1977 to 1978, team physician Dr. Bob Murphy and athletic trainer Billy Hill helped undo withholding water from football players during games and practices. Buckeye head football coach Woody Hayes from 1951 to 1978, who loved his players and students, agreed with the change. In the late 1970s, football players were encouraged to drink fluids before, during and after games as needed. Withholding water, however, still took years to go away in many football programs.

In many ways, inadequate water hydration has not fully disappeared in sports and elsewhere. Sudden deaths from heat illness associated with high school and collegiate sports are not disappearing. Despite the advertising hype for hydration with "sports drinks," fatalities are increasing. A 2012 task force from the National Athletic Trainers' Association (NATA) and the National Strength and Conditioning Association wrote that we have an unfortunate culture that prizes toughness, discipline and success at all costs in athletes. It has led to increased collegiate deaths and serious injuries from practice and conditioning routines.[7]

According to the 2016 Annual Survey of Football Injury Research, they found 14 heat stroke deaths at all levels of football from 1987 to 1996. Deaths increased to 24 in the next 10 years, from 1997 to 2006. Over the last 10 years from 2007 to 2016, there were 30 heat stroke deaths, and they are preventable. Well-rounded educational efforts have had a modest dampening effect over the last 3 years from 2014 to 2016 with 6 deaths, which is 2 per year or a rate of 20 per 10 years.[8] Clearly, "sports drinks" are not the best answer in light of their heavy use and promotion during the last two decades. The problem of how much hydration and what, if anything, to add to water remains. It varies with the individual, the sport or activity and the environmental conditions.

Drinking water intermittently before, during and after exercise is important. Replacing the salt we lose is also very helpful by using foods such as crackers or soups that contain salt (sodium chloride). Adding carbohydrates is good, but

[7] Douglas J. Casa, Ph.D., ATC, Scott A. Anderson, ATC, Lindsay Baker, Ph.D., Scott Bennett, MS, Michael F. Bergeron, Ph.D., et al., "The Inter-Association Task Force for Preventing Sudden Death in Collegiate Conditioning Sessions: Best Practices Recommendations," Journal of Athletic Training, August 2012, Volume 47, Number 4, page 477, www.ncbi.nlm.nih.gov/pmc/articles/PMC3396308/, accessed May 9, 2018.

[8] Kristen L. Kucera, MSPH, Ph.D., ATC, David Klossner, Ph.D., ATC, Bob Colgate, Robert C. Cantu, M.D., "Annual Survey of Football Injury Research, 1931–2016," University of North Carolina at Chapel Hill, National Center for Catastrophic Sport Injury Research, March 2017, Report #2017-01, pages 13–16 and 28–29, nccsir.unc.edu/files/2013/10/Annual-Football-2016-Fatalities-FINAL.pdf, accessed May 9, 2018.

highly advertised "sports drinks" are not better than adequate water hydration, normal foods and a normal diet. Common sense approaches for coaches and athletic trainers to prevent or decrease heat illness are available from the National Athletic Trainers' Association. These include medical screening, time for acclimatization to heat, activity modification or cessation with other illness or high humidity and hydration to keep weight loss less than 2 percent after exercise.[9]

Comparing a current weight with the pre-exercise weight gives a good estimate of the remaining water weight deficit. Water, nutrition and electrolytes are easy to replace in many ways, and we do not need highly processed, costly products. We must consider all symptoms, signs, weight and urine color when doing 2 hours or more of training, competing or heavy work. For all of us, urine color should be clear at least once per day, most days.

After our family moved back to California in the early 1980s, I was an assistant scoutmaster for our Boy Scout troop. In that assignment and later as an adult leader for other ages of scouts, I attended many summer camps in the Southern California San Jacinto and San Bernardino Mountains. When we traveled from home to camp, we went from an elevation of 900 feet to 5500 feet in 90 minutes. The local lay knowledge at our scout camp was that if a scout felt bad in any way or was not acting right, tell him to "Drink water!" That hydration guidance was usually right. Daytime summer temperatures in the mountains are often in the 90s. Twelve-year-old scouts and even some older scouts were too busy exploring new things to be concerned about drinking water. When I got a headache at camp, drinking more water made it go away. After a few years, I noticed that if I purposely drank water before I left home, I did not get headaches in the mountains at all.

---

[9] Douglas J. Casa, Ph.D., ATC, Julie K. DeMartini, Ph.D., ATC, Michael F. Bergeron, Ph.D., Dave Csillan, MS, ATC, E. Randy Eichner, M.D., et al., "National Athletic Trainers' Association Position Statement: Exertional Heat Illnesses," Journal of Athletic Training, September 2015, Volume 50, Number 9, pages 986–1000, natajournals.org/doi/pdf/10.4085/1062-6050-50.9.07?code=nata-site, accessed May 9, 2018.

The Miracle of Pain

In the early 1990s, I was a varsity coach for our local unit of the Boy Scouts. We took our 14 to 18-year-old scouts on High Adventure waterski and fishing outings in August at Lake Mead in Nevada. We brought our shade, water and food. We prepared well and taught our scouts how to survive in the hot, dry desert. Our shade consisted of heavy dining flies that we tied down securely because of the afternoon winds. With our runabout ski boat, we transported water and supplies. We kept our water in a 55-gallon drum that was set in 3 feet of water at the edge of the lake. The lake's constant 80-degree water temperature kept our drinking water at the same usable temperature of 80 degrees, despite air temperatures in the 100s. Ice and ice cream were rare treats, 8 miles away by boat at the Callville Bay marina. We had a wonderful time but learned to stay well hydrated.

Also in the 1990s, I noticed that I was gradually taking more over-the-counter decongestants for the allergy symptoms of sinus headaches and a runny nose. When I went to the desert or mountains for Boy Scout outings, I had no allergy symptoms and did not need any medication. Because dust and dirt were everywhere when camping and hiking, I thought it was strange that I had no allergy symptoms there. I joked with my wife that I might be allergic to home. I started drinking water more consistently at home and at work. The need for all medications gradually went away. Since 2001, I have not needed decongestants for allergy symptoms. Except for some occasional sneezing, drinking more water resolved all the headaches and allergy symptoms.

I started teaching my scouts to prevent headaches and other dehydration related problems by drinking more water. I encouraged them to stay away from sodas, soft drinks, "electrolyte drinks," "sports drinks" and "power drinks." What is wrong with good, simple food and water? It seems that they are two of the best kept secrets in our high-tech world. Water is best for hydration and tap water is usually the best kind of water. It is the least expensive. For most water districts and municipalities in the United States, tap water is more regulated and is as good as, or better than, bottled water.

In about 2005, occasionally when I was taking a patient's history in the office, I had afternoon drowsiness. It made me think that I was getting old or developing a problem with narcolepsy or hypoglycemia. Nodding off a little was embarrassing. Patients probably wondered if I was not interested in their history or if I needed a nap. After a few months of struggling with it, I excused myself from the exam room for a short break and a little water. After returning to the exam room, it surprised me how quickly a few sips of water solved the drowsiness and fatigue. The symptoms did not return the rest of the day.

In a humid climate, sweating is less effective for a cooling mechanism of the body, so water losses are higher. Even in cold temperatures, water losses are higher in humid climates. In Southern California, usually humidity is not an issue. To get enough water and stay hydrated sounds easy, but it is not. I must remember and work at it like anyone else. Even though you might think that I would know better, I have to use all available signs to keep enough water in me. Because weight scales are not always easily accessible, common signs for mild water dehydration are 1) urine color not clear at least once per day, 2) ear popping or congestion, 3) nasal or sinus congestion (mucus), 4) throat congestion (phlegm), 5) dry or cracked skin or lips, 6) occasional headaches.

Is it possible to overdose on water? Yes, but drinking too much water is hard to do. When it happens, we call it water intoxication (hyponatremia). It can be fatal, but it is uncommon. It occurs from too much water, too little salt or a combination of both extremes. If your urine is clear several times in a row, decrease your water intake. Add salt to food to taste if you do not have high blood pressure. Do not use salt tablets for cramps or dehydration because too much salt is also a problem.

Through the mechanisms of appetite, taste and smell, our bodies are normally able to tell us when they need more or less salt. The body is also able to tell us when we need more or less water. Unfortunately, our abnormal habits can sabotage those natural body defenses. Too much salt is a common dietary habit from fast foods and also from processed or prepared foods. It contributes to high blood pressure. So, if we have problems with high blood pressure, we should try decreasing our salt intake.

Learning to control our appetites and passions is a good thing. Too much of a good thing is often a problem for many of us. Taking mega doses of a vitamin causes specific, known, severe illnesses (hypervitaminoses). Fruit and vegetable juices are not a solution for hydration and nutrition. They lack the full structure of the fiber needed in our diet that minimizes constipation. Believing internet, TV or radio ads can often be dangerous. Chewing is a normal function that helps digestion. When will we learn to consume enough good things, stay away from unnecessary things, control overeating and drink adequate amounts of water? With a few exceptions, advertising for simple, good things and habits has not been very exciting.

With mild chronic dehydration, our body is an accident waiting to happen. As a result, pain and many other disorders can occur in various parts of the body. With experience as a doctor and as a patient, associated conditions include headaches, earaches, allergies, nasal congestion, runny nose, sinusitis, dry lips or skin, halitosis, altitude sickness, frostbite, seasickness, narcolepsy, constipation and kidney stones. Other associations like sleep apnea, tinnitus, asthma and angiospasm leading to heart attacks and strokes are possible. The risks for problems with dehydration increase with an abnormal diet, obesity, alcohol and other drink fads. Remembering that we are 60 to 70 percent water, depending on our age, is helpful. Like we must stretch until we die, we must drink water until we die. With good water hydration and a normal diet, the many challenges our bodies must weather is easier.

Another learning experience for me occurred after retiring in January 2010. I had endured an inguinal hernia for 4 years. It went away for weeks at a time. However, for 6 weeks before the surgery, the hernia was continuing to hurt and stay more often. On March 28, 2010, I had hernia surgery. After the surgery, my surgeon told me that it was, "the hernia from hell." He said that he found a racquetball-sized benign fatty tumor associated with the hernia defect. Repairing it took 2 hours, twice his usual time.

At the site of the surgery that night, the numbing medication wore off (local anesthetic). The pain was tolerable without any medication if I was lying down. After a day or two, the pain increased. A single Tylenol Extra Strength pill (acetaminophen 500 mg) helped enough. After that, I did not need any other medication. Occasionally, I held the surgical dressing with my hand. I rested flat often because the pain was less. Two days after the surgery, I thought my allergies were going crazy, so I drank more water than usual.

Hydration helped, but the nasal congestion, sore throat and constipation kept getting worse. I felt terrible with muscle spasms from my neck to the back of my thighs. I wanted to throw up, but I was afraid to damage the hernia repair. I could not sleep. I wondered briefly if I was going to die. The surgery or the general anesthetic could not account for all the symptoms. Then, I remembered having a mild sore throat before the surgery that morning. I thought the soreness was only a dry throat from sleeping on my back with my mouth open. Three days after the surgery, the viral illness became obvious.

Trying to recover from a viral illness and surgery at the same time is not a good idea. For years when I saw my patients preoperatively, I warned them not to have surgery if they had a cold, flu or other viral illness. I did not want them to have to recover from two things. We also did not want them to expose our staff to a contagious virus. I was experiencing firsthand the reason for the warning I gave to my patients. It took me several weeks to recover from the viral syndrome. During that time, I had to rest in horizontal positions a majority of the time. I became really bored. Because I was feeling useless, I learned the Morse code. Later, I had fun teaching it to our scouts in Boy Scout troop meetings.

On May 9, 2010 while recovering, I wrote to my immediate family, "I am not 100 percent, but I am way better than 4 days ago. I can now think straight." Two weeks later, I wrote to my extended family about the family reunion my wife and I were hosting in July. I wrote, "…doing much better and have recovered from surgery and a viral flu illness, thanks to many prayers and the mercy of God. My retirement since January 1st has been 'interesting.'"

In June 2010, I wrote in my journal, "I am now able to spend more time writing and less time recovering from something. I am thankful to be doing well now but almost feel guilty because of it. Herman Ah Sue, a very good friend of mine at church, suddenly passed away this morning. He was in his forties and had helped with many of our scout outings as a parent and as an adult scout leader. He was also enjoying recreational bike riding and was increasing the biking distances with his wife and sons. He had become comfortable with rides up to 65 miles and was losing the weight he had planned."[10]

I continued, "Life is so precious. At times, it is so temporary and fragile. Understanding it, at times, is hard. Our bodies are similarly precious. They are also temporary and fragile. At times, they are hard to understand, and at other times they are so resilient. How can I complain about my little, inconsequential, transient pains? I have been blessed with knowledge and, so far, with an ability to recover. I hope not to die, if God is willing, at least until I have written and passed on to others some of what I have been privileged to learn."

Our imperfections, gifts, possessions and challenges that we have been blessed with during our lifetimes all have purpose. How much will we learn without them? Sir Robert Baden-Powell, a dynamic British leader and founder of the Boy Scouts, said it this way, "Be glad of what you have got, and not miserable about what you would like to have had, and not over-anxious as to what the future will bring."[11]

---

[10] His name is used by permission and with the encouragement of his wife.
[11] William Hillcourt with Olave, Lady Baden-Powell, Baden-Powell, the Two Lives of a Hero, The Gilwellian Press, New York, 1992, page 312.

❧ *Chapter 6* ❧

Pain is Always a Warning Sign

For more than 30 years, I have been looking for an exception to my observation that pain is a warning sign. Pain mechanisms vary widely from sprains and nerve injury to disease and cancer, but I have found no exceptions. A big red warning flag is severely abnormal pain with burning or stabbing (dysesthesia). I have noticed a disturbing trend with patients and physicians wanting to cover up pain with medications. They see no useful purpose for the pain.

I treated an increasing number of patients who had been cared for elsewhere and did not know what to do for their pain. They became dependent on or addicted to medication and still struggled for relief. The same result comes from masking pain in any other way. It can be from drugs, drinking alcohol or using a TENS unit on the skin (transcutaneous electrical nerve stimulation). Masking the pain lessens warning signs and the ability of a patient to learn from pain and get over it. Ignoring pain also diminishes the learning capacity of a patient.

Without pain, we would always be overdoing things, and our bodies would break down. The skin of the feet of a person with diabetes mellitus can wear out and form ulcers. Many of them have limited sensation in their feet (peripheral neuropathy). Some diabetic patients with a broken ankle have difficulty healing the fracture (neuropathic fracture). They may come to an orthopedic surgeon several weeks after the fracture with little pain, but they have a displaced, crumbling joint (neuropathic arthropathy). The destroyed joints in those patients are nearly impossible to repair. To fix them, healing a bony fusion of their foot or ankle joint is an ordeal.

Many incorrectly assume that poor healing in diabetics is due to poor blood flow in the small arteries (end vessel disease). That is one reason diabetic feet have been amputated too often for a chronic nonhealing ulcer. The main difficulty in diabetic healing is from the limited protective sensation, especially in the legs. Other less common conditions with no protective sensation have similar end results. Examples are idiopathic peripheral neuropathy, peripheral nerve injury, congenital absence of pain, leprosy, syringomyelia and tabes dorsalis from syphilis. The continued use of the feet in spite of small injuries that they cannot feel cause bigger problems that do not heal. For example, pressure spots on the skin easily become blisters and then ulcers. If treated properly, blisters, ulcers, fractures and bony fusions of joints in diabetes can heal with non-weight bearing. Then, we can salvage a functional leg or foot.

For the rest of us who have normal sensation and nerve function, what if we ignore or mask pain? Patients are often tired of the pain. After a while, pain is easier to ignore. To an extent, somehow the body accustoms itself to pain. Whether pain is only a nuisance or a real bother, is there anything bad that can happen from ignoring pain or masking it? The answer lies in understanding what is going on in the body part causing pain. Is it constructive or destructive? Pain means that something bad is happening in the soft tissues, such as ligaments, tendons, muscles, fibrous connective tissue (fascia), fibrous bone coverings (periosteum), fat, skin, blood vessels or nerves. There are no nerve endings in bone itself. Fractures hurt because of nerves in surrounding soft tissues.

Ignoring or masking pain always produces negative consequences. It gives a false sense of security. Impulses from a TENS unit are distracting to the pain pathways of the body. A TENS unit does not contribute anything to healing. Medication for pain also has no capacity to help healing, except for relaxing muscles for a few days after an injury. On the other hand, in the right settings, we can see dramatic healing with specific medications. Good examples are ibuprofen, aspirin, other non-steroidal anti-inflammatory drugs (NSAIDs) or some steroid medications (corticosteroids).

Mechanical helps for healing such as elevation, supports and motion can be just as dramatic. For that reason, we should primarily use specific medications and mechanical helps. We should use pain medications, heat and TENS units secondarily. We should use secondary helps for 3 months or less. The patient should discuss any exceptions to this time limit with a physician. In doing so, the physician should give honest answers, not dismissive replies, to questions about treatment. Responses such as, "It can't hurt," are a disservice and belittle the learning capacity of a patient. Especially if a patient is interested, we can discuss the pros and cons of each medication or treatment, not merely the risks. Describing the pros of a treatment is delightful because it gives hope. But it takes time to explain the cons of a treatment that include dependency and diminishing benefits over time.

Patients who tell me that they have a "high pain tolerance" often imply that pain is not important to them. They seem to want to be tougher or more courageous than others. A parent will sometimes tell me that their child has a high pain tolerance. When a patient or a parent tells me that, I tend to believe them. High tolerances for pain are a pattern or characteristic for some patients. That pattern may change with different injuries in the same patient if an injury or pain becomes chronic.

High pain tolerance has some advantages and some disadvantages. The advantages are that a person can sit, stand or run longer than average. Some have a tremendous capacity to focus on a task for extended periods of time or until they complete it. However, disadvantages of a high pain tolerance are real. It allows injuries and reinjury to accumulate. At the very least, it sets up patterns of stiffness or hyperflexibility that increase the probability of reinjury.

Over time, consequences of a high pain tolerance will always be negative. The most common is pain lasting 3 months or more. In patients with a history of high pain tolerance, it predisposes them to prolonged recoveries and complications. Some patients with chronic pain syndromes, such as fibromyalgia, claim that they have a high tolerance for pain. I tend to believe them as well. Perhaps it is part of what contributed to their pain vicious cycle in the first place. Pain is always a warning sign!

The following three paragraphs show pain mechanism examples in bone and soft tissues of the body. I have sorted the examples into immediate, delayed and accumulated onsets. Immediate and delayed mechanisms are acute, and an

The Miracle of Pain

accumulated mechanism is chronic. Pain that lasts less than 3 months is acute. Chronic pain lasts 3 months or longer. There is no clear dividing line between immediate and delayed onsets of acute pain. Pain mechanism examples are listed with specific medical examples in parentheses.

Immediate acute pain mechanisms are sudden: a cut by a sharp object (skin, tendon or nerve laceration), a cut by blunt force (skin avulsion, skin stellate laceration), stabbing penetration (skin puncture wound, artery laceration, collapsed lung), scrape (skin abrasion, scratch, road rash), blunt force blow (soft-tissue contusion, spleen rupture, brain concussion, rib fracture), twisting force (knee meniscus tear, spiral tibia fracture), overstretch (muscle strain, ligament sprain, joint subluxation or dislocation), expansion (intestinal gas, bloody joint effusion, toe infection, intracranial bleeding), compression force (hand or foot crush injury, vertebral body compression fracture), sudden blood vessel obstruction (muscle spasm, frostbite, venous thrombosis, pulmonary embolism, stroke, heart attack), obstruction of urine (kidney stones or infection), excessive heat (heat exhaustion, first, second or third degree burn).

Delayed acute pain mechanisms are slower: sustained or repetitive pressure (red skin pressure point, skin blister, broken skin blister, skin callus fissure, skin ulcer, nerve irritation, lumbar radiculopathy, ear ache), excess fluid (ring finger swelling, swollen black eye, leg pitting edema, ankle swelling, prepatellar bursitis with effusion, knee joint effusion), soft-tissue inflammation (knee joint synovitis, ankle tenosynovitis, wrist tendinitis, shoulder subdeltoid bursitis, hepatitis, gastritis), excess soft tissue (trigger finger, knee joint synovial impingement, rotator cuff tendon impingement, carpal tunnel syndrome), stiffness (frozen shoulder, hamstring muscle tightness), muscle irritability (calf muscle spasm, tension headache, foot cramp, vitamin D deficiency, Lyme disease), strength overuse (biceps tendinitis, foot stress fracture, inguinal hernia), expansion (spinal disc herniation, neck abscess, osteomyelitis, metastatic spine cancer, constipation, diarrhea), gradual blood vessel obstruction (thigh deep vein thrombosis, brain transient ischemic attack), mechanical insufficiency from disease or tumor (spinal osteoporosis, femur pathologic fracture), pain that is out of proportion to the injury (disuse, reflex sympathetic dystrophy, causalgia, malingering).

Chronic pain mechanisms accumulate slowly: overuse reinjury (tennis elbow, rotator cuff tendon tear), easy reinjury (sore thumb, recurrent ankle sprain, chronic lumbar strain), chronic stiffness (spinal ankylosing spondylitis, knee contracture), soft-tissue degeneration (Achilles tendinosis, biceps tendon rupture, shoulder calcific tendinitis), bone and joint inflammation and deformity (elbow contracture, rheumatoid arthritis of the hand, knee and hip arthritis, hammertoe, great toe bunion), muscle or joint inflammation (myositis ossificans, rheumatism, psoriatic arthritis), soft-tissue inflammation (panniculitis, dermatitis, lupus erythematosus, psoriasis), failure of bone healing (delayed union, bony nonunion), chronic venous obstruction (varicose veins, brawny pretibial stasis dermatitis, skin ulceration), chronic disuse and unknown (chronic fatigue syndrome, fibromyalgia, fibromyositis).

There are many variables, but pain tends to warn us when we have gone too far and are testing limits beyond the capacity of our body. When carelessly cutting vegetables, pain occurs when a knife tests the limits of our skin. If we are searching for something sharp in a pocket or a purse, we tend to be cautious. If we have no protective sensation in one of our fingers from a prior nerve injury, we will be more susceptible to injury from something sharp. If a bee stings us as we walk barefoot on grass, the memory of pain may nudge us to wear shoes, or it may keep us off the grass.

Patients see abrasions of the skin and understand them easily. Bruises, muscle strains, ligament sprains and tendinitis are inside the body, however. Because patients cannot see them, many misconceptions occur. Internal organs such as the heart, kidney, gallbladder and spinal nerves are even more misunderstood. They have pain that radiates to other places such as the back, shoulder, arm or leg.

The mnemonic and acronym RICE is appropriate for pain with most acute arm and leg injuries in the first 48 hours. It means rest, ice, compression and elevation. These 4 tools can slow and often stop the unseen internal bleeding from a soft-tissue bruise. Rest means to stop the aggravating activity. Compression may be pressure from a hand or an elastic bandage (Ace bandage). It can directly limit internal bleeding. We can minimize both pain and the amount of bruising by immediate, gentle, firm, frequent pressure. Cold or ice, on and off, along with frequent elevation also helps minimize bleeding, bruising and pain.

After the blood from an injury clots in the soft tissues, it spreads over a period of days as the body breaks it down and recycles it (metabolizes it). Old blood may take days to come to the skin surface as black, green or blue colors. Hidden bleeding in the abdomen from a ruptured spleen or in another cavity such as the chest or skull can be life threatening. We should avoid heat, aspirin or ibuprofen in the first 48 hours for all injuries. They will increase bleeding and swelling.

A strain is an injury to a muscle and a sprain is an injury to a ligament. Pain from a grade I muscle strain or ligament sprain is from a tear of a few fibers. A grade II injury can be many fibers but not enough to cause displacement or instability with stress testing. A complete tear or rupture is grade III. If we deal with all these injuries appropriately, the pain will resolve, and they can heal. That means rest, a controlled amount of motion in the right directions or surgery for some of the grade III injuries.

The good news is that grade I injuries heal in a few days to a few weeks. Grade II injuries heal in 6 to 8 weeks. Both of them should take no longer than 2 to 3 months. Grade III injuries will take 3 months to heal and a year to reach full maturity for maximum tensile strength. Any grade of injury can persist and become chronic. If any injury takes longer than the times listed above, patients are reinjuring themselves, often without being aware of it. When they stop reinjuring it, chronic pain from injuries dealt with in the right ways will usually be better in 3 weeks and a lot better in 3 months.

Pain always accompanies a broken bone. With intact skin, we call it a closed fracture. A nondisplaced or stable fracture may only hurt when moved or stressed. If the pain from an injury persists or if other signs of a broken bone occur, the patient needs an x-ray. Orthopedic surgeons have the greatest amount of experience with all fractures, except the head. They should see the patient if there is any uncertainty about the treatment of a fracture.

Orthopedic surgeons take care of most fractures without surgery. When we find a fracture, we should avoid all NSAIDs, such as ibuprofen or aspirin. They inhibit new bone formation (bone callus). Acetaminophen is okay because it is not an NSAID and does not cause added bleeding. A broken bone with a cut or hole in the skin connecting to the bone is an open fracture (compound fracture). It should be seen by an orthopedic surgeon immediately.

A hand or foot crush injury causes immediate pain from damage to all the soft tissues and often from bone fractures as well. All crush injuries have a higher incidence of chronic pain, stiffness and disability even though the skin and bones may not be broken. These injuries are a challenge to treat because the pain level is often more than we expect for the damage we find. Both patients and doctors tend to over treat with ice, immobilization and medication. Early after the injury, NSAIDs will cause more bleeding and therefore more swelling. We also have a tendency to underutilize elevation and motion. Both would help pain, swelling and healing.

Blisters of the skin after hours of work in the garden may cause delayed pain. They can occur if skin thickness and toughness is not sufficient. A common mistake is to pop a blister. Stopping early or changing the work that is causing the blister is better. It is also better to hold the area of the blister with the flat surface of the hand. Applying broad, gentle, frequent pressure minimizes blister fluid accumulation. Testing full motion of the nearby joints also minimizes blister fluid. Within a few hours, these techniques used on my own hands have resolved pain and blister fluid. After that, the top layer of the skin (epidermis) heals like a perfect skin graft without any visible residuals. If a blister breaks before 3 days, it can hurt and get infected. If a blister breaks after 3 days, the new skin underneath has usually healed, and there will be no pain or risk of infection.

It may take hours to feel pain from delayed mechanisms such as swelling, stiffness and muscle irritability. The delay gives us a window of time for simple tools to minimize the damage and pain. Ice on and off for the first 48 hours after an injury will help minimize bleeding and swelling. After 48 hours, ice will not help swelling. Ice will not help neck or back sprains because they do not bleed. Ice may numb things temporarily, but it will tighten up the muscles. For any injury, compression will help us minimize bleeding and swelling. For delayed pain that occurs from muscle irritability, easy movement of a joint or range of motion in the right directions will help. Massage or other warm-up tools in the right amounts will also tend to help.

If the onset of strains, sprains and tendinitis is gradual, we find an accumulation of pain, swelling and other delayed warning signs (repetitive or cumulative trauma). A great deal of misinformation exists about common accumulation injuries though we can easily detect them by pain. Damage to muscle, ligament or tendon fibers from overuse may occur slowly. Both sudden and gradual injuries can produce a wide spectrum of injury and pain, from irritation to a complete rupture of these structures.

If we want our body to heal from painful conditions, we must learn patience, especially with the acute or chronic pain from vicious cycles of disuse syndromes (dysuse). Patience is a learned character trait and an attitude that allows learning to continue despite the challenges of persisting pain. Pain is a reliable indicator of physiologic responses to abnormality. When dealt with inappropriately, physiologic responses cascade into a vicious cycle that can become worse and are not easy to get out of. When pain is out of control, patients tend to grasp at straws and the negative consequences are real.

The more recurrent a strain or sprain injury is, the more easily the pain reoccurs, which also leads to chronic pain. I have diagnosed pain at 2 months to be chronic when the speed and direction of the patient's recovery were not right. Despite having worked with them for 2 to 3 weeks or more, it seemed unlikely that a full recovery was going to happen within 3 months. Chronic pain does not mean that it must be permanent or cannot heal. The term "chronic" indicates that the injury has had time to heal, but it has not and will not unless something changes. Chronic pain will take longer than acute pain to turn around when we finally put our body in the right circumstances to allow it to heal. Even with a disease, however, our pain can be less by keeping the stiffness out and avoiding heavy or prolonged use. An example is rheumatoid arthritis of the hand.

Pain from tendon overuse injuries usually takes days or weeks to accumulate. Tendon damage has a wide spectrum of injury like other structures. Irritation (inflammation) of the tendon itself occurs with or without tendon fiber damage (tendinitis). Irritation of the surrounding tendon lining (tenosynovitis) can also occur without tendon fiber damage. When the tendon fibers are worn, degeneration occurs (tendinosis). The degenerated tendon fibers may form a lump in the tendon or associated bursa with or without painful calcium deposits. In the shoulder, it can be in the rotator cuff tendon or subdeltoid bursa. From proper angles, we may see calcium deposits on shoulder x-rays. Any tendon thickening may make rotator cuff tendon movement in its bony channel painful (rotator cuff impingement).

The Achilles tendon at the ankle has no bony channel, so the need for surgery is much less likely. Doing things to resolve pain in the Achilles tendon will allow it to heal and will also lessen the thickening or knot that occurs with Achilles tendinosis. Without healing, if tendon wear compromises many fibers, the tendon may rupture suddenly. If a tendon injury has not yet ruptured, it will heal if we put it in the right environment such as rest and a controlled amount of motion in the right ways. Tendon rupture with a gap between the two ends of the tendon usually needs surgery.

The Miracle of Pain

The results of disuse and accumulated mechanisms of pain such as chronic sprains, reflex sympathetic dystrophy or fibromyalgia are difficult to treat. Initial treatment consists of helping the patient to understand what the diagnosis is and what is contributing to it. We can alleviate each of these conditions. It is reassuring when pain lessens even if only temporarily. Ruling out disease and cancer is also reassuring. Disuse pain in the extremities involves areas that are trying to heal, but they are struggling because the patient is tending to go in the wrong direction. Disuse pain means not doing enough of the right things to help healing and doing too many of the wrong things that retard healing.

A common mistake is to walk too far because it takes time to get going. Then, when we finally warm up, it is also hard to want to stop because it feels good. Then we suffer for it afterwards when things cool down. Another mistake is to not move often enough. For disuse syndromes, we need to move much more often than normal. We tend to stay in one position too long watching TV or using a computer, and we tend to not move until the pain reminds us. Another mistake is stretching until it hurts. Keeping the distance and repetitions shorter is better, so pain does not occur at the time or afterwards. Then, come back to it more often.

Pressure from cancer cell growth is another mechanism of pain that physicians worry about when patients come in with pain, a mass or swelling. A chronic strain or infection can mimic cancer and may also cause pain, a mass or swelling. The diagnosis and treatment of cancer should not be delayed. In the presence of cancer, some of the principles for treatment of pain will still help to lessen pain and decrease dependence on pain medication. Many of these principles are common sense such as rest, limited activity and motion but are forgotten, assumed or ignored.

In 2002, I learned more about pain limits when I was a venturing crew advisor for our older Boy Scouts, including my son. We went to Beaver High Adventure Base for our annual summer camp. It is in the rugged Tushar Mountains of southern Utah. Among the daily activities for our 16 to 18-

year-old young men were rappelling, rock climbing, shotgun shooting, archery, wilderness survival and mountain biking. After breakfast on the second day, we rode mountain bikes starting from our base camp at an elevation of 9,000 feet. We went down to Three Creeks Reservoir at 8,600 feet, then up narrow dirt trails. We crossed a dry stream bed to get to a dirt road that followed Lake Stream. Then, we kept going up.

Occasional shade and water helped, but the climb was long and steady. The 21 gears of the mountain bike helped. When we reached State Highway 153, we followed it north a short distance. We turned northeast using the dirt road on the west side of Puffer Lake at nearly 9,700 feet elevation. North of the lake, we stopped at a lush, green meadow and water spring. The water was refreshing, and the simple sack lunch was energizing. We had climbed 1,100 feet in 4 miles.

Our camp trek leader then gave us a choice. We could go down the trail we came up, or we could bike up higher on the paved highway. The reward of more bike climbing, he told us, was the nearly straight, steep, downgrade afterwards. Cars or trucks were rare on the highway at that time in the summer. We chose the highway. In the next 0.7 of a mile, we climbed to the top of the pass, over 10,000 feet elevation, then down to cross North Fork Three Creeks and then back up to 10,000 feet. We headed downhill, easily going 45 miles per hour past a quiet Elk Meadows Ski Resort. After the resort, a highway sign warned us about the 10 percent downgrade. We could go as fast as we wanted, down to a flat stretch of road. The vertical descent was over 1,000 feet. The thrill of going downhill for 2.5 miles made up for the pain of going uphill.

When we reached the dirt road turnoff leading back to our base camp, we followed, instead, a narrow path east of Three Creeks Reservoir. On the left were hills and thick brush. On the right, a cliff down to the water seemed to narrow the path. We moved quickly through the beautiful terrain. Then finally, we rejoined the dirt road leading to our base camp. We finished the 10-mile trek without injuries, and I was grateful for that. The normal muscle tightness resolved with changing positions, a cool-down and some time that afternoon.

The Miracle of Pain

I learned that physical preparation with hiking or biking once a month, some at high elevations, built enough endurance to safely complete the day's trek without pain. We enjoyed the downhill rides. Since then, extreme mountain bike races fascinate me. The July 2011 inaugural, "Crusher in the Tushar," started an annual event. It is in the same mountains our Venture Scouts and I rode our mountain bikes in 2002. The 70-mile race starts in Beaver, Utah and has 10,400 feet of climbing. It ends at Eagle Point Resort (Elk Meadows Resort before 2010). I admire those who enjoy it. For me, an extreme bike ride is not necessary to have fun.

Pain will always be a warning sign. When we do enough good things or when we recognize and change our mistakes, feeling less pain is very reassuring. Then, we know that we are going in the right direction. The same direction must continue longer and at higher levels to develop a period without pain. The next step is longer periods of time without pain. It sounds easy, but it is not. Doctor Paul Brand, a British trained orthopedic hand surgeon, wrote emphatically about pain being a warning sign. He wrote, "…Pain is not the enemy, but the loyal scout announcing the enemy."[12]

Diverse levels of pain are like various levels of baseball. At each level, including T-ball, little league, pony league, high school, college, professional double A, triple A, major leagues and the World Series, players have different lessons and habits to learn. Few players can ever actually be on a team that wins the World Series. However, most of us can fortunately and eventually reach a level of no pain. To do that, we should always value and respect pain as a warning sign to learn from.

---

[12] Paul Brand, M.D., Phillip Yancey, <u>Pain: The Gift Nobody Wants</u>, HarperCollins, New York, October 1993, page 187.

Chapter 7

The Canoe Adventure

On a Sunday morning in early August 1993, I knew I was in serious trouble when I could not get out of bed to get to the bathroom. There was severe pain in my low back every time I tried to sit or stand. The pain was worse if I tried to walk. The pain inhibited me from being able to use my back and leg muscles when upright. Crawling lessened the pain enough for me to get to the bathroom. As I crawled, I put up with mild pain because I did not want to wet the bed. It surprised me when the pain eased up a little as I first stood up in the bathroom. Because standing there for a minute or two was okay, I was surprised again when I tried to walk. I could not walk without the same severe pain I had before. So, I crawled back to bed. I had no idea what I had done to bring on this predicament.

As I was lying there in bed that morning, I reflected on all the things I needed to do in the next few days at church and at work. I also thought of my obligation as a Boy Scout varsity coach that was coming up in 16 days. We had organized a 5-day High Adventure camp with a 62-mile canoe trip on the Colorado River between the Davis and Parker Dams. We had 25 young men and 5 adults going on the trip. At that time, our council in the Boy Scouts of America (BSA) required a BSA Lifeguard certification for water activity tour permits. At the time, I was the only adult with the certification in our Boy Scout units. Without me, they could not go.

I did not make it to church and could not get to work for 2 days. Then the pain began to ease off. I was applying at home what I was teaching my patients at the office, and it was working, though slowly. I was happy with the improvement, but a week before we were to leave on the canoe trip, I was still having constant, mild pain. I worried that the trip might make the pain worse. Prolonged sitting for many miles in a canoe would not be good for my back. I feared getting stuck out there on the river in the wilderness areas. I might have the same severe pain that I had at home when I could not move or walk. I decided that I could do most of the things on the trip

59

that I tell my patients to do. I would stretch; I would move, and I would avoid heavy lifting.

So there would be no misunderstandings and fewer unknowns, I also would let others know. I called my assistant leader for the trip and let him know what I was dealing with. We decided that we could not do much at that time, except go ahead with the trip as if everything was okay. We both felt that if the trip was going to happen, the snags would work out. If I stopped improving, we could still call it off at the last minute. A multitude of other things also needed to fall into place to allow the trip to happen anyway.

The morning of the trip came on a Tuesday, and I was stiff that morning as usual. I could move and loosen up, but the pain was still there and was still constant. The pain was less after I warmed up. The 230-mile, 4-hour drive to the Colorado River was another challenge with the prolonged sitting. I drove my 1989 Chevy 2500 extended cab, long bed truck and 21-foot runabout ski boat on a dual axle trailer. It was like driving a train. The boat trailered well, and the steering felt solid.

While driving with cruise control, I squirmed, wiggled and stretched often in the driver's seat with careful, small amounts. I stayed acutely aware of my back and paid attention to it often. I had some of our scouts with me in the truck cab, but I could still stop when I needed to, which I did once for gas. The pain was no worse when I pulled up to the boat storage facility at Moabi Regional Park, near Needles, California. Loading and unloading the supplies went well. I was careful, very careful. Again, the pain was no worse, though still constant.

After our outfitter, Jerkwater Canoe Company, transported us to Bullhead Community Park in Bullhead City, Arizona, it was time to climb into the canoes. We had 15 two-man canoes. My canoe partner was Justin Berry, one of our 25 young men. I told him that I was going to take breaks from paddling, and he could too. I could not ask him to paddle more than I did. All of us had practiced canoe paddling techniques ahead of time. But learning from the Canoeing Merit Badge pamphlet and a little practice with a canoe in a swimming pool did not make us experts with the J-stroke or keeping the canoe in a steady direction. With time on the river, however, we improved. The wind forced us to become more efficient by keeping the bow of the canoe going in the right direction and into the wind.

We were traveling downstream, and the water was flowing with us at about 3 miles an hour. But we could not keep up the pace with the others by coasting. Similar to our hikes, we had leaders in the front and leaders in the rear to keep from losing anyone. That was reassuring. All the supplies in our canoes were in double plastic bags. That was also reassuring. There are dangers on the river with overhanging trees, submerged rocks and a few jet skis. Capsizing would have been a lot of work, a catastrophe that I did not want to think about. Moving slowly in the canoe was a necessity for stability.

Because I was so concerned about my back in the canoe, I stretched often. Every few minutes, I slowly stuck one or both of my legs over or under the canoe cross bar to straighten my knee. I also moved one of my knees towards my chest, often. By raising my ankle and toes, I stretched my calf. If I stretched gently before I stood, it made standing up in the canoe easier. Also, stretching or standing was easier if I did not wait too long.

We were leaving civilization, and we kept paddling. I kept doing the back and leg exercises often. I started to think about trying to sleep that night and what I could do to help the pain and stiffness by altering my sleeping habits. I brought with me three firm, thin, foam pads to sleep on in the tent. As I paddled, I wondered if that was enough to keep me out of trouble. There was not too much else I could do at that point.

Purposely that night, I tossed and turned cautiously and often. It did not help much. It lessened the pain for a few minutes at a time, but my pain was still constantly there. Because I was in a tent by myself, I did not have to worry about disturbing anyone else while changing positions. I wondered if I could get any sleep that night. We had a long day in the canoes the next day to get past Needles, California and then camp at Park Moabi. The morning air was cool as I got up for breakfast. My muscles were tight, and I had to move slowly. I felt that I was no worse for the wear because the pain was about the same after the first night in the tent with little sleep.

In the afternoon of the second day, the wind picked up, and we were mostly heading into the wind. The distance between the canoes spread out as some canoe teams had different amounts of endurance and resolve. I continued to squirm, stretch and change positions often. I was still worried that I might not be able to finish the trip. After a long day, that night in the tent I again tossed and turned often on the foam pads.

We had planned waterskiing for the next morning, and my ski boat was the only one. Passing the helm of the boat to someone else would have been difficult for me. I loved to drive the boat and loved to teach others how to waterski or cruise on a wakeboard. About a year before, our family bought a new wakeboard. Getting up on it was much easier than a skurfer, an earlier version of the wakeboard. The wakeboard was less buoyant but thin, broad and flat. It had a small tail fin. The bindings then were loose, comfortable straps. They allowed for comfortable cruising. Since then, the boots and bindings have evolved to be tight and rigid. The boots are not comfortable but allow tricks in the air off the wake. I still just like to cruise.

When morning came, I felt better and was pleasantly surprised that I had no pain. I was stiff, but that also seemed to dissipate easily as I helped with breakfast and prepared the ski boat for a day of waterskiing and wakeboarding. I felt that I could drive the boat, but I did not know yet whether I could last all day like I usually do. During the day, I did not need to stretch as often and noticed I was forgetting at times that I even had a problem.

We changed the 9 passengers in the boat several times. Late that afternoon, our scouts and adult advisors had worn themselves out having fun with both skiing and wakeboarding.

Just before sunset, one of the adult leaders with me in the boat asked if I wanted to ski. Yes, of course, I wanted to ski. I did not ski too often on scout outings because I wanted the young men to have every opportunity to learn and experience the thrill of getting up on the water.

Time was short, but no one else wanted to go. So, why not go for it? I felt fine, and my muscles were not even tired. The other adult leader was responsible and had some experience driving a ski boat before. A brilliant, orange sun was just above the western horizon with a slightly purple cast to the clouds. The air was still, and the water on the river was like glass. How could I pass that up? The next day might be different. I got up easily on the wakeboard and the boat gradually worked up to a speed of 21 knots. As the sun slipped over the horizon, I cruised back and forth over the wakes. I had no desire to get air, but stopping was hard.

Right after sunset, I dropped the tow rope outside the wake and coasted to a stop, sinking slowly into the nearly still, cold river water. As I climbed into the boat, I still felt good. I did not have any pain or stiffness. There had been no pain the entire day. The sky was almost dark as we glided back into the marina at 5 miles per hour with our running lights on and with no wake behind the boat. After covering and securing the boat for overnight and checking on dinner assignments, I began to wonder what I had done to resolve the pain.

What could I learn from what I had experienced? Would the pain come back tonight or tomorrow? Was I going to be able to drive the boat tomorrow again? We had one more day of waterskiing and wakeboarding in the same area before canoeing down the river through Topock Gorge. The long, narrow gorge is usually the most difficult stretch of the 60-mile trip. Travel is usually against a stiff wind. That section of our trip was also the most scenic. The terrain is part of the Havasu National Wildlife Refuge.

That night, I tossed and turned again but this time out of habit. I was awake most of the night because I was so excited about the relief of pain and stiffness. As I rested, I thought about what I had done to resolve the pain and tried to learn from it. I determined several things. First, the tossing and turning at night can help resolve pain. Second, the stretching, changing position and paying attention to pain more often than I thought helps. Every few minutes is okay. Third, doing things that challenge the pain may be okay if paying attention to the pain often enough. Fourth, do not ignore the pain to get things done.

The other adult scout leaders stopped asking me if I was okay. They could see I was able to do everything and felt fine. The many challenges that occurred on the canoe trip with the young men during the rest of the week were no problem because the pain was gone. Because the pain was gone, I also wondered if I could figure out what had happened to cause the pain. I did not want to go through that nightmare again.

After sorting through the prior 3 weeks, the best I could come up with was that the back problems probably started with sleeping wrong. That means staying in one position too long during the night. Then, when I woke up, I must have moved or turned too far or too fast, creating low back pain from a muscle strain and muscle spasm. I learned to teach patients to stretch in smaller amounts and more often. I had been telling them to stretch, but previously I had no idea how often they could do it. I started quantifying my stretching recommendations with the degree of stretching, number of repetitions and frequency.

The pain in my back did not return. For me, the adventure was challenging, but I learned a lot. We finished the canoe adventure at a beach just south of the London Bridge on Lake Havasu. The 5 days with our scouts was awesome. The drive home was quiet, peaceful and without a problem. Everyone was tired. They had worn themselves out learning new things and having fun with new challenges. I also had new insights I could share with my patients.

Chapter 8

Why the Practice of Medicine?

The practice of medicine is a common expression. Why is it called a practice? What does that mean? Are physicians, who are dealing with patients with disease, injury or pain, learning as they go? That might be scary, but there is some truth to it! Disease evolves, epidemics defy and each injury is a little different. Does the phrase mean that physicians should read, take classes or go to medical meetings? Does it mean that physicians should learn from peers as we compare cases? Does it mean that we should listen to our patients and their family members? Do we learn from each one of them as we help them deal with their concerns and the patient's pain? The answer to the last five questions is "Yes!"

If we must go to a medical meeting, why would we go to an uninteresting location? Physicians must continue to learn during their careers. Learning should, however, be void of fads. We should fill our minds with solid evidence and conclusions from well thought out scientific studies by investigators, respected for their honesty.

The term "practice of medicine" is not an invention of modern medicine. The terminology has been around for thousands of years. The concepts of "medical practice" as an "art," as well as many medical terms, date back to at least 400 B.C. with Hippocrates. Another physician, Jewish rabbi and philosopher, Moses Maimonides who lived from 1138 to 1204 A.D., wrote about the practice of medicine in the twelfth century. He was born in Cordova, Spain, lived in Cairo, Egypt and wrote, "Medical practice is not knitting and weaving and the labor of the hands, but it must be inspired with the soul and be filled with understanding and equipped with the gift of keen observation; these together with accurate scientific knowledge are the indispensable requisites for proficient medical practice."[13]

Many years ago, when I read that, I recognized that not all physicians practice the principles that Hippocrates or

---

[13] A small framed plaque, courtesy of Sandoz, Ltd., 1990.

The Miracle of Pain

Maimonides taught. Because of evolving government and insurance company payment schemes, gradually more physicians do not take the time to listen and understand their patients. As described by Maimonides, his "labor of the hands" applies to orthopedic surgery. But if our hands are all we use, the patient stays lost in a world of darkness. With compassion for all who ask for help, we as physicians can be "filled with understanding" if we listen to our patients and to their families.

We should also keep current with good, honest medical science. But keeping up-to-date with the "latest and greatest" fads that are here today and gone within a few years, satisfies only our selfish desires and our pride. That kind of knowledge is not dealing justly with our patients. Many of our patients demand the "latest and greatest" treatments. Part of keeping current is knowing enough about the fads to be able to talk patients out of them. Some patients will go elsewhere, but that is okay. Sadly, they will suffer the consequences of their choices.

William Carlos Williams (1883–1963), a poet, essayist and physician who practiced in Rutherford, New Jersey, wrote in 1955, "It's the humdrum, day-in, day-out, every day work that is the real satisfaction of the practice of medicine... I never had a money practice."[14] A money practice is run by a doctor whose primary motive is money. They have always been around. Be wary if a physician has a high volume of surgeries or patients.

In our prideful, technology driven world, in some ways we have lost knowledge. We have not treasured truth of past ages that is right. Our medical community has lost some types of knowledge over several decades because of dishonesty. It affects all parts of health care. What I call "economic research" is when we allow the sponsors of research to influence our knowledge. Because the sponsors are selling something, it is a dishonest pseudoscience. Before starting the

[14] William Carlos Williams, "The Practice," from his autobiography in On Doctoring, Stories, Poems, Essays, edited by Richard Reynolds, M.D. and John Stone, M.D., Simon & Schuster, 1995, page 68.

research, they know what they want to prove. A hypothesis is different, and it requires curiosity and honesty. We have not spoken out enough against dishonesty and those who want to control and limit good health care choices. A better direction would be more opportunities for health savings accounts.

Vitamin and nutritional supplement industries have been rife with dishonesty for years. Prescription medication and orthopedic surgery equipment industries have gone over the edge with abuse of their advertising and marketing power. Since the 1990s, ads on TV directed at the patient have become common place for those industries. The disclaimer is, "Ask your doctor if it is right for you."

In about 2001, one orthopedic equipment maker told all the orthopedic surgeons on staff at one of our local California hospitals that they could "legally" give us "shared income" if we used their company products for surgeries on our patients. They requested a meeting at the hospital with those who would be interested. That was an odd request, and I had never heard that before. It sounded unethical or illegal. I did not attend the meeting. I do not know if other orthopedic peers at our hospital pursued the offer.

Murky choices did not end there. In 2005, a former administrator at the same local hospital wrote a letter to all the orthopedic surgeons on the medical staff informing us about a program to reduce costs. They wanted to restrict us to using three companies, Stryker/Howmedica, Depuy and Zimmer, for total hip and total knee replacement surgeries. What concerned me was the "gain sharing" aspect that the letter described for physicians. To me that part of the program had the look of a kickback. We were told to sign up for it and undergo training within 5 months to do the procedures. To reassure us he wrote that he sent the plan for approval to the federal Office of Inspector General (OIG).[15]

I felt that the program and the plan were plainly unethical. I did not attend that meeting either. I did not want

---

[15] Established in 1976, the OIG is part of the U.S. Department of Health and Human Services (HHS).

to be a part of it. I kept doing total hip and knee replacements at the hospital as I had in the past. The hospital did not want me to start scheduling my surgery cases elsewhere. Hospital medical staff doctors and hospital administrators will always have an ever-present win-win struggle as we deal with the prevailing medical challenges and economic forces.

Since the 1990s, advertising, dishonesty and arrogance permeate many university medical institutions. Wanting to refer patients to them is harder. They are often less reliable in following up with patients. Elitism is one way to describe it, but it is an abuse of power and a form of bullying. Any medical institution that advertises heavily is suspect. Hearing radio and television ads or seeing magazine advertisements for university medical facilities is sickening. Be wary of any facility whose physicians are always in too big of a hurry to listen or to clearly explain what the diagnosis is and what can or cannot be done. There still are good physicians, hospitals and universities, but choose wisely.

Medical ads were illegal before the 1980s. Since then, ads by academic tertiary care centers have created hype for some questionable new treatments. They own an awkward competitive edge against private physicians in the community who do not belong to the institution. Many private practice physicians have better practical experience and judgment because they experiment less with the "latest and greatest" fads. There are good and bad physicians on both sides.

Depending upon personal ethics, some physicians may be less inclined to listen to patients because of ancillary personnel. They are known as physician extenders and are an efficient barrier between a physician and patient. They include a medical assistant (MA), nurse assistant (CNA), nurse (RN, LPN/LVN), nurse practitioner (NP), physician assistant (PA), medical student, medical intern (MD) or medical or surgical resident (MD). The powerful economic squeeze from governments and insurance companies affects all physicians.

Before the year 2000, the atmosphere between academic and private doctors was more collegial. A spirit of cooperation, learning and education flourished. Now many academics have an attitude that they are doing physicians in private practice a great favor by accepting patients needing tertiary care. Some also have an attitude that the referring physician has done something wrong. It is a self-serving attitude that has replaced serving patients and peers, feeding the need for advertising. Academic physicians are not immune from misinformation. Humility, a desire for truth and gratitude for a source of referrals is becoming harder to find.

Politically correct terms from academic and other large institutions may sound good, but be careful. They may describe health care as using a team approach, having user-friendly quality or having integrated cost-effective models. What do those words mean? In health care, a team approach conveys the excitement of sports and refers to several exams from different vantage points. User-friendly designs are for computers. Integrated systems are for business managers and engineers. A model is a toy airplane or ship that I built as a child. The above terms are feel-good terms. They conjure up images that we are comfortable with and are meant to be reassuring. Many feel-good terms, however, have hollow promises attached. Without further medical care specifics, they tell us little.

Private practice physicians are not immune from poor or limited verbal skills. They may also be under the wrong influences. Peer pressure from partners and sales pressure from various sources is real. Pharmaceutical and procedure equipment sales are often lacking in honest science. Some government regulation and monitoring has helped but will never be the best answer. Word of mouth referrals from physicians and from patients are still the best sources of help. It is like the word of mouth referrals for other professions and trades. They are still the best defenses against poor physicians, businesses or contractors. Online referrals do not come close to being the same. With word of mouth, we consider the source honestly when we talk to each other and take stock of the opinion.

There are many useful sources of medical knowledge. We should be willing to learn from all good sources. Learning from the experiences of patients is not the least of those sources. Learning from the experiences of my peers in the community is a wonderful source. In the private practice of orthopedics, a partner's experience and their patients, though different than mine, offer other vantage points. Another major source of medical knowledge is from the study of interesting medical journal articles from reliable authors or institutions that we grow to trust.

Among the multitudes of new medications and procedures that are created every year, a few are appropriate and helpful. Medical schools have taught for years how to discern good, honest, medical journal articles. We can say the same for new helpful drugs and appropriate procedures. Practicing physicians dismiss most new treatments for good reason. We have seen variations of many of them before with all their failings. A practicing physician must evaluate all new treatments considered for use with a critical eye. The intuition and experience of an honest physician goes a long way to shield patients from unscrupulous purveyors and proprietors who have been around for thousands of years.

When knee joint arthroscopy first came out in the 1970s, using the instruments was thrilling for me.[16] I knew it would be around for a long time. Seeing that arthroscopy was good was exciting because the benefits were easy to see. The fiberoptic instruments allow us to see a meniscus cartilage tear in a knee better. The visualization allows a precise removal of the small torn part of the meniscus (partial meniscectomy). The icing on the cake was that we could do it as an outpatient with much smaller incisions, each less than ⅜ of an inch long.

The old procedure used a 3-inch open incision (knee arthrotomy). The surgeon could not usually see the torn part of the cartilage piece until they removed the entire meniscus and examined it outside the body (meniscectomy). They, therefore, also removed normal parts of the torn cartilage. Patients

---

[16] Arthroscopy is an outpatient surgical procedure, first done in the knee in about 1975. We use an arthroscope, a fiberoptic instrument about the length and thickness of a pencil, with two to four small incisions. We do arthroscopic surgery most often in the knee, followed by the shoulder and ankle.

needed to stay in the hospital for 2 to 3 days for pain control until they could be up safely on crutches. When video cameras became smaller, we attached them to the fiberoptic arthroscope. They allowed us to have even more flexibility in safely seeing the pathology. When visualization is better, good things can happen, and we can avoid problems. Arthroscopy made sense then, and it still makes sense now.

After studying it, the first knee arthroscopy I performed was in 1979. I was an orthopedic surgery resident at Riverside Methodist Hospital in Columbus, Ohio. Some surgeons were still doing open knee arthrotomy procedures. The contrast with arthroscopy was stark. Arthroscopy patients had much less pain. They were comfortable being treated as outpatients. They had significantly decreased recovery times. The results for all patients were good about 95 percent of the time. Over the years since, I have had a few patients with severe pain before surgery, who told me afterwards that they had no pain and did not need any pain pills.

We also have other good procedures that have grown out of knee arthroscopy. One example is shoulder arthroscopy for abnormal thickening of the rotator cuff tendon or of the bursa (tendinosis or bursitis). When there is not enough room for the tendon in its bony channel, the rotator cuff becomes painful (impingement). Shoulder arthroscopy can resolve pain by removing some of the thickened bone and bursa to create more room for tendon movement.[17] If calcium deposits are in the shoulder rotator cuff tendon or bursa, using a needle to break up the calcific deposits can also resolve pain without doing anything else (aspiration under x-ray control).

Small incisions are not always better. Each part of our anatomy is unique. Many proponents have invented ill-conceived, ill-advised procedures, hoping to succeed, based on the strength and success of arthroscopy. When a procedure such as microdiscectomy of the low back gives a surgeon bragging rights for a smaller incision for a herniated disc

---

[17] This surgical procedure is shoulder arthroscopic subacromial decompression with anteroinferior partial acromionectomy and bursectomy.

removal, risks are higher. Dreadful things can and do happen when a surgeon is not seeing well in a small incision.

Also, for a while, use of similar fiberoptic instruments was faddish in the spinal canal (spinal endoscopy). However, it never made sense for mechanical reasons. There was a real danger to the movable, free floating nerve elements in the spinal canal. When some surgeons tout small incisions as better, be careful. New instrumentation allowing better visualization and smaller incisions may make sense. Check with a doctor whom you can trust.

In my second year as a general surgery resident at Ohio State University (OSU) in 1978, I saw an exciting opportunity and switched to orthopedics at OSU. For years after that, I teased my general surgery colleagues that I might perform an appendectomy with my arthroscope "pretty soon" if they did not. Because the use of a fiberoptic scope made sense, I knew it was only a matter of time before general surgeons would start doing appendectomies with fiberoptic instruments. Since the 1990s, they use them fairly routinely for removal of the appendix (laparoscopic appendectomy).

For doctors in medical practice, Continuing Medical Education (CME) requirements have become the domain of each state in the United States for purposes of licensing. To practice medicine in California, state laws and regulations have since December 1976 required that licensed physicians complete 25 hours of CME credits per year, "as a condition for relicensure." CME hours are a valid effort to push doctors to stay up-to-date, especially as economic constraints on a doctor's time have increased.

Fine-tuning in 2003 by California lawmakers made 12 hours of CME mandatory for, "pain management and the treatment of terminally ill and dying patients." These CMEs have done nothing but worsen the epidemics of pain and pain medication abuse. California then followed 4 other states, allowing assisted suicides with an End of Life Option (EOLO), effective June 9, 2016. This is directly against the Hippocratic Oath, which says, "To please no one will I prescribe a deadly drug, nor give advice which may cause their death." The

California Medical Association changed its stance against assisted suicide in May 2015, stating that they are "neutral." Being for assisted suicide would not look good for them. However, their neutral position makes them complicit in assisted suicide, which was a felony until 2016.

CME credit hours at some medical meetings are worth the time attending, and some are a waste of time and money. Some medical journal articles are well worth reading, and some are not. Finding good articles in a respected medical journal is less time consuming and less expensive than going to a medical meeting. For many years in the United States, we could not earn the required CME credit hours by studying credible orthopedic articles from respected journals. The Journal of Bone and Joint Surgery (JBJS) and Journal of the American Academy of Orthopaedic Surgeons (JAAOS) solved that. Since 2003, the JBJS and then the JAAOS, since 2010, offer 10 CME credit hours for reading 6 journal volumes, completing an exam and paying a fee.

Learning by practicing, studying and helping patients deal with or eliminate pain are normal parts of a doctor's medical practice. It has always been so and always will be in this world. This aspect of the medical profession is, by far, the most satisfying. CME credits are only a tool and are a good reminder. The best learning is from listening to and examining patients, reading good journal articles and consulting with trusted peers. Learning depends on a desire to learn and a willingness to spend time with patients and their families.

Useful scientific studies are based on the honesty, morals and ethics of the researchers involved. Likewise, honest assessments, diagnoses and treatment recommendations by medical doctors will continue to depend upon their ability to stay honest and practice freely. Limited interference from government and insurance companies can allow a level playing field for the exchange of solid ideas and treatments.

Chapter 9

Epidemics of Misinformation

We often see misinformation about medical basics confuse patients in our high-tech world, and it can inhibit a patient's recovery. Simple things like the use of heat and ice for injuries or for pain are turned upside down and distorted. Many people have the false impression that they should use ice for all injuries. Misinformation has contributed to the use of ice for back or neck injuries. It might feel good temporarily, but ice is only numbing the area, and the pain will keep coming back.

Because most injuries of the spine do not have swelling or bleeding, there is no good reason to use ice on them. If swelling or bleeding happen, they are usually far enough inside that ice cannot help. Without ice, the surrounding muscles will reflexively tighten anyway to splint the area. That contributes to involuntary compression that lessens any tendency for bleeding. If local swelling in a muscle occurs, it usually means a spasm or cramp is in the muscle, which would be worse with ice. Ice would also increase the gap between the two torn ends of a muscle rupture.

Misinformation has also led to the use of ice on injuries for many days or weeks at a time. In addition, some use ice several weeks after an injury for persisting pain or swelling, "to help the swelling," or they say, "to stop the pain." Using ice in these ways will not help the swelling. In many patients with ongoing pain, ice will diminish the pain only because of the temporary numbing effect that masks pain. In that setting, ice is no more effective than a mild pain pill. Using ice alone more than 48 hours after an injury offers no benefits for healing but has many disadvantages.

In some patients, ice will increase their pain. However, the greatest adverse effects from ice are stiffness, increasing muscle tightness, decreasing blood flow in the veins and, therefore, increasing venous stagnation (venous stasis). These effects increase delayed pain and decrease the ability of the muscle to recover. They increase the risk of muscle strain, vein clots (venous thrombosis) and dangerous, mobile clots (venous thromboembolism). The dangers of clots in leg veins are higher with too little or too much activity, especially after surgery. Do not use ice by itself more than 48 hours following an injury or surgery.

A frequent question is, "Should I use heat or ice?" Because of prevalent misinformation, it is a good question. I have a good, easy answer. For the first 24 to 48 hours after a closed arm or leg injury, use ice for 20 minutes at a time, on and off. In that first day or two, it inhibits bleeding and swelling. If the skin is cut, care for the wound and then use layers of plastic and cloth to keep ice condensation and additional bacteria away from the wound. Pressure with a hand or compression is very helpful for bleeding and swelling. For fingers and toes, the use of gentle pressure becomes more important and the use of ice has more risk because of diminished blood circulation.

Contrasts are 5 minutes of ice followed by 10 minutes of heat, every hour, or more often. They are useful after 48 hours for arm or leg injuries without fractures. When ice alternates with heat, the body increases the blood flow to the injured area. The evidence for this is redness of the skin. We can use contrasts for weeks. The body then reflexively dissipates the heat or cold to surrounding areas to prevent more injury from the heat or cold. The disadvantages of contrasts are the inconvenience and the time that they require. Many athletes are intensely focused on recovering quickly. They do not mind putting in the time it takes to do contrasts. Because the athlete is doing something productive, it helps limit the temptation of too much activity, too early.

Though it almost always feels good, many patients underuse local heat because of misinformation. Heat is good for all arm and leg injuries without a fracture after 48 hours. Its use should be intermittent, up to 20 minutes at a time, in conjunction with 3 other tools, elevation, movement and compression. Heat helps muscle relaxation, swelling and stiffness. Elevation at or just above the heart level can also always help swelling, but patients do not use it enough. Elevation is the hardest of the tools to utilize because it is limiting, inconvenient, boring and takes time. Motion can be helpful for swelling when done in directions that do not stress the injury in the wrong directions. Compression with an elastic bandage inhibits swelling, but it does not stop swelling.

Using heat within the first 48 hours after an injury can increase the swelling and bleeding. Also, use of heat with a cast or a splint at any time is not a good idea because of the real danger of increased swelling inside the cast or splint. With tight back muscles and aggressive movement, the hot water in a shower can relax all the muscles too well. Then, the lack of muscle support may create bigger problems with a sprain, then muscle spasm and sudden severe pain. Moving slower or showering later in the day may eliminate that risk.

Because a hot tub or Jacuzzi feels good and helps muscles relax, many patients ask if they can use it. Unfortunately, when the injured part is a leg, heat will accentuate swelling because it is below the heart level (a dependent position). Even without an injury, if there is already swelling in the legs, the same accentuation of swelling occurs. If 10 minutes or less in a hot tub helps movement by loosening up the joints and muscles, then the movement may help swelling. The temperature should be 98 degrees Fahrenheit or less and the time in a hot tub should be 20 minutes or less. Many ask, "If it feels so good, why can't I stay in there longer?" The body cannot disperse the damaging effects of heat to other areas when the heat is generalized. Common lay knowledge is to avoid staying in a hot tub too long, but many of us have not thought about why.

The problems with short, high levels of heat from fire or scalding hot water are obvious. On the other hand, what happens with prolonged, low levels of heat? When we cook meat in a crock-pot or slow cooker, we end up with meat so tender that it falls off the bone and falls apart. A low level of heat for prolonged periods damages the proteins of muscle and of the surrounding supporting ligaments and fibrous layers (denaturization). We do not want that for our muscles. It can happen with a hot tub or with a heating pad (generalized or local heat). Early damage from prolonged exposure to various levels of heat is manifested by burns, muscle tension or tightness, inability to tolerate heat, muscle irritability, heat exhaustion and heat stroke. Late heat damage includes increased skin pigmentation, muscle stiffness or weakness, muscle shrinkage (atrophy), joint scar tissue (adhesions and contractures) and brain damage.

I have seen each of these problems with heat injury in patients who were treated elsewhere. They often have severe pain or chronic pain syndromes. The patients did not know what else to do for their pain besides heat. The medication, exercises and other things they were trying were not helping. We need to remember that an injured body part is more susceptible than normal to additional injury from any stress. It can be heat, cold, vibration or use.

In proper situations with an appropriate level and duration, heat can help to relax muscles and improve blood circulation. It can help the body fight skin and other soft-tissue infections. When heat is right and feels good, it is okay to come back to it often. In some situations, under the direction of a doctor, longer periods of low-level, local heat can be useful. Temporary use of a heating pad for 1 to 2 hours at a time 4 to 8 times per day is very helpful for vein clots (phlebitis and deep vein thrombosis). Prolonged local heat is also good for some arm or leg infections.

More than 48 hours after an injury, rarely heat does not feel good even for short periods. If heat does not feel good, do not use it. If so, heat is making irritable muscles more irritable. The muscles are heat intolerant. That happens when the muscles cannot tolerate any added stress. They will not respond well to heat, which tries to force them to relax. Use heat again after a few days or a few weeks. When heat is right, it will feel good, and the muscles will relax.

Trying to force a muscle to relax with either stretching or heat when it is not ready is a mistake. The muscle will rebel with pain and spasm becoming worse. To say, "just force it more," is misinformation. In many ways, muscles are like teenagers. Muscles need to be taught, encouraged and usually not forced. We should respect, love, appreciate and not abuse them. Muscles must be allowed to learn over a period of time. We have to be patient with muscles and remember that they can heal and do better when they are ready. We should give them some time and attention. Sometimes we should leave them alone. Muscles will relax but on their own time frame. When we help them to be in the right conditions, they will often respond better and sooner than we think.

Worry and misinformation affects our choices if we believe that we will quickly lose our muscle training and aerobic capacity. We will tend to do too much instead of resting to take care of an injury. Many say that there is "muscle memory." That is true. It means that the muscle does not completely forget its training. Both muscles and teenagers are learning all the time. We need to spend time with them, teach them and train them. They are learning to make choices, which helps them do things independently in the future. Teaching consequences of their choices is powerful.

After resolving pain, an injured muscle will come back and surprise you with how well it does despite the trauma it has been through. Muscles and teenagers have a mind of their own. They will do good things, often when you do not expect them to. They need a variety of positive influences to recover fully from trials and mistakes. When they are taught correct principles and choose to do good things on their own, they can accomplish amazing things. My wife and I had five teenagers, and we survived. Those times were often perplexing, but the memories are good. There were rays of sunshine along the way. We learned new things, especially patience, in dealing with the challenges.

Be patient with your muscles. Trust that they can heal if you help by putting them in appropriate conditions. When the pain is gone and after a reasonable recovery time, muscle memory and aerobic capacity return relatively quickly. The muscles decide when they are ready to relax, recover and improve. When done in the right ways, encouragement will help. A little heat in short amounts a few weeks after an injury, like hugs for a teenager, often helps muscles having trouble relaxing.

Heat is also very effective for many infections. For a boil (a localized skin infection or abscess), using moist heat while showering with soap and water is often sufficient (generalized heat). If the boil is painful or not improving, it is more helpful to use moist warm compresses for 15 minutes at least 4 times a day (local heat). Within a day or two the boil is often gone, especially if moist heat is used early and frequently. More often is better. Longer than 15 minutes is not helpful. Using 30 minutes twice per day is not as helpful as 15 minutes 4 times per day even though the total time is the same.

A quick and effective way to apply a moist warm compress is to use a washcloth that is folded twice. Run hot water on the center corner of it in an apple-sized area. When comfortable on the skin, place it on the boil. Cover the wet area of the washcloth by unfolding the dry parts of it for insulation to keep the heat from dissipating too quickly. The warmth will last about 15 minutes. Do not lift it to check it. Simply hold it in place for the full 15 minutes. If you check it after 15 minutes and it still feels slightly warm to the touch of your other hand, the warm soak was still helping the entire time.

The softening of the skin from moist heat allows the pus of the skin boil to come to the surface or resolve without damaging the surrounding skin or soft tissues. It relieves pressure, which lessens the damage and pain. Pushing on or poking an infection with fingers or a needle will cause a bigger problem. Because it pushes bacteria into the surrounding soft tissues, it is like pouring gasoline on a fire. If a boil or any infection is not improving each day, see a doctor immediately for possible antibiotics or surgical treatment.

Warm water soaks are also effective for a painful ingrown toenail that may or may not have pus associated with it. The water does not need to be terribly hot or have Epsom salts. The softening of the toenail and skin with moist heat allows the offending toenail spike to move or grow over the skin without damaging the skin or other soft tissues. It relieves the pressure and pain. Especially if done early, 15-minute soaks in warm water at least 4 times per day are extremely helpful within a day or two.

For mechanical help, after each soak we can lift the toenail a tiny amount using only a fingernail. With a frequent, gentle lift, the ingrown toenail will grow over the skin and resolve more quickly. However, we can create a bigger problem and split the toenail by lifting with too much force when the toenail is soft. "Digging out the ingrown toenail," is never a good idea and can cause a serious infection. We should not cut the toenail until it is long enough to be over the skin. The nail should have a white, free edge at the end of the nail. When cutting a nail, leave some of the white edge.

In summary for ice and heat, remember that good tools have a high rate of success when used properly. We can misuse all good tools, and when that happens they can create more problems than they solve. If heat feels good, in the right circumstances we can use it often. In conjunction with heat, we can use other mechanical measures such as movement and limitation of activity. One useful tool should not be relied upon exclusively because one tool will often not be enough to solve pain and finish recovery.

Another example of an epidemic of misinformation is the idea promoted by many people and physicians that we need to walk farther to decrease the risk of clots. After most surgeries and leg injuries, movement is good, but walking too far will get us into trouble. Walking distances that we are not ready for will cause swelling, muscle tightness, muscle spasticity, venous congestion and leg clots. The swelling and tightness contributes to and perpetuates a vicious cycle in the muscle. Swelling may then continue in different ways. The consequences vary and include varicose veins (venous insufficiency), increased skin pigmentation (venous stasis dermatitis), leg ulcers (venous stasis ulceration), leg blood clots (phlebitis, venous thrombosis, deep vein thrombosis) or clots that move to the lungs, which may be deadly (pulmonary embolism).

A "walk farther" mentality therefore, does exactly the opposite of what we are trying to accomplish. Walking too far is easy to do. Because we have warmed up, walking may even feel good. Unknowingly, we are increasing the risk of leg clots after surgery or injury. Clots in deep veins of a leg with swelling from the ankle to above the knee are known to be dangerous. For that, we immediately put patients in the hospital for bedrest, tests, low levels of local heat, leg elevation and blood thinners (anticoagulants). The local heat relaxes muscles and helps blood flow, decreases swelling and increases the body's ability to dissolve the clots in the deep veins (clot metabolism). If the swelling is not above the knee, we can usually use the same methods without blood thinners successfully at home.

A corollary of the "walk farther" error is the hesitation of patients and their physicians to use rest. Their impression is that if patients rest, they will be at greater risk of leg clots and pain. The opposite, however, is true. Patients resting horizontally with their legs frequently elevated above heart level have less risk of leg clots, swelling and persisting pain. Resting and moving can prevent and heal problems. The necessary resting time and frequency depends on the problem and the swelling that is already there.

Though horizontal rest is best, patients often worry that others will see them as not trying. Others may see them as lazy or wimpy. We can use various horizontal positions. Horizontal rest does not mean that patients should be sleeping or merely lying there, doing nothing. They should be paying attention to the pain and moving often in accordance to what decreases the pain. Doing other things, like reading, is a distraction from what they should be doing.

Resting in a chair or recliner is okay occasionally, but it does not count towards the benefits of elevation or horizontal rest. A recliner limits hip motion. Side to side turning is harder and therefore inhibited. Prolonged sitting in any chair when the legs are not higher than the heart gives us no prophylactic protection from clots. Clots are less common in the arm and occur with overuse or after injury or surgery. Although arm clots occur much less often than in a leg, they occur in the same way when we ignore early warning signs.

Actively changing horizontal resting positions often is important. We should use many comfortable side positions and various positions on the back as well (lateral decubitus and supine). Lying on the stomach for short periods can be a comfortable option (prone position). Moving all joints in normal directions is also helpful for blood circulation of the arms and legs. It also helps keep the muscles, tendons, joints and nerves less tense in all areas. Tension inhibits blood circulation and leads to clots.

In about the year 2002, I saw a perfect opportunity to test my theory of the forgotten benefits of horizontal rest. I took care of a 76-year-old female patient admitted to the hospital from the emergency room for a left hip fracture. She also had a chronic left leg ulcer from bad veins. She said she had always had the leg ulcer, and she was afraid that the hip fracture would make it worse. The 2-inch by 4-inch ulcer on the front of her shin was down to the fatty layers of the leg (subcutaneous layers). There was no evidence of healing in the wound (no red granulation tissue). She had surrounding skin damage with increased pigmentation (venous stasis dermatitis). I knew that the hip fracture would force her to rest. If I could change some of her habits, I felt she might be able to heal the leg ulcer.

I boldly promised her that because of the hip fracture, she had also bought the cure for her leg ulcer. I explained that she needed to continue doing at home what I encouraged her to do in the hospital. I also explained that I wanted her to use horizontal rests more often than we would normally do for a hip fracture by itself. After the planned hip surgery, she could get up with a walker and physical therapy as usual. She needed to be partial weight bearing as usual, but we would keep the time for sitting and distance for walking shorter than normal. I showed her the mechanical tools for leg clot prophylaxis with toe, foot, ankle and knee motions. She would use them every few minutes on the left leg and less often on the right. She did not have clots, and we would not use blood thinners. She gladly agreed to the plan after I discussed the options with her.

She was already in a skin traction boot for the left hip fracture. I asked her to start the small left leg motions I taught her before I left the room. The hip surgery with metal hardware went well (open reduction and internal fixation with large hip compression screw and plate). I gave the physical therapist the same instructions with sitting and walking limited to 10-minute intervals. I thought that the ulcer could heal, but how quickly it healed surprised me. Before I discharged her from the hospital, 5 days after the surgery, the ulcer had healed well enough that it no longer needed a dressing. Her body's speedy ability to heal proved to me again that many things will heal when we put them in the right circumstances. This was an elderly patient with a chronic ulcer! Fortunately, after her discharge from the hospital, the patient continued horizontal rests often enough that her leg ulceration did not come back. Her hip fracture also healed, and she resumed her normal activity.

The proper use of frequent horizontal rests during the day will enable healing of many orthopedic problems, including severe back pain. Patients should not feel guilty about resting. Patients should not feel guilty about taking care of themselves. When facing significant challenges, they must learn how often to rest and how long to rest at a time. Any prolonged position while resting or watching TV, including horizontal positions, can be counterproductive. The use of a laptop computer also tempts us to stay in a prolonged, counterproductive position.

If I could convince a patient with back or neck pain to use horizontal rests often, it became much easier to help them improve. That means rests at least 4 times per day, usually for 10 to 15 minutes at a time. They may have had a herniated disc or large bone spurs in the spine. I did not expect the abnormal disc or bone spurs to disappear. They improved by having less muscle spasm, less nerve irritation and a partial healing or solidification of the abnormal disc. When pain and spasm are very bad, horizontal and upright position changes are the only truly natural things that can help. Paying attention to whether pain is getting better or worse over a few days gives us a sense of direction. During recovery, a sense of direction helps determine the number of daytime horizontal rests to use.

Both misinformation and fear have become epidemic and are the lifeblood of "alternative" treatments. These treatments become more appealing when patients become overly fearful of surgery or other well established medical treatment. I fear surgery as well, especially if I am the one in need of the surgery. However, I am not overly fearful of surgery and have needed it several times. It has been successful each time. As a surgeon and as a patient, I have a genuine respect for what surgery can and cannot do. As a medical doctor, I can say the same for medication.

If we recommend elective surgery, there may be a waiting time to see if the patient really needs surgery. During the wait, the patient should do simple things at home or also at physical therapy. They should not use "alternative" treatments that have marginal or little benefit. What to do and what not to do is the foundation of effective home care or nonoperative treatment. If the patient's pain is not continuing to improve after injuries have healed, physical therapy with a prescription by the doctor and a specific diagnosis can usually help. Though uncommon, if physical therapy causes more pain, we should modify or stop it. If the patient cannot travel to physical therapy without hurting more, they should wait, rest often and go later.

Some describe "alternative" treatments in ways that sound good, easy and popular. They include many marginal disciplines. There are better ways to deal with acute and chronic pain, especially back pain. These disciplines often have small amounts of truth. By adding misinformation, they morph into fashionable schemes. Stretching and traction by themselves are good tools and may have wonderful benefits. They also have disadvantages when misused or their extremes are encouraged. A common result of the extremes is a chronic strain with recurrent pain. Many "alternative" care providers promote accompanying misinformation such as "nutritional supplements" and the recurrent use of ice that provide false hope and no healing.

There can be relief with some "alternative" treatments, but the provider often leaves the patient with no realistic idea of what is wrong and how to prevent recurrent problems. The benefits may be short-lived and may induce dependency. They frequently cause distractions from the real diagnosis and may make the patient worse. The risks for persisting, recurrent or chronic pain are real. A delay in the correct diagnosis is a frequent problem.

Expensive upside-down home traction machines, so-called inversion tables, have also been popular on and off. Patients who buy them usually find them sitting in their garage or their closet after a few months. If the position of being upside down is of benefit, why not go outside and find a monkey bar or a tree limb to hang on upside down? It would be a lot less expensive. If the patient finds any benefits from the machine, it usually gradually stops working within a few weeks. Better ways that work just as fast are safer and are not upside down.

Even when some benefits of "alternative" care occur, recurrent usage will allow negative repercussions for the muscles to accumulate. How would you like it if you were the muscle and someone kept overstretching you? Would you like it if they kept poking you with their fingertips or a needle? Irritation is the least that happens to the poor, abused muscle with recurrent "alternative" treatments.

We can say the same for recurrent injections of any kind. Scarring of the muscle and chronic recurrent pain in the muscle are resulting long-term effects. The longer the abuse of muscle occurs, the greater are the effects that accumulate. Even after years of recurrent abuse, however, those results are not necessarily permanent. To make improvements, the environment for the muscles must change. We should recognize and avoid popular, widespread misinformation.

~~ *Chapter 10* ~~

Epidemics, Addictions, Dependencies

The wide use of and dependence on pain pills are epidemic. Many voices promote the use of pain medications. They contend that many patients, especially the elderly, are undertreated. Experience has taught me, however, that elderly patients are easy to over treat with pain medications after a hip fracture. Like children, they usually need less for pain. Even average doses often will aggravate or precipitate acute episodes of confusion or disorientation (dementia). This can be dangerous when the confusion leads to combativeness because both the patient and the nursing staff are at risk for injury. Many times, I have had to decrease the pain medication ordered by the patient's internal medicine doctor. Afterwards, the confusion resolved. Then, when I asked the patients how they were doing, they denied having any pain. They were cooperative again. For them, less treatment for pain was the right answer.

The misguided efforts of many groups, including hospital accreditation agencies, some academic professional associations and some state medical boards, put significant pressure on physicians to over-prescribe. Note the following narcotic (opiate or opioid) pain medication recommendation by an academic group. They admit a low quality of evidence to support it. They tell us that every patient suffering from, "moderate to severe pain, pain-related functional impairment, or diminished quality of life due to pain should be considered for opioid therapy (low quality of evidence, strong recommendation)."[18]

On the other hand, other state and federal government entities look for and prosecute physicians who over-prescribe pain medications. Going back to no regulation would be

---

[18] American Geriatrics Society Panel on Pharmacological Management of Persistent Pain in Older Persons, "Pharmacological Management of Persistent Pain in Older Persons," Guideline Recommendations, Opioids, VIII, Journal of the American Geriatrics Society, August 2009, Volume 57, Issue 8, page 1342, John Wiley and Sons, © 2009 Authors Journal compilation, © 2009 The American Geriatrics Society.

difficult. Trusting physicians to do what is right and what their mentors have trained them to do is missing. It is hard to trust a physician who spends little time with the patient or family. If that is true, we can look for another physician or health plan.

Health Maintenance Organization (HMO) and Preferred Provider Organization (PPO) health care insurance contracts save patients or their employers money. But they also squeeze providers so much that they cannot easily spend enough time with the patient or family. To sustain or improve income, many physicians speed up visits and surgeries. That creates problems, including frustrated patients, omissions, mistakes and cranky doctors. I have often heard patients say, "My doctor won't talk to me," referring to their previous doctor or a current family doctor. Many patients are not even seeing their doctor and see a physician assistant or nurse practitioner instead. The constraints of time on physicians create a pervasive attitude of, "good enough for government work." What kind of "health maintenance" is that?

The pressures from HMOs and PPOs on physicians are not on a level playing field. Federal anti-trust laws are enforced against physicians who are not in an HMO. But, because of an exemption in the McCarran-Ferguson Act of 1945, federal anti-trust laws have not been enforced for insurance companies, including HMO plans. Huge medical insurance companies are able to bully physicians who are not in large groups. Real negotiating does not occur during the contracting process. With sparse competition, insurance carriers have a take-it-or-leave-it attitude and get away with it. That explains why physicians tend to join large groups. Very large is not better; it simply has more power.

The PPO and HMO limits on physicians contribute to mediocrity and a decline in initiative. We see increasing limits of honest innovation in health care since the 1990s. Changes in the laws of many states, including California laws in 1982, allowed insurance companies to contract with individual physicians. Managed care grew exponentially thereafter, especially PPO's in the 1980s. Managed care includes both HMOs and PPOs and is not health care managed by your doctor. Managers of health care use prepaid (capitation), pay-for-performance and other contracts to manipulate payments in their favor. Taking control away from patients and their doctors is never a good idea. Real insurance keeps the patient and doctor in control of medical care.

Many features of PPOs have grown out of HMOs. Some examples are "utilization review" by non-physicians and lists of "cost-effective" drugs (formularies). Utilization review hinders and frustrates doctors. It increased business overhead by more than one full-time employee for our office of nine physicians. Patients found their health insurance premiums and out of pocket costs were lower but only at first. Even with utilization review, use was higher because of huge discounts in out-of-pocket costs for patients.

Control of medicine became solidly under the power of insurance providers that include both state and federal governments. Workers' Compensation, Medicare and private insurance began slowly cutting back payments to health care providers. They cut slowly to avoid upsetting the system and losing their power. They keep a percentage for "management cost." The assault by "managed care" had begun with failed justifications that it holds back health care costs and improves care. Obamacare (The Patient Protection and Affordable Care Act), enacted in 2010, has not and will not help the quality, affordability and availability of health care. It has markedly accelerated the cost of and financial stress of the private practice of medicine that was already going the wrong way.

Because of leadership in the wrong direction for decades, we see less honesty in all areas of medical care. Electronic medical records (EMR) sound good, but they are laughable because of a, "garbage in, garbage out," mentality. Going in the right direction will take changes in state and federal laws. We need state and federal executive branches that enforce the law. Does HMO medicine measure up to fee-for-service medicine, found in PPO and indemnity insurance? Because of the power of insurance carriers, PPOs in many ways have become like HMOs, settling for mediocrity and the do-less HMO mentality. An early study found a significant difference for chronically, physically ill elderly and poor patients with HMOs not doing as well.[19]

We have dishonest or misinformed government and academic leadership. Resulting economic realities produce medical fads that sound good but come and go within a few years. Instead of more and better medical innovation, we often have economically incentivized research marketed to the public or physicians. In a 2006 monograph to physicians, one article cites less knee pain using a combination of chondroitin sulfate and glucosamine. But it admitted that limitations of the study were a significant placebo response rate. It also cites other trials with similar responses to a placebo.[20]

The ongoing glucosamine and chondroitin research and marketing is an example of a pattern of economically based studies. They promise pills that offer joint comfort, health and mobility for an active lifestyle.[21] A product label for another pill with glucosamine and chondroitin says that it is not a medication and not meant to treat joint ailments, but it has vital molecules for joint tissues. It also says it has three essential ingredients.[22] Supplements often sound too good to be true.

Patterns of dishonesty are not new. Con artists over the past few thousand years have had the same patterns. Snake oil salesmen in the 1800s were often known as medicine show hucksters and many had accomplices in the audience. But,

[19] John E. Ware Jr., Ph.D., Martha S. Bayliss, MSc, William H. Rogers, Ph.D., Mark Kosinski, MA, Alvin R. Tarlov, M.D., "Differences in 4-year health outcomes for elderly and poor, chronically ill patients treated in HMO and fee-for-service systems, Results from the Medical Outcomes Study," Journal of the American Medical Association, October 2, 1996, Volume 276, Number 13, page 1039, jamanetwork.com/journals/jama/article-abstract/408692, accessed May 9, 2018.
[20] Orthopedics Today, "Chondroitin Sulfate: Mechanisms of Action and Clinical Response in Osteoarthritis," a monograph to physicians, May 2006, "Chondroitin sulfate combo effective in moderate-to-severe pain," pages 8–9, Slack Incorporated, supported by Bioiberica SA and Nutramax Laboratories, Inc. its U.S. distribution partner for CosamineDS.
[21] Nutramax Laboratories Consumer Care, Inc., www.cosamin.com, accessed May 9, 2018, federally required note at bottom of webpage in bold capital letters: "These statements have not been evaluated by the food and drug administration. This product is not intended to diagnose, treat, cure, or prevent any disease."
[22] HSN, Inc., www.hsn.com/products/glucosamine-and-chondroitin/10069061, ProCaps Laboratories, View Product Label, accessed May 9, 2018.

then and now, after someone unknowingly buys a dishonest remedy, they may justify it by saying, "It couldn't hurt," or "It might help!" They do not want to look foolish afterwards because they bought it. They may rationalize it for years. In a 1962 television episode of Gunsmoke, a peddler claimed that he used to serve as the personal surgeon of King Santo del Rio. He also claimed that Professor Eliot's Wonder Medicine cures, "all disorders of the human race."[23]

Medical schools have trained medical doctors for years to honestly evaluate new medications coming to the market. Honest physicians effectively evaluate studies and their sources. Good medical doctors are usually not the first to prescribe new medications. Clinical trials study medications in various parts of the world. Drugs released in the U.S. market always have new adverse effects that come to light after their release. Different populations do not account for the increased adverse effects (adverse reactions or side effects).

New drug "innovation" makes us mistakenly think that all the new medications are a wonderful advance in medical research. The problem is that they may be poorly tested. Nearly one-third or 71 of 222 new drugs approved by the Food and Drug Administration (FDA) from 2001 to 2010 required 123 significant follow-up actions. During a follow-up period of 9 to 14 years, they made 3 drug withdrawals, 61 warnings and 59 safety communications.[24]

Similar to drugs, our wide use of and dependence on procedures are also an epidemic. An injection procedure in the 1980s used a papaya extract (chymopapain). We injected it under x-ray control into the soft-tissue center of a low back bulging spinal disc (herniated nucleus pulposus). An enzyme

---

[23] Gunsmoke, Season 7 Episode 34, "The Boys," CBS, May 26, 1962.
[24] Nicholas S. Downing, M.D., Nilay D. Shah, Ph.D., Jenerius A. Aminawung, M.D., MPH, Alison M. Pease, BS, Jean-David Zeitoun, M.D., MHPM, et al., "Postmarket Safety Events Among Novel Therapeutics Approved by the U.S. Food and Drug Administration Between 2001 and 2010," Journal of the American Medical Association, May 9, 2017, Volume 317, Number 18, pages 1854–1863, jamanetwork.com/journals/jama/article-abstract/2625319?amp%3butm_source=JAMALatestIssue&utm_campaign=09-05-2017, accessed May 9, 2018.

in it shrunk the disc. It had a 70 percent success rate in the operating room. There was only one "little" problem. It had a 1 percent incidence of a severe allergic reaction that had a real risk of death (anaphylactic shock). Within a few years, we replaced the procedure with another better, outpatient surgery. The newer procedure also had a 70 percent success rate. Under x-ray control, it used suction to remove the soft-tissue center of the offending low back disc with a tiny incision and a 3-mm diameter probe (percutaneous discectomy).

We used the suction procedure for a little longer period than chymopapain. The right reason for the procedure was a herniated disc from 3 to 5 mm. That size is a narrow window. Changing the indications to other sizes of disc herniations was tempting for surgeons and their patients. Because doctors and patients used increasingly poor indications, the 70 percent success rate for the procedure deteriorated. It accumulated a poor reputation among patients. If many spine surgeons and their patients had not overused poor indications, we might still be doing it today. Another cause of its decline was the excellent 90 percent success rate with a small incision for a standard inpatient open discectomy.

For pain control, some doctors are also overusing series of corticosteroid epidural injections.[25] These spinal injections can help sciatica. But we should not use them as an automatic series of three, 1 injection each week for 3 weeks. We should use them one at a time at judicious intervals. The needle tip should be directed to the spot in the spine causing the pain. If the pain is a lot less after the first injection, we should do the second injection only if needed later. If no relief occurred or if pain increased after the first injection, we should avoid the second. If there is limited pain relief, we can consider a second injection in a few weeks. A third injection may also help, if needed, after another few weeks. The benefits decrease after

---

[25] An epidural injection is done with a long needle under x-ray control in the operating room using a local anesthetic in the skin and soft tissues and includes an injection of synthetic corticosteroid and local anesthetic into the epidural space of the spinal canal, outside the dural sac. Epidural anesthetics are temporarily very effective and have been used for many years for the delivery of a baby.

three injections in one specific area, and the risks increase. We should only rarely repeat a series of three injections again.

Contributing to the epidemic of opioid use, many writers and entities support their increasing use. Prescription opioid pain pills are narcotics. In 2009, a pharmaceutical company sent an advertising letter to me for the prescription medication tramadol (Ultram ER). The letter emphasized that it works for 24 hours and relieves moderately severe chronic pain allowing patients to stay active. It admitted that patients can abuse tramadol like other opioids.[26]

Masking pain so patients can do more is not a good idea. It causes patients to become dependent on pills and is one of many causes of chronic pain. A local magazine article, also in 2009, implied that there is a level of safety in the use of prescription opioids. The author recognizes that the use of opioids for noncancer chronic pain is a radical choice of treatment. But incorrectly, it states that a growing acceptance of them is occurring among doctors, including for severe low back pain and other non-life-threatening conditions.[27]

Many physicians, fortunately, share my alarm about the increasing use of prescription opioids for chronic pain. The use of opioids in chronic pain is not consistently safe. After injections and other procedures by pain management doctors have not worked, acceptance of opioids may occur because they do not know what else to do. On the other hand, many physicians see the results and risks of masking pain.

The authors of an article in a throw-away medical journal expressed a goal for opioid therapy.[28] They say that it should improve patient function and pain control with no excessive opioid physical signs. However, they write that the amount of opioid medication prescribed is less important. They admit that highway patrol officers have a tough job enforcing laws for influence of opioids. Signs of opioid excess must be present on physical examination, arranged with a drug

[26] Ortho-McNeil-Janssen Pharmaceuticals, Inc., Business Letter, March 2009.
[27] Inland Empire M.D. News, "The Safety of Opioid Therapy," by Brianne Carswell, June 2009, page 23.
[28] We refer to free journals sent for a signature as throw-away medical journals.

recognition expert. The article brazenly concludes that they see no reason for a maximum opioid dose.[29]

The need for more opioids is a sign that the pain and the warnings are worse or that the body is becoming used to the drug (tolerance). Opioid use is an epidemic and is too easy of an answer for the complex problem of chronic pain. Using more opioids always has consequences, 100 percent of the time. They also increase the risk of larger problems. If the body is becoming more tolerant, that is a wonderful opportunity to wean the patient off the medication. At the very least we should keep the level of the opiate the same. That forces the patient to deal with the pain in better mechanical ways as the drug becomes less effective.

Opioid chronic pain control without physical signs of excess sounds good but is at best an elusive, quick, temporary help. Some make it sound easy. Because of patient variability and omnipresent adverse consequences, it is not easy. These adverse effects are impaired judgment and reaction times and the inability to learn from pain. I am not against using opioid pain pills. I have prescribed them in a limited way for selected chronic pain patients. At their first visit, many of my acute and chronic pain patients were already trying to get off the pain pills prescribed by others. I merely had to help them along in the direction that they already knew was right.

Because of health plan disincentives, primary care providers refer less to specialists, especially in HMO settings. They deal with patients having pain though they may be uncomfortable with it. Some use variations of opioid prescribing in our country to justify practice guidelines. Many professional, academic and government entities have offered opioid prescribing guidelines and warnings for decades. Regardless, an increasing epidemic of opiate use and abuse is proliferating. It will not abate until patients have more responsibility and individual physicians have more say.

---

[29] Forest Tennant, M.D., DrPH, and Jeffery Reinking, M.D., "Appropriate Opioid dosing for Activities of Daily Living," Practical Pain Management, November/December 2008, pages 15–16, 18.

In March 2016, the United States Centers for Disease Control and Prevention (CDC) described an "overdose epidemic" instead of calling it what it is, an opioid abuse epidemic. It seems that they want to show that physicians are to blame for it and that patients are not. The CDC issued their opiate guideline for primary care providers.[30] Later the same month, the FDA issued their opiate recommendations and warnings. The FDA called it an epidemic and a "public health crisis."[31] As if the government and some academics have all the answers for pain and opiates, both want to give physicians and patients more "education." Have they discovered new things? I believe they have forgotten something old.

Giving physicians and patients more power to control their decisions has not yet been in open discussions. We have had an ongoing, increasing atmosphere of government control of health care for several decades. The attitude of our government has been to never let a crisis go to waste without spending other people's money. They love giving it to their friends and gathering power. This continuing corruption of medical science will never solve the problem of chronic pain or the abuse of medications. Was there more government response in 2016? In July 2016, the U.S. government enacted the Comprehensive Addiction and Recovery Act (CARA). They felt a need to do something but did not know what else to do. The law spends more money for the problem, up to $181 million every year.[32]

---

[30] Centers for Disease Control and Prevention, US Department of Health and Human Services, "Guideline for Prescribing Opioids for Chronic Pain – United States, 2016," Deborah Dowell, M.D., Tamara M. Haegerich, Ph.D., Roger Chou, M.D., Morbidity and Mortality Weekly Report, Recommendations and Reports, March 18, 2016, Volume 65, Number 1, pages 1–49, www.cdc.gov/mmwr/volumes/65/rr/rr6501e1.htm, accessed May 9, 2018.

[31] Food and Drug Administration, US Department of Health and Human Services, "FDA announces enhanced warnings for immediate-release opioid pain medications related to risks of misuse, abuse, addiction, overdose and death," March 22, 2016, www.fda.gov/newsevents/newsroom/pressannouncements/ucm491739.htm, accessed May 9, 2018.

[32] Community Anti-Drug Coalitions of America, Policy Priorities, Comprehensive Addiction and Recovery Act, (CARA), www.cadca.org/comprehensive-addiction-and-recovery-act-cara, accessed May 9, 2018.

Others have added to the false worry that there is no real hope. A magazine article in 2007 declared that chronic pain is a widespread and unresolvable medical condition, afflicting 20 percent of Americans. It lists baby boomers, cancer patients, retired football players, civilians and soldiers as participants in a growing epidemic of chronic pain. The article has scientific drawings of pain pathways, but it gives a false hope that newer narcotics have less of a stigma of addiction. The article correctly admits that new morphine derivatives can also create a dependency.

The same article then repeats an incorrect but popular saying that pain in chronic conditions is "no longer useful." They say that it is a malfunctioning or a disease of the nervous system. They feel that there is nothing you can do about it. Then, the article dolefully states that scientists do not know why chronic pain occurs in some and not in others. It describes a connection of medications, injections and early aggressive therapy with possible less chronic pain. It is true that early proper treatment is always better for any injury or disease. Yet the author concludes with histrionic advice for mild pain from a sprained ankle, "If you want to avoid chronic pain later, you might need serious therapy, and right away."[33]

When an epidemic such as chronic pain occurs, it is usually a problem that we as fallible humans have created. We often overlook or ignore obvious problems we create because solving them is not popular, or it requires work. To recover from an acute or chronic injury, take good care of it! That is what an ankle sprain, other injuries or many sources of pain need. What happened to rest, range of motion in the right directions and limited exercise without pain? Not a word about those things was in the above article though it said that patients are afraid of exercise because it hurts.

Of course, exercise or physical therapy that hurts is bad. The pain does not mean that we should not try to move or exercise in the right ways. It does means to learn from what

---

[33] Newsweek, "The Changing Science of Pain," Mary Carmichael, June 4, 2007, pages 40–47.

we feel, modify what we are doing and not keep making the same mistakes. Limited exercise that does not hurt is almost always good, especially if done easy and often. Exercise increases should usually be slower than we would like. What will heal is amazing when we put it in the right circumstances. Yes, pain from an ankle sprain will take longer to resolve if it has been there more than 3 months. But if we take better care of it, pain will go in a better direction, and the ankle will usually heal.

Epidemics of chronic pain, obesity and insulin resistant diabetes (type 2) are flourishing in our modern world. Health misinformation and quick, misleading cures bombard us daily. Overeating can be an addiction, but it is at least a dependency. Short walks, frequent rests, a balanced diet and reasonable calorie intake are not glamorous. But they are effective for a multitude of conditions. Many of us ignore or forget simple, effective helps, yet we glorify exercise. Overdoing exercise is tempting and exciting. If we do something that hurts when we exercise, we may incorrectly justify it by saying, "At least I am doing something."

Others around us feed into an exercise mindset by wrongly judging us and may say, "You have to do more." We may also ignore little things that do not hurt and can help us. We might say, "That cannot possibly be helping because it is too easy." It is also easy to feel guilty when doing small amounts of things. We may be tempted to exaggerate by saying, "I cannot do anything." In doing so, we are missing the important, little things we can do.

Does ongoing complaining help us feel better? Does ignoring pain help? Widespread misinformation fuels these mistaken approaches and attitudes. It is fueling an epidemic. I believe that a large majority in the United States are honest and have no interest in taking advantage of others. Even so, because of corruption among us in all cultures of the world, misinformation and fads can mislead each of us if we are not diligent.

✑ Chapter 11 ✑

What is Wrong?

When we feel pain, a diagnosis helps to explain what is wrong. The problem can be in the structure of the body (anatomy). Or, it can be in how parts of the body work together (physiology). Abnormalities can also be in the metabolic processes of the body (biochemistry). The problem can be in one or multiple areas of the body (regions). Problems can be in tissues that are fluids, soft tissues or bones (systems). The story of symptoms and their characteristics is a history. It includes what happened before, during and after symptoms started. The history may be from the patient or from the family if the patient is unable to give it. A good history taken by a doctor points towards a diagnosis. The doctor should listen carefully and then should question the patient or family further for pertinent details. Then the doctor should think of a preliminary diagnosis.

During the physical examination, a doctor looks at (observation) and touches the patient (palpation) to finish establishing the preliminary diagnosis. Blood or urine tests, microscopy, x-rays, CT scan, MRI scan, nuclear medicine bone scan, biopsy or other tests may help turn a preliminary diagnosis into one or more final diagnoses. Multiple diagnoses are common in orthopedics (comorbidity). Studies of what is wrong with patients with similar diagnoses and end results (pathology) gives doctors ideas for treatment (therapeutics). Treatment or sometimes just time may lessen or solve pain.

Signs of a diagnosis are occasionally something that we cannot see on exam, tests, x-rays or an MRI scan. Normal tests create anxiety in some orthopedic patients. They ask, "Are you telling me that nothing is wrong?" A doctor should explain the diagnosis to the best of their ability in easy to understand ways. A diagnosis that is not verbalized or explained and is only on the medical record does not help. A probable or an uncertain diagnosis still means that some understanding or help for it exists. We may know less about a diagnosis such as fibromyalgia than we would like. That does not make the pain and other symptoms less real. When body regions and systems do not work together as they should, symptoms are warning signs like the engine warning lights in a car.

Since the early 1980s, to have a valid claim for payment, doctors in the United States were told to provide a diagnosis code. Governments, health plans and insurance companies, for their own purposes, required an ICD-9-CM four or five-digit code (International Classification of Diseases, 9th Revision, Clinical Modification). Why didn't those who want coding do it and pay for it? They had the economic and political power to mandate it, and doctors had no power to object. The tedious ICD-10-CM coding scheme, required as of 2016, intensifies the problems.

The American Medical Association (AMA) gave a superficial objection to the above unfunded coding mandate. Because they sell coding books and guides, they have a conflict of interest. The AMA has not represented my best interests for years, and I do not belong to it. Many physicians in California feel the same way.[34] Making the doctor give codes for a diagnosis gives no real benefit to the patient. And there are significant disadvantages. It increases the office overhead and wastes time. Coding tends to have a dumbing down effect on diagnoses. A doctor or an office assistant will tend to put down numbers they already know or have listed on a cheat sheet. Then, they might not look up another diagnosis or an odd part of the diagnosis unless it helps payments.

The words of a diagnosis by a good medical doctor can reflect a description of findings, a pattern of symptoms or a mechanism of injury. Where appropriate, it should include the body part, location and side of the body. It should not be a regurgitation of symptoms the patient gave the doctor. If the diagnosis is specific enough, it will help us determine initial treatment. When patients know what is wrong, they are better equipped to turn things around. If they know more about what is wrong, they will have more perspective to know what to do

---

[34] An informal phone and online survey by me on October 31, 2014, showed that of 954 medical and surgical MDs in Riverside, California and San Francisco, California, only 6 percent (59) of the 954 were members of the American Medical Association, with similar numbers in each location.

and what not do each day. Do you remember the diagnosis a doctor gave you or a family member? If the diagnosis is difficult or lengthy, is it written or printed somewhere? Is the diagnosis a printed description of a nonspecific diagnosis code? Is the diagnosis understandable? Do you understand how it causes pain?

A medical doctor is trained and licensed to determine a diagnosis. As doctors, we should be able to make it as understandable as possible. We are trained to know how to investigate and find answers where possible. There will always be things doctors do not know about the body. If you push a good medical doctor to tell you things they do not know, they will admit that they do not know. Asking for an educated guess is okay, but they will acknowledge it as a guess. For the best result, information should come from the best sources.

A Registered Physical Therapist (RPT) is also trained and licensed to sort out what physical things the patient should do. Their treatment and advice should be based on the diagnosis by the doctor and the doctor's comments on the therapy prescription. The diagnosis and types of treatment on the therapy prescription should be as specific as possible. If they are not, the physical therapist must do more than they are trained and licensed for. Communication between the doctor and the physical therapist is critically important. Advice that each professional gives the patient should make sense. It should give them a sense of comfort and direction.

For a doctor, the diagnosis gives a statement of what is wrong and a sense of what to do about it. For a patient, the diagnosis gives a sense of hope that things will heal. That is true even if the diagnosis is cancer because we have found what is causing the problem. A doctor who gives a diagnosis of "Back Pain" is not really giving a diagnosis. They are regurgitating a symptom or a complaint. Capital letters of the diagnosis may make it look important, but it is nonspecific. It does not address where the pain is coming from, what is causing it or what to do about it. It is a descriptive diagnosis, and it gives the patient no hope. After the doctor visit, the patient knows nothing more than before. If the diagnosis is nonspecific, delayed, uncertain or always in question by the doctor, it is more difficult for a patient to have hope. This happens when a doctor does not give an impression or initial diagnosis on the first visit. If they continue in the second and third visits to run tests without giving the patient the benefit of a most likely diagnosis, having hope is hard.

If a doctor never definitively states and explains the obvious diagnoses to a patient's satisfaction, the patient will stay uncertain or confused. To be alert for other unusual diagnoses is good. There can be more than one thing wrong. However, to avoid saying the obvious things that are wrong, such as a back sprain, is a disservice. Telling the patient gives them hope and, suddenly, things to try. When we have a diagnosis to try to understand and do something about, sooner is better. The patient can then begin to test what to do and what not to do from the things the doctor has said. If improvement occurs during treatment, it adds weight to the diagnosis. If the findings on physical exam change or evolve during treatment, the changes may add certainty to the diagnosis, or they may disprove the diagnosis. A doctor watches the overall progress, but they are also charged with checking the symptoms and findings along the way.

Because physicians and patients tend to think more in structural or concrete terms, we think of the diagnosis more often in terms of anatomy. Which soft tissues or fluids are involved with what is wrong? Which parts are involved? Are the bones involved as well? Many sources of pain are more in the physiology of the body than in the anatomy. Pain and healing functions of the body are miracles. Their interaction is fascinating. How the anatomy and metabolic pathways work together to help the body heal is amazing physiology. We often poorly understand them in their roles contributing to pain and healing. Our activities and how we treat our bodies affects healing positively or negatively. Many other variables also affect how our bodies heal.

An example of abnormal physiology is the swelling that occurs from prolonged, upright positions after a leg injury. It often leads to a vicious cycle in the soft tissues and muscles of the calf with increased soft-tissue pressure and muscle tension. The vicious cycle causes things that are more noticeably wrong such as extra swelling, varicose veins, dermatitis, leg clots or recurrent muscle strain. Earlier symptoms, which we can often ignore for a while, are also manifestations of abnormal physiology. However, the sooner we pay attention to them, such as swelling or pain, keeping them from becoming a bigger problem is easier.

An unstable broken leg bone is abnormal anatomy that also has abnormal physiology with pain, swelling and muscle spasm. The muscles cannot effectively rest. The muscles reflexively contract to support the bone, but that causes movement and pain at the fracture site, which sends muscles into muscle spasm. Immobilizing the fracture with splinting or casting helps pain because the muscles can relax. Movement at the fracture site is less.

Abnormal anatomy by itself may not cause symptoms at all. A bone deformity after a healed fracture may not be visible or cause any symptoms. If a bone deformity is visible, but not near a joint, it may also not cause any symptoms or limitations. Another example of abnormal anatomy that can have no symptoms or limitations is a lipoma, a benign fatty tumor. They may be small or not near enough to skin, nerves or blood vessels to irritate them.

Another example of a diagnosis that may not have symptoms is a malignant cancer. The cancer may not yet be pressing on or doing any damage to surrounding structures. Doctors are well aware of the potential presence of cancer, whether there are symptoms or not and do their best to detect it early. Though pain is common with cancer, pain is not always present. The same is true for many other diagnoses. If pain is persisting or gradually increasing, a doctor's concern for the possibility of cancer is higher. However, there are many patients who have persisting, severe or increasing pain that do not have cancer.

Patients without a cancer diagnosis are sometimes disappointed because they do not know what the source of their pain is. It is always good news if pain is not due to cancer. But patients without cancer still need to hear their diagnosis and the most likely cause of pain. Without destructive diseases or injuries and without cancer, patients will likely heal. However, they must put their body in the right situations to allow healing. Secondary diagnoses may limit the healing capacity of our body, such as hyperactivity, bipolar disorder or obesity. They can slow healing and have complications that stop healing. A diagnosis of depression is also well known to delay healing and accentuate pain.

Some diagnoses are very common, such as a chronic strain and osteoarthritis. Some are less common, such as rheumatoid arthritis and fibromyalgia. Many diagnoses are much less common, such as systemic lupus erythematosus and reflex sympathetic dystrophy. There are also many rare diagnoses. Each field of medicine has thousands of diagnoses. "Acute" or "chronic" are modifying terms that can be a part of a diagnosis and add perspective.

Acute pain is pain that has been present for only a few hours, days or weeks. It goes away in a reasonable time for the type, level and intensity of the injury or the cause of pain. Chronic pain refers to pain that has been present for 3 months, even if it comes and goes. Chronic pain from an injury is pain that lasts longer than it should. The body has had a chance to heal, but it did not within the usual time frame. That often means that reinjury has occurred many times without the patient being aware of it or paying enough attention to it.

These concepts about chronic pain also apply to pain associated with disease. How well we deal with chronic pain from a disease greatly affects its severity. Pain from diseases such as rheumatoid arthritis and lupus erythematosus is less predictable than injury. There can be flairs and remissions. More issues are playing a role in the duration of pain from a disease. Most patients with rheumatoid arthritis find that they hurt less if they keep stiffness out with limited exercise. They move, but they avoid heavy or prolonged use.

Even patients with severe crippling rheumatoid arthritis who have deformed joints of the hands and wrists can use the same principles and some of these patients hurt amazingly little. Some of the same concepts apply to cancer pain fueled by the growth or extension of the cancer cells. Cancer pain mechanisms are like those for injury and disease though we may have less control over them. Often, cancer pain is chronic pain, yet there may be cures and remissions.

For each diagnosis, the amount of control we have over pain is different. Osteoarthritis or degenerative joint disease is a common disease and another source of pain that tends to come and go with flairs and remissions. We may have more control over pain associated with osteoarthritis than with cancer. But we may have less control over osteoarthritis pain than with pain from an injury. With more control, keeping the pain away from becoming chronic is more likely.

In about 1994, I received a call from Adam Tyler, a friend who lived nearby. He said that he was in trouble with back and leg pain. His call came in the middle of the week, and he had a heavy schedule as an attorney. He asked me if he should go to the emergency room. I told him I could call ahead for him, so they would know that he was coming. He then asked, "Is there anything else I can do now?" I told him that if he described what was going on, I could give him a few ideas he could try before going to the emergency room. That was a bold change for me at the time. For patients, friends and family before then, I held on to traditional exams. To be sure I did not short change anyone, I did a history, physical exam and x-rays. Then, I gave a diagnosis and described treatment.

When Adam asked me if he could do anything else, I decided to let him try some simple things. In my office, I had been giving many simple things for back pain patients to do after a full exam and the usual x-rays. I gave the same instructions over and over. I encouraged him to go to the emergency room if he did not steadily improve within 1 to 2 days. He agreed, and then I asked him a few questions. He had no numbness. His worsening pain over the last 3 days was going down to one of his calves. He was in a sitting position and was having trouble lying down without increasing the pain. He gave a history of a few previous, similar painful episodes, but they had resolved years ago. He said that his current pain was much worse.

The most likely diagnosis was recurrent acute low back sprain with radiating leg pain from nerve irritation (a presumptive diagnosis of lumbar sprain with radiculopathy). I asked him to do some simple motions designed to confirm the diagnosis as far as possible and to test the level of function and disability. I asked him to slide the foot of the uninvolved leg out on the floor slowly until he felt tightness or pain and to go no further (knee and hip extension). Next, I asked him to do the same on the involved side, to go slower and to describe how far he got, compared to the uninvolved side.

On the involved leg, he could only straighten it out half of what he could do on the uninvolved side. He could not straighten his knee out fully on either side. I said to him that he had just done one of the exercises that I needed him to do. Except, he was to go only half way to the point of tightness or pain, each side one at a time. In other words, he was to go only half as far as he had stretched. I asked him to use 4 or 5 repetitions at a time.

The second exercise I asked Adam to do was to bring his knee up towards his chest with the help of his hands on the front of his knee. He said he could do that on each side without any problem, except the involved side was a little tight. I asked him to do both exercises at least every hour if he could do them without pain. Again, he was to use 4 to 5 repetitions at a time on each side. I asked him to lie down when he could do it without pain. He was to keep it short, change horizontal positions often and sit up again when he needed to or before he needed to.

If he was worse or no better, I told him again to go to the emergency room that night or come to my office the following day. I would do a full exam, take x-rays and give him a diagnosis and recommend further treatment. I did not hear from him until he called 3 days later. He said that he was doing fine and was working. He had no back or leg pain. His back was only occasionally tight, and the exercises were helping nicely.

I again explained to him that if the pain reoccurred, he could come to my office for an exam. That was to cover all bases since many odd things can happen. For friends and family, odd things happening seems to be especially true. All orthopedic surgeons are aware of the possibility of tumors, infection, disc herniations or other underlying problems. My friend said that he felt fine. He reassured me that he did not need any further evaluation despite my hesitation. Adam continued to do well and had no further problems.

His phone calls taught me several things. First, I could be more aggressive in evaluating what was wrong over the phone. Second, with the information available, I learned not hesitate to make a most likely diagnosis over the phone. The diagnosis is only probable anyway. Common problems usually need common solutions. Worry about exceptions does not need to delay obvious solutions. Third, I learned to describe better what I wanted patients to do for the diagnosis, including specific, simple exercises for rapid improvement. Becoming free of pain, feeling less pain and knowing how to keep improving often proves the diagnosis indirectly.

When diagnoses accurately describe a patient's clinical picture, both the doctor and the patient benefit. It is easier for the patient to understand what to do and what their limitations are. The next time the doctor sees the patient, remembering what is going on with the patient is also easier. With the help of a clear, concise and accurate medical record, the doctor can guide the patient more efficiently. Other doctors seeing the patient will also have a clearer view after reading the record.

After time and testing, we hope that a single diagnosis can explain all the symptoms and findings. Those patients are usually easier to treat. They have not waited too long to have things checked and taken care of. For those who have waited longer, having multiple or complex diagnoses is common. When the symptoms are widespread or present for a longer time, multiple diagnoses are more likely.

An example of multiple simple diagnoses would be acute right knee sprain, acute neck, mid and low back strain, mild degenerative disc disease, osteoporosis and obesity. An example of multiple complex diagnoses would be chronic mid and low back sprain with severe degenerative disc disease, radiculopathy with tingling in the foot, possible herniated disc, left knee degenerative meniscus tear, vitamin D deficiency, insulin resistant diabetes mellitus (type 2) with foot ulcer, morbid obesity and depression. I have had many patients at a first visit with 7 or more diagnoses causing problems for which they were seeking treatment. After sorting through diagnoses, we should treat the problems that are the most significant and bothering the patient the most.

Delayed diagnoses occur for many reasons. Among the reasons are symptoms that masquerade as something else. Other delays for a diagnosis occur because there is no pain or because of complex abnormalities. More reasons for delays are health plan, insurance company and government disincentives for doctors to be thorough. Also, patients may have a fear of seeing a doctor, a fear of mentioning a symptom or a fear of surgery. Some patients seek "alternative" care and others have inattentive doctors. Malpractice lawsuits have not and will not solve any of these problems. Some patients may simply neglect to say if their symptoms are on the right or left side. Some doctors neglect to ask or document the side that the symptoms are on.

We will always need diligence by all those who are concerned for the patient. For a full, correct and early diagnosis, patients, their families and doctors should be conscientiously working together. We should remove the distractions of time constraints, government policy, health plan practice guidelines and insurance restrictions. We are then more likely to experience the full benefits of the miracles of modern medicine.

∽ *Chapter 12* ∾

Is There a Need for Surgery?

We have few indications for emergency orthopedic surgery except for some spinal cord damage, infections, swelling, open fractures and motor vehicle accidents. The patient or family and the physician need to deliberate more carefully on all other orthopedic surgical procedures. When the location and type of symptoms are right and the correct findings are significant enough, surgery may make sense. Choosing the right procedure is critical for any problem. Each procedure has specific risks and benefits.

The correct surgery is more likely to permanently resolve pain. If pain is in the left leg and a herniated disc of the low back is on the right side, surgery will not help. The pain is coming from somewhere else. The symptoms must match the findings to expect good end results. Except for emergency surgery, the indications are often better after the patient has used the time-honored practice of, "Give it some time." That is usually a few weeks or months.

Severe back and radiating leg pain and numbness in the right areas is often a large herniated disc with nerve irritation or compromise (lumbar radiculopathy). We can take out the disc bulge in surgery with a small open incision of the low back (hemilaminotomy and discectomy). With 90 percent good to excellent results, the improvement should be significant. That means complete or significant relief of pain, so the patient is glad that they had it done. Therefore, 9 out of 10 patients will do well with that surgery. Another 9 percent have some pain relief, but they and I wish they had more relief. The last 1 percent of patients has slight change, and fewer patients may be worse, about 1 in 1,000. For any procedure, a surgeon should give an estimated percentage of good to excellent results. They should also outline the risks based on all the known factors in the patient.

Other spine surgeries can have similar, high percentage, good to excellent results. An example is surgery to achieve bony healing across a single disc level for moderately severe disc space narrowing in the neck or low back with surrounding bone spurs (spinal fusion for degenerative disc disease). The incision is on the front side of the neck or the back side of the low back. It should be without plates or screws for a single level. It is a gold standard, and we measure all procedures by it for that diagnosis. Bone from the patient's pelvis stimulates the best healing (iliac crest autograft). Only for rare reasons should we do the surgery with bone from a deceased person (cadaver allograft). Despite popular worries, pain at the bone donor site is not an issue when we close the incision well and protect it as it heals. Worries of donor site pain give surgeons an excuse to use cadaver bone. It raises payment though the fusion has a higher risk of not healing.

After a bony fusion using the patient's own bone for bone graft, the need for repeat surgery at the same level is significantly less. Using cadaver bone, bone substitutes or growth factors has been fashionable (orthobiologics such as bone morphogenic protein-2). However, they often create a less robust bone healing response (atrophic fusion). Your own bone is always the best, and the available amount is usually enough. The likelihood of healing is better, and the risk of infection is less. Each fusion level that we add multiplies the risk of bone not healing at one of the levels of the surgery (nonunion). This is true for both the neck and the back. In the neck, the use of a plate and screws is good for fusing more than one disc level. In the low back, hardware with rods and screws also makes sense for more than one spinal disc level.

A degenerated joint level of the spine will occasionally spontaneously fuse by itself. It happens when bone spurs around a joint get large enough to grow together. That happens most often in the mid back, but it can happen in the neck or low back and rarely in other joints of the arms and legs. These spontaneous fusions are what gave surgeons the idea of doing fusions in the first place. For most joints, the body is not able to finish the bony fusion on its own. When we do a surgical fusion, we are finishing what the body has not been able to do. Pain in the degenerated joint goes away when the joint fusion heals by itself or with surgery. Since the surrounding joint levels of the spine are at risk for similar degeneration, patients may want to be more judicious with activity or exercise. We are all getting older, and parts of our body do wear out.

In the spine, fusions are still a better choice than disc replacements. Some joints of the body do better with a joint replacement, and others do better with a fusion. Spinal disc replacements are controversial. They only address one of the three degenerated joints at each spinal level. If a disc joint is severely degenerated, the other two joints are usually severely degenerated as well (facet joints). A spine fusion relieves pain reliably because it solves the problem with all three joints. With a solid spine fusion, most patients do not lose motion because the degenerated joint is already stiff before the fusion.

Good to excellent results can also occur in 90 percent of spinal fusions with metal implants for other diagnoses such as chronic spine fractures (spondylolisthesis grade I defects of the pars interarticularis). The correct surgical procedure deals with the findings that are painful (pain generators). Fusions get rid of pain and muscle rigidity from associated spasms. Then, the surrounding joints may move better. It is not science when authors with an economic interest distort surgical results or when surgical implant companies influence research. We do not trust those who distort the truth for notoriety or money unless they admit their dishonesty, and they change.

Time and effort by the patient and the doctor with good nonoperative tools before surgery are needed for good surgical results after surgery. Nonoperative treatment is important especially with mild findings because most of the time it works. Marginal nonoperative therapy is not good enough, and "alternative" treatments are inadequate. Watch out when a surgeon says, "If nonoperative treatment fails, surgery is always a last resort." It sounds good, but if it is a ploy, their marginal nonoperative treatments will be a halfhearted effort.

Failure of nonoperative treatment, by itself, is never a reason for surgery. Surgery is not always a last resort. A chronic back sprain will never benefit from disc or fusion surgery. If temporary improvement for it with surgery occurs, is only from the rest needed to recover from the surgery. It is the equivalent of a sham surgery (a placebo effect). We need significant symptoms with corresponding findings before we can expect good to excellent surgical results.

Trial use of a low back brace is a helpful tool (lumbosacral corset with stays). It suggests to the patient and the orthopedic surgeon the amount of relief that we can expect with low back fusion surgery. How does a bracing trial work? It partially immobilizes the location where the pain is coming from. If the brace helps the pain a lot, we can delay surgery. The patient can use the brace 1 hour at a time until they need surgery later. They should usually not wear it longer than an hour at a time because they will become dependent on it. Constant use causes the muscles to become stiffer and weaker.

If pain or discomfort returns when the brace is off, the patient should lie down or at least change positions. The patient should not wear it when lying down. Horizontal rests intermittently are always a help. Pain with a brace trial is an indicator of muscle irritability and foreshadows a poor surgical result. If the pain is better while upright in the brace but then worse in 15 minutes, keep the brace on less than half that time, which is 7 minutes or less. Later, increase the time with the brace on slowly up to an hour over a period of several weeks if it feels good. If the pain is worse when the patient puts the brace on, they should not wear it. The muscle irritability can lessen and resolve with good nonoperative care. After a few months, if the brace feels good and helps the pain for an hour at a time, then we can again consider fusion surgery.

Another surgical procedure of the spine that has good to excellent results is a procedure that removes bone spurs and thickened ligaments. We use it for low back spinal canal narrowing (decompression for central spinal stenosis). The bony holes become narrowed from arthritic bone spurs, thickened ligaments and thickened joint capsules (lateral stenosis from ligamentum flavum and facet joint hypertrophy). Making more room for the nerves as they exit the spinal canal through bony holes and travel down the thigh is part of the procedure (foraminotomy). This procedure is also a gold standard. It gives good to excellent results for moderately severe or severe central and lateral spinal canal narrowing.

Back and leg pain may limit walking distances to less than 4 city blocks (neurogenic claudication). Indications for this surgery are usually in patients 55 to 85 years old. After 60, the spine is already stiff enough, so patients do not need a bony fusion with the surgery.

Many patients have become hesitant to accept spine surgery because of "war stories" they hear. Poor results are more common than they should be. There are many reasons for occasional poor surgical results. They tend to fall into four categories. First, are technical reasons that relate to the diagnosis, indications, procedure or timing. Second, are patients not doing what they should. Third, are surgeons not doing what they should. And fourth, good people occasionally have complications that cannot be avoided.

Patients talk to each other and "word of mouth" works well for both good and bad experiences that patients have with their medical care. It works especially well if patients have options to freely choose their physicians. Most HMO patients must choose their doctors only from a list (closed panels). Because of the vested interest in their health plan, patients are less likely to say anything bad about their doctor. It blunts the value of a word of mouth referral. Some doctor referral websites help with the doctor's age, education, credentials, location, hours and interests. But be cautious with anonymous ratings and criticisms. They are much different than a verbal recommendation from a known and trusted friend. Many individuals in our world ruin the reputation of others by complaining inappropriately or unnecessarily. Some websites give them an unfortunate platform.

Some family physicians become hesitant to encourage surgery because they see the results from the surgeons they must refer to in their large group or HMO. Other doctors find and trust good surgeons and specialists who diligently care for their patients. If the family doctor is a partner of the HMO, the doctor has a financial incentive not to refer and not to say anything negative about marginal surgeons they might refer to. We all, however, are still able to judge between good and bad doctors with first, second and third impressions.

Insurance companies are expected through mandates of state law to screen the doctors they sign up on their panels. The "credentialing" of doctors by insurance companies does little to weed out bad physicians. The insurance carrier credentialing process is famously slow. It delays good, young physicians in the start-up of their practices for months, or years in some cases, making business risks outside of HMOs higher. Hospital medical staff organizations are better at credentialing and more efficient because they get to know the physicians.

Word of mouth is still the best and probably always will be. It is why poor or marginal physicians in the past could not maintain a practice. They had to move on elsewhere or do something else. Now, in contrast, marginal physicians can merely sign the PPO or HMO insurance contract and accept the payments. Even with a mandated medical director, insurance companies do not have the capability or medical judgment necessary to discern between bad and good doctors in the local community. They have a tough time turning away a doctor who wants to accept their discounted payment. Contracting with enough physicians in all specialties is hard for insurance carriers. Good doctors want to spend time with patients and do not want to compromise their standards. However, higher office overheads and insurance payment cuts push them.

Because greater numbers of patients are using Workers' Compensation claims for back and neck surgery, the rates of good to excellent results have deteriorated. The patient receives a larger benefit for having a greater disability. Therefore, a disincentive for getting better exists when using Workers' Compensation insurance coverage. It is widely known among doctors and attorneys as "secondary gain." In spite of efforts to combat fraud, overly generous employment benefits tend to increase the problem. Patient support from family, responsible local charitable organizations and laws that promote responsibility and self-reliance will tend to decrease the problem. Many patients do not want to be stuck in Workers' Compensation coverage, but they do not have a choice if they claim their injury happened at work. Many common orthopedic procedures have had good to excellent results in the 95 percent range such as total knee replacement. They also have deteriorating results when influenced by Workers' Compensation insurance benefits.

Success rate deterioration is more evident for surgeons who do not painstakingly wait for good indications for surgery. Mild findings and marginal indications will always degrade surgical results. Over a period of years, I noticed a trend for new patients who came to my office with severe knee arthritis and clear indications for a total knee replacement. They knew a friend with bad results from surgery done elsewhere. They hesitated to accept surgery even after they had already tried everything else. However, if they knew me or one of my patients, they simply wanted to know when I could schedule the surgery. The pattern was similar for patients who needed a total hip replacement. We should not be doing surgery too early. But waiting too long when surgery is right is not good either.

Other surgical procedures with deteriorating results include knee arthroscopy, foot surgery, carpal tunnel surgery and spinal injections. What do all these procedures have in common? All have adverse factors which contribute to their overuse. For each, usage of government health care programs and Workers' Compensation claims have increased. We see more dishonesty in research for new approaches, especially for expensive instrumentation. Patients have more impatience. They do not wait to let the body heal and say that they, "just want to have it fixed." This occurs even though what is wrong may be minor or may heal with more time. Surgeons may have impatience as well and not wait for the right indications.

When we read about the results of a medical treatment or a surgical procedure, we usually see the term "outcomes." Why has the word "outcomes" replaced the terms "results" and "findings" for medical research? Outcomes grew out of the need to try to justify substandard contract medicine and prepaid company doctors. These were approaches of the 1970s that formed the beginning of managed care. Proponents of managed care made outcomes sound good by saying that it means to find end results with a humanistic approach. Using cost-benefit data, advocates of "outcomes research" have an agenda to control medical and administrative decisions, policies and protocols.[35] Many academic institutions are also proponents and justify their position by selling policymakers health care outcomes to "improve" health care quality.[36]

 Surgeons are easy targets for managed care. Procedures are more easily watched than illnesses. Surgeries are big ticket items and include many services bundled in one price set by the insurance carrier. Insurance companies knew their data was inadequate for making decisions about individual physicians. So, they asked physicians to send "outcome data" to them to justify their contracting positions. Physicians soon began adjusting their data to impress the insurance companies and obtain better contracts. The origin of outcome data is therefore not based on science. Research about outcomes is not the same as scientific end results.

 The word confusion game is real. Soon everyone was using "outcomes" with the allusion that they are longer term results. That is a desirable connotation, but orthopedic researchers were already using the longest feasible follow-up periods. Nothing changed, except the word "results" changed to "outcomes" with a false premise and a false promise. Outcomes research is an agenda driven term and has become a pseudoscience with proponents promoting themselves. Though the term has attracted a great deal of research money, outcomes research has not saved money or improved quality of health care. Insurance companies and especially managed care entities have tremendous power by virtue of contracting laws. Because physicians have so little power, the term "outcomes" became politically correct and fashionable. It is comical now when many researchers and writers use the word "outcomes" for preliminary or short-term results.

---

[35] Academy of Managed Care Pharmacy, Concepts in Managed Care Pharmacy, "Outcomes Research," approved by AMCP Board April 2012, page 2, www.amcp.org/outcomes_research/, accessed May 9, 2018.
[36] Johns Hopkins Medicine, General Internal Medicine, "Outcomes Research," www.hopkinsmedicine.org/gim/research/method/outcomes.html, accessed May 9, 2018.

Governments and their contracted companies began doing what insurance companies were already doing with their digital patient care data. They started looking at their data to see what they could do to further their agenda to gain power. One of the favorite types of studies for "outcomes research" looks at combinations of studies to amass tens of thousands of patients to boost the "significance" of their findings and "importance" of their opinions (meta-analyses). Unfortunately, drawbacks to these statistical studies are known serious biases, such as publishing bias and agenda bias. Different studies when combined with varied controls and various definitions create lots of room for misinterpretations.

Another example of interference from the interplay between government and insurance companies began in the late 1980s. Medicare unilaterally decided not to pay for a doctor visit and a physical therapy visit on the same day, even if the patient was coming from out of town. Within a few years, private insurance companies were following Medicare's bad example and doing the same. A more recent outgrowth of this trend for government and insurance company interference is "pay-for-performance" (P4P), a pilot project of Medicare in 2005. The program name sounds good, but in practice it allows the government to change a payment to an individual physician. Federal contractors decide payments based on artificial targets.

In the early 1990s, under the influence of socialized health care, professors at McMaster University in England invented the term "evidence-based medicine." The words sound good, so watch out. Where it is based on real science, there may be limited merit. Its overt purpose was to develop a standard cookbook approach to minimize variation in different practice locations. Its real purpose is to control and, therefore, to accumulate power. The California State Legislature adopted a form of it in 2003 for their Workers' Compensation system. As a result, the use of many "alternative" treatments lessened for a few years. In 2007, the California Administrative Director of the Division of Workers' Compensation, however, added acupuncture specifically back in, despite the lack of evidence for doing so.[37]

Of the many drawbacks from evidence-based medicine are stifling innovation and limiting allowances for patient variation. It also misuses science by ignoring or twisting it when governments or insurance companies have enough power to do what they want. Through managed care "treatment authorizations," the State of California, health plans and insurance companies are making decisions for physicians about individual patients as well as groups of patients. This is despite the illegality of the corporate practice of medicine in California since the state Medical Practice Act of 1980.[38]

Since the early 1900's, to prevent profiteering and quackery by prepaid company doctors, most states have some form of prohibition on the corporate practice of medicine. It limits financial relationships with licensed physicians. Federal law has exempted HMOs from this law and similar laws since 1973. More control by insurance companies and governments creates mediocrity in the practice of medicine in addition to less innovation. Laws forbidding the corporate practice of medicine were designed to protect patients and physicians from that kind of influence. However, many states inconsistently enforce these laws and also have many exemptions.

In the early 1990s, I saw trouble coming to our surgical practice from "evidence-based medicine." Our office was required to start calling for "authorizations" from insurance adjusters to get something done for PPO patients. Within a few weeks of that starting, my medical assistant told me that we could not get a custom knee brace for a patient who tore an anterior cruciate ligament (ACL). When I asked why, she said

[37] State of California, Division of Workers' Compensation, Medical Treatment Utilization Schedule, History, June 15, 2007, www.dir.ca.gov/dwc/MTUS/MTUS_RegulationsGuidelines.html, accessed May 9, 2018.
[38] The Medical Board of California, "The policy expressed in Business and Professions Code section 2400 [within the Medical Practice Act] against the corporate practice of medicine is intended to prevent unlicensed persons from interfering with or influencing the physician's professional judgment," www.mbc.ca.gov/Licensees/Corporate_Practice.aspx, accessed May 9, 2018.

that the insurance adjuster denied it. I called the adjuster on the phone. After I explained why the patient needed the brace, she said, "No, I am still going to deny it because my husband had a knee injury, and he did not need a brace."

I could hardly believe what I had heard. The insurance adjuster was making things up to deny medical care. She was making decisions that directly and negatively affected my patient. She could not examine the patient and did not have a license to practice medicine. I explained to the patient what had happened. He could appeal to his insurance company or pay for the brace himself. That was only the beginning because the abuses continued to get worse. Soon, they did not answer their phones, and then they did not return phone calls.

Within a few years, insurance companies made policies that required physicians to appeal decisions of insurance adjusters formally in writing. Again, it increased our office overhead. The patients could not appeal. Even if science is used correctly, the cookbook approach of evidence-based medicine minimizes advances in medical care. It demeans experience and sometimes common sense. It is a disservice to patients who have unusual or complex conditions, which are common in orthopedics. In the last few years of my office practice, about 40 percent of the new patients I saw had unusual or complex, chronic conditions.

An example of an unusual condition is moderate to severe knee joint surface damage in a young adult (articular cartilage chondromalacia). Many patients less than 30 years of age have benefitted from arthroscopy to trim out knee joint surface flap fragments. They have symptoms that mimic meniscus tears. These patients came to me after having their first arthroscopy by another orthopedic surgeon. The knee joint surface has a chance to heal after removing these fragments down to a stable base with a small mechanical trimmer. The procedure has produced dramatic long-term results (arthroscopic chondral debridement).

Unlike an isolated meniscus tear, those patients do not usually experience a rapid and permanent resolution of pain after arthroscopy because their condition is more complex. It

117

takes at least 3 months—and a lot of patience by the surgeon and patient—to allow the remaining joint surface defect to heal. The healing is slow, but the time taken is worth it. Showing patients what to do and what not to do before and after the surgery is critical. If the patient does not do what they should, the joint surface can develop more defects or degenerative joint disease (osteoarthritis).

In 2007, UnitedHealthcare, a large health insurance company in the United States, unilaterally told doctors in a policy statement that they would not pay for arthroscopy to remove knee joint fragments for a diagnosis of osteoarthritis.[39] We do not do that procedure for generalized osteoarthritis. We do it for localized joint surface fragments (chondromalacia), which is a different diagnosis code. However, because the diagnoses are related, will the procedure be covered by the insurance carrier now or in the future? They did this, perhaps, because a few doctors abused the procedure. Instead, they should warn the culprits or, if necessary, not renew their contracts.

At the time of a surgery, we may find partially attached, widespread, loose fragments of the knee joint cartilage surface (femoral condyle chondromalacia or early osteoarthritis). If so, it takes more time than usual to do a decent job at the time of arthroscopic surgery. Removal of loose fragments has helped many patients avoid ongoing pain and the need for more surgery later. The insurance company policy statement suggests that they may not want to pay for such a procedure. It adds an element of misgiving in a surgeon's mind, "Am I wasting my time because I will not get paid anyway?" For a patient, the insurance company decree creates doubt about the motives of surgeons.

The policy statement from UnitedHealthcare did not make it clear if they would pay for other related procedures. One is arthroscopic loose body removal if the first diagnosis is a loose body and the second diagnosis is osteoarthritis. Loose body removal by arthroscopy is a gold standard procedure that

---

[39] UnitedHealthcare Network Bulletin, September 2007, Volume 21, page 5.

has been around for many years. The results are 95 percent good to excellent.[40] But the results are less dramatic if osteoarthritis accompanies the loose body. That is where the judgment and experience of an orthopedic surgeon is critical. We should not relegate decisions to a cookbook approach, practice guidelines or corporate policies.

The UnitedHealthcare mandate takes away some incentive for physicians to do a thorough job with the findings at the time of surgery. Should the surgeon merely get the loose body out and go on to the next case? When the fee is the same, why would they care about washing out many cartilage fragments in the joint, known as chondromatosis?[41] Residual fragments make the need for a total knee replacement more likely down the road. If your health insurance creates burdensome restrictions on your doctor, be wary. If your surgeon has a high volume of surgeries and is proud about being very fast in surgery, be careful.

The studies on knee joint surface fragment removal I have reviewed do not pay attention to the basic detail of the fragment removal and the specific exercises of physical rehabilitation. Those are two critical, basic deficiencies. With the wrong exercises, patients in large or small studies will never show benefits. Surgeons may do an adequate fragment removal in one area and then ignore the rest of the joint because insurance reimbursement is the same. If multiple areas need help, doing what the joint surfaces need may take us an extra 30 minutes or more. Cartilage fragmentation of the joint surface often accompanies a meniscus cartilage tear in the same area of the knee. Orthopedic surgeons know that insurance companies will only pay for removing the torn meniscus. They will not pay for joint surface fragment removal in the same compartment of the knee.[42]

---

[40] A joint space loose body is a slippery rounded piece of bone covered with cartilage, also called a "joint mouse."

[41] Synovial chondromatosis is uncommon and varies from several floating cartilage pieces to many thousands, with a blinding, whiteout "snow storm" like appearance.

[42] Knee joint space main compartments are, 1) around the kneecap (patellofemoral), 2) inside (medial tibiofemoral) and 3) outside (lateral tibiofemoral).

In 2011, a friend Thomas Christian reminded me that I had done a repeat knee arthroscopic surgery for him in 2009. He expressed gratitude for the improvement in his activity level after surgery, and he still had no pain. When I first saw him in the office, he had painful, obvious, mechanical knee problems, both by history and on physical exam. After a first knee arthroscopy by another orthopedic surgeon elsewhere, he complained of persisting knee pain. A repeat MRI scan had nonspecific findings, but the mechanical clunking on exam was significant. I could hear it and feel it. We decided to go ahead with a second knee arthroscopy.

During his outpatient surgery, I trimmed a few cartilage fragment flaps from the joint surface down to a stable base on the inner side of the knee joint (arthroscopic debridement for localized medial femoral chondromalacia). In the same area, the meniscus was degenerated with a small, movable, meniscal flap. I also trimmed it back to a stable base (partial medial meniscectomy). The joint surface fragments were the biggest problem holding him back. The frayed meniscus tear may have also been a part of it. At the first postoperative office visit, he said that he could already feel a difference. Thomas later said that his end result was completely different than his first knee surgery. His pain resolved quickly.

Other types of knee surgery can also be extremely satisfying for the patient and the surgeon when the indications are right. One of them is a reconstruction of an anterior cruciate ligament (ACL). For the patient to notice a significant improvement, before surgery the ligament must be lax enough (2 to 4+ out of 4+ on physical exam by an orthopedic surgeon). If the ligament is not very loose, a custom knee brace is a good answer for most, including athletes at many levels (trace to 1+). Making a knee too tight with an ACL reconstruction can, in less than 8 to 10 years, contribute to arthritis (degenerative changes). When the surgery and rehabilitation are done well, the results can be dramatic.

The 2014–15 college basketball season was the first season back for Kyle Collinsworth after an 8-month absence for ACL reconstructive surgery. During the rehabilitation and that first season back, Kyle worked hard. He built his endurance gradually and used a custom knee brace wisely. That season, as a junior at Brigham Young University (BYU), he set an NCAA single season record with 6 triple-doubles (double-digit points, assists and rebounds). That also tied the NCAA career record. The next season, he added 6 more triple-doubles for a NCAA career record of 12 total.[43]

A hands-on physical examination is still necessary, despite amazing x-ray, CT and MRI scan technology. Skillful history taking and listening by the physician are just as important, if not more important. Electronic medical records will not solve deficiencies in these areas. A medical assistant or a physician assistant may help within their scope of practice. But an orthopedic surgeon is obligated to take a proper history and do a physical exam, especially if he is thinking about operating on the patient. If the doctor does not listen to you or touch you, walk out and find another doctor. Seek the best if you want the best result.

I am not alone in having concerns with the dishonesty and shortcuts among my peers. In the internationally respected The Journal of Bone and Joint Surgery, an orthopedic surgeon Dr. Shelbourne from the Midwestern United States lamented in 2010 that he had increasing concerns about the direction of orthopedic practices.[44] In discussions with his peers, they also had concerns about the lack of adequate knee exams. Some orthopedic surgeons do not touch the patient, do not spend enough time doing the exam or do not ask the patient about pain or other symptoms. It takes courage and time out of a busy schedule for a doctor to do what is best for their patient though there may be less income. As a profession, I know we can do better. The negative influence of some state and federal laws and HMOs is real.

---

[43] Brigham Young University Cougars, Kyle Collinsworth, 2015–2016 Senior Year, byucougars.com/athlete/m-basketball/16194/Kyle-Collinsworth, accessed May 9, 2018.
[44] K. Donald Shelbourne, M.D., "The Art of the Knee Examination: Where Has It Gone?" The Journal of Bone and Joint Surgery, August 4, 2010, Volume 92-A, Number 9, page 1909, journals.lww.com/jbjsjournal/toc/2010/08040, accessed May 9, 2018.

Dr. Shelbourne also had concerns that some doctors send patients to have an MRI scan before the physical examination of an orthopedic surgeon. He observed that our dependence on x-ray, CT scan, MRI scan, laboratory tests and other surgical technology is decreasing our capacity to reason and may therefore decrease our ability to be good doctors. Instead of treating the patient and their symptoms, the trends to do quick exams and to treat findings on an MRI scan are too common. Is there a valid need for surgery? Yes, for the right reasons and by the right doctor, there can be.

Hand, wrist, knee, ankle and foot surgery are areas of expertise that most of us orthopedic trauma surgeons are very comfortable with. Many elective procedures in those areas consistently have 90 percent good to excellent results and are a joy to do. For example, ganglion cysts are especially common in the wrist and hand. Before surgery, rest, splinting, anti-inflammatory medication, passive range of motion and needle aspiration with a corticosteroid injection are worth trying. Cysts can resolve spontaneously. Passive range of motion uses the help of the other hand or something else. And we can use it often. We can remove a cyst surgically if pain persists or if they keep growing bigger. A Baker's cyst in the back of the knee is larger. Knee arthroscopy usually takes care of the problem in the knee joint causing the swelling of the cyst.

Another common problem is trigger finger, which is annoying and painful. It occurs most often in the thumb, middle and ring fingers. Triggering occurs when the tendon cannot fit through the tendon pulley sheath without popping or getting stuck. It occurs with slight flexor tendon swelling from use, age or tendinitis. If the finger or thumb is not popping all the time and is not hurting, gentle passive range of motion is worth trying first for a few weeks. The passive motion has a 60 percent rate of good to excellent long-term results. Outpatient surgery with a small incision in the skin crease of the palm easily cures the triggering with a 98 percent good to excellent end result. Waiting to do surgery until the finger locks and stays locked is not a good plan. That will compromise the results with stiffness and other problems.

In the foot, a patient needs surgery when the great toe has a moderate to severe bunion deformity and when pain persists. Surgery on the bunion can prevent cascading deformities of other toes on the same foot. The gratifying results include 90 percent good to excellent pain relief, correction of deformity and easier wearing of shoes. If other toes of the foot already have deformity, surgery can solve that too. If the patient has rheumatoid arthritis, the results are not as good but are still about 80 percent.

When I was in high school, a cousin of mine was a podiatrist, and he encouraged me to go into podiatry. I studied the options. They care for the foot and do surgery on the foot, but they are not medical doctors. They have their own colleges that grant Doctor of Podiatric Medicine degrees (DPM). I found that Medical school with a Doctor of Medicine degree (M.D.) is a better education in anatomy, physiology and all other medical sciences for the whole person, including the foot. I wanted the best education I could find. Years later, during my orthopedic practice, I saw my cousin's name on a disciplinary notice for the State of California licensing board. I have always been glad, but especially then, that I had chosen to go to medical school. It was a well-rounded education that has helped me continue to learn. Orthopedics incorporates all areas of the arms and legs, including foot surgery.

The right symptoms, the right findings, the right indications, the right doctor and the right reasons are all important. No hidden agendas on the part of the patient or the doctor are also important. Long-term results of surgery for most musculoskeletal problems should be good to excellent. There should be complete or significant relief of pain in a high percentage of patients.

Chapter 13

A Deposition from Heaven

In 1998 during the night, I had a dream. That morning, I could not remember much about the dream. It left me with an impression that I needed to write a book about pain. I also knew what the title of it should be. It was to include what I was learning about pain from my orthopedic surgery practice. However, I had no time to write a book! Commitments to family, church and work were important to me. I did not even know how to start. The only real writing I had done before were weekly letters to three of my children, who were abroad at various times on 18 to 24-month church missions. I worried about the overhead in my orthopedic surgery private practice. Economic forces on small medical group offices were causing increasing risks. Regardless, I knew that I needed to start writing.

Before that, our practice partnership decided to decline an HMO contract that would have stretched us thinner with the local Independent Practice Association (IPA). It would have increased our patient volume while decreasing per patient the reimbursement. We could not have taken care of patients as well as we wanted. Overhead margins were already becoming thinner with cuts in PPO contracts, Workers' Compensation contracts and Medicare. I needed to continue working hard to keep up with our business overhead. I could not take time to sit down and start writing a book.

Yet, I found ways of using my experiences and the things I was learning from my patients about pain. Though I had not yet written any down, I began sharing experiences with friends who asked for advice and with a few patients. As I used those experiences, not only did I improve my ability to communicate, I found more ways to apply the principles I had learned. I remember praying and asking God for help to find a way to start the book if He wanted me to do it.

In 1999, I walked into a scheduled deposition in our company conference room. I assumed that it would be like any other deposition. As usual before the deposition, I studied my medical record for an hour. The patient had made a California

Workers' Compensation claim. Seven months before, I had examined the patient once and functioned as an agreed medical evaluator (AME). I had given my diagnosis and treatment recommendations in the report I had sent to both parties (applicant and defense). I had not given any treatment, and nothing unusual was in the record. So, I did not know what the attorneys were going after.

As usual, two representatives and a court reporter were present for the deposition. One attorney represented the patient, and another was there for the insurance company. The attorneys usually argue about issues influencing the monetary amounts of a Workers' Compensation case. Before swearing me in, however, they told me that this deposition would be different. I thought to myself in cynical disbelief, "Oh sure, they all want the same thing." I did not say anything, but I must have looked skeptical. Both attorneys reassured me, "No really, we just want to know what you know about reflex sympathetic dystrophy." They explained that when I saw the Workers' Compensation patient about 7 months before, I had given the patient in my report a diagnosis of right foot and leg reflex sympathetic dystrophy (RSD). Other physicians had not agreed with my diagnosis, but within a few months, the diagnosis of RSD became more obvious. Then, the attorneys told me, the other physicians agreed that my diagnosis was correct.

I was sworn in under oath for the deposition. When one of the attorneys asked the first question, I could tell that they were being honest with me. It stayed that way. Both attorneys were true to their word. This deposition was very different from any other deposition before or since then, and I have had my deposition taken for hundreds of Workers' Compensation cases. They only asked questions to understand. That is, of course, different from asking questions to confuse the issues or create controversy. It is also different than asking accusatory questions or questions with a built-in opinion or bias such as, "I can't believe that..." It is also different than asking questions with a gang mentality with the interrogator pretending that he has like-minded persons, "We see that you

..." Or they may ask, "We cannot believe that..." I am well accustomed to answering and deflecting questions from attorneys by answering with facts from the records, based on the truth and consistency of the record.

Asking questions to understand, reflects an approach that has an attitude of learning. "Wow," I thought to myself, "I have two attorneys who want to learn." In the deposition from there on, I could give facts, opinions, ideas and beliefs without worrying about them trying to twist the facts or opinions. For me to continue candidly, I had to trust that they would not change what they had said their approach was going to be.

I did not normally keep a copy of my depositions. Because I recognized that this deposition would help me start putting things on paper, I asked if I could keep a copy of the deposition for the book I wanted to write. I knew then how to start writing. When I received the certified deposition copy 2 weeks later, I carefully filed it away at home. I felt that the deposition was an answer to my prayer. The deposition stimulated me to begin writing the experiences I was having with pain.

Within a few months, I started writing at 5:30 AM every morning except Sunday for 30 minutes. I wrote most of the book before I retired from active practice in 2010. I knew that I would forget many things after retiring. In 2008, I looked for the deposition copy at home. I had not seen it since filing it away 9 years before. I only found a thick, manila file folder filled with journal articles, labeled with the title of the book. After looking through the folder multiple times, I could not find the deposition. I was in disbelief. After looking in all my files and trying to find it for a few weeks, I was very discouraged. I could not believe that I had lost the deposition copy. My wife and I said a prayer together and asked God for help finding the copy of the deposition. I could not remember the name of the patient. I tried searching my deposition schedule at the office. I could not remember his name or find the date of the deposition to locate the court records.

Then, nearly 2 years later and a few months before retiring in January 2010, my wife and I were looking through my files for our passports. In one of my filing cabinets, I noticed a thin file folder labeled "Writing Ideas." In the folder was the certified deposition copy! What a relief. For me, finding it was another answer to prayer. Somehow, I had missed it though I had looked through all the files in my filing cabinets at home and at work several times. As I read the deposition, the words on paper were reassuring. I was grateful for what was already there.

The ideas described by me in the deposition are simple. They are what I learned to do to help patients with reflex sympathetic dystrophy. First, I help them understand the diagnosis in terms that anyone can understand. Second, I help them understand what to do and what not to do to help them get better. Many of the concepts I described in the deposition were helpful for coping with and resolving other types of pain. Over the last 10 years of my practice, they helped the healing and recovery in many different musculoskeletal areas.

I noticed many transcription errors by the court reporter in the certified deposition copy. Errors are common in medical deposition transcriptions. I have reviewed thousands of them over the years. Fortunately, when I notice the errors, most of them are easy to sort out and correct. Many of the errors are phonetic words or spellings. As an example, "alignment dissatisfactory" should have been transcribed as "alignment is satisfactory." I have corrected many of the transcription errors in the edited digital version of the deposition that follows in the next two chapters of this book. Another example of an error in the transcription was when I spoke the word "induration." It means a firm area of swelling. The court reporter incorrectly transcribed that word once as "in racial" and twice as "interracial." Another correction was the word "whether," incorrectly transcribed twice in the same paragraph as "rather," changing the meaning both times. I have marked the error corrections with brackets.

The questioning in the deposition continued for 1½ hours. In the 35 years of my active surgical practice, this deposition was more peculiar than any other. Both attorneys continued what they promised at the first of the deposition.

They just wanted to try to learn. They were not trying to prove anything, and both kept their honest approach. As I taught them, I reflected on the similarities in teaching my patients with this disorder.

When I teach a patient with reflex sympathetic dystrophy or chronic pain similar things and guide them, a few will not improve at first. More than half will improve to some extent by the first follow-up visit. Most do not understand or remember more than half of what I tell them at the first visit. If I answer their questions and patiently repeat some of the things they need to know, they will learn more each visit. The more specific a question is, the better it is, especially if it is about something they have tried. They may learn some things easily and struggle to learn other things, no matter how well I explain things to them.

After I explain a patient's pain and the consequences of their actions, they notice their choices more in the next few weeks. They tend to find similar characteristics in other areas of their lives such as impatience and impulsiveness. Then, it becomes possible for them to continue learning. When they come back for follow-up visits, I ask them questions. Discerning what they learned and what they missed is possible with the right specific questions. If their symptoms are less and the findings on exam are improving, they are going in the right direction. Though their progress may be slow, some progress is also occurring when the area of pain becomes smaller or the pain is less intense. When the patient begins to notice short periods of time with no pain, they can gradually begin to make faster progress. Resolution can only occur if the patient learns well enough to cultivate and create longer and longer periods without pain.

If a patient does not learn anything between visits, then I worry about them more. Fortunately, about 90 percent of my RSD patients will go in the right direction within 3 months. The right direction does not mean that it cures them. It only means that they are making some improvement. That means that they can notice a significant difference in the pain. It also means that risk of the pain worsening again is less. How much improvement they make afterwards is variable and impossible to predict. Many variables are dependent on the patient. The amount of improvement depends on the patient's motivation, desire, consistency and determination to learn.

Physical therapy can be of help with some RSD patients. If the therapy is causing more pain or if the patient's pain is continuing with no improvement, we should stop physical therapy. Improving range of motion with the pain staying the same is not a good reason to continue physical therapy. Without improvement of pain during the course of treatment with physical therapy, the patient will usually lose any improvement in range of motion after we discontinue physical therapy.

Movement is not the only answer for RSD. If it were, its resolution would be easy, and patients would not have to come in for help. They could sort it out and get better on their own. Movement, however, is important and the patient must do it carefully, slowly and after an appropriate warm-up. If a joint is moved too far or too fast, more than it is ready for, the pain will become worse. At the very least, the pain will keep coming back. The answer is to do the opposite of too far or too fast. They should move more slowly and with smaller amounts of motion (smaller excursion). Keeping the number of repetitions for a patient small, means less than 5 to 10 at a time. If a patient is struggling, they can move in an easier direction first.

Resting is okay, but the longer a patient stays in an immobile position, the more stiffness will accumulate. The answer is to do the opposite. Move more often but well within the limits of pain. In other words, the patient should stop before feeling the pain. If the pain is constant, stop before the pain increases. Another way to think of it is to go only half of what it takes to cause pain. That sounds easy, but it is not. Using small amounts often takes a lot of patience and practice before getting it right, so the patient can do it often without getting into trouble.

Warming up means to do things to the muscles that enable them and the surrounding joints to move without pain.

An example is dressing warmer in cooler weather. Another is covering a body part that hurts with a blanket or another body part such as the hand. If the pain is in one of the hands, then a patient can use the other hand. If both hands hurt, then they can use something else such as the armpits. Holding gently but firmly is okay because it usually feels good, and it inhibits swelling. Even if a warm-up feels good, patients should not keep doing it for too long. They should not do the warm-up for more than 5 to 10 minutes at a time. Instead, they can come back to it often.

Rubbing is okay as a part of warming up if it feels good. If rubbing feels good, a patient should not continue for sustained periods of more than 2 minutes at a time. Patients can come back to it frequently. They should not do deep muscle massages, which will irritate the muscles. Even if they make the muscles relax, they will tighten back up readily. Patients should do rubbing easily, lightly but firmly. We should not do rubbing repetitiously, which means we should not do it in one direction or in circles. It should feel good. Better rubbing motions are random. If rubbing does not feel good, a patient will have to wait until later when their muscles are not as irritable. They should not scratch because it will eventually damage skin. The itch will keep coming back anyway. Holding is better and relieves itching.

If heat does not feel good to a patient, their muscles are too irritable, and they should not use it (heat intolerance). If heat feels good, we can use it to help the warm-up process if we keep it short enough, 5 to 10 minutes at a time. Patients with RSD should not use ice even if it feels good. Ice is only numbing things up. It tightens muscles and will, because of the numbing effect, fool the patient into thinking they are better than they really are.

If they feel good, cool structures in a house such as a tile counter top or tile floor may be okay. The patient should keep time on them short initially or less than 2 to 3 minutes at a time. Cool tile, a warm blanket or small differences in air temperatures are good to experiment with because they will help the body acclimatize to weather changes. The next winter will not be as much of a struggle if we expose our injured body part to changes in the climate a little at a time.

When a storm front comes in, the barometer goes down. When the barometer goes down, the air pressure all around us is less. Because of less air pressure, things in the body that tend to swell will swell more. A bag of potato chips taken from sea level to the mountains at an elevation of 6000 feet reacts in the same way. The bag gets bigger because the air pressure is less at a higher elevation. That is true for a joint with arthritis, a finger with infection, an ankle sprain or a leg that has swelling from poor veins (venous insufficiency).

All the diverse tissues of a body part, such as the hand, are involved with reflex sympathetic dystrophy. Most will tend to swell. We must be kind to the skin, fatty tissue, bones, nerves and blood vessels as well as the joints and muscles. Elevation can feel good and be helpful for swelling or fullness. Elevation should not be prolonged. Instead, we can come back to it often. Stiffness of all the soft tissues and joints subsides with movement. Because each of the soft tissues gets rid of the stiffness at different rates, movement is not easy. Irritating one of the many soft tissues is easy when we move them. Gradual light use of the body part and limited exercise can be helpful for warming up and lessening stiffness of the joints and muscles. However, they are very tempting and easy to overdo. Most RSD patients know that strengthening will cause trouble.

Patience is mandatory at each step or level of recovery. Most everything we can think of that feels good should not be prolonged. Prolonged use will usually turn a good tool into a bad tool. A heating pad and pain medication are two examples of good tools that patients often misuse. Those good tools will become problems if we use them for more than 2 to 3 months. In the long term, the most natural tools are position changes, movements and exercises that consistently feel good. These are usually the most important tools, and they are less likely to become bad tools.

Chapter 14

The Attorneys Wanted to Know

"Before the Workers' Compensation Appeals Board for The State of California, Deposition of David E. Smalley, M.D., at 4444 Magnolia Avenue, Riverside, California, 10:15 AM, Wednesday, February 17, 1999.[45]

"David E. Smalley, M.D., called as a witness by and on behalf of the Defendants, and having been first duly sworn by the Certified Shorthand Reporter, was examined and testified as follows:"

"Q. BY MS. SMITH: Good morning, doctor. I suspect you have a C.V. [curriculum vitae][46] with you."

"A. Yes."

"Q. We can waive qualifications. I may want to attach that to the deposition transcript. I may have a few questions later on pertinent (sic)."[47]

"MR. HERNANDEZ: I will stipulate to that."

"Q. BY MS. SMITH: We're here today because the parties selected you to examine Donald Watson in the capacity of agreed medical examiner, and you did so July 5th, 1998. And you wrote a report bearing that same date. And in your examination of Mr. Watson, you diagnosed a condition called chronic reflex sympathetic dystrophy [RSD]. What is that condition generally?"

"A. It's recovery-phase problems with injuries as well as surgeries. There are several things that can stimulate it, but it causes sometimes short-term, sometimes long-term problems. It depends on how it's treated. It depends on how the patient deals with it as well."

"Q. What are the criteria for a positive diagnosis of that condition?"

---

[45] The dates and names are changed to protect privacy. The name of the insurance company attorney (defense) is changed to Ms. Smith. The name of the patient's attorney (applicant) is changed to Mr. Hernandez.

[46] Words in brackets [abc] are added for gross error correction or clarity. Empty brackets [ ] are added for words or letters of a word that were deleted for clarity. Punctuation is corrected for clarity. All changes are faithful to the original meaning.

[47] A (sic) notation shows where errors in the deposition transcript are not corrected.

"A. It is a very multi-faceted problem. When it's very obvious, it can include limitation of joint motion. It can include atrophy. It can include skin and vascular changes. When it is very subtle, it can include things such as pain [that is out of] proportion to the findings. It can also include stiffness. It can also include muscle pain inhibition."

"Q. I'm sorry, muscle pain inhibition?"

"A. Yes. Those are just examples of the extremes of the diagnosis. And there [are] many variations of that."

"Q. Do some people get it and some don't? Is there a predisposition?"

"A. Yes."

"Q. And what would that be?"

"A. Previous history of RSD would certainly be one. Patients that have [a] history of prolonged recoveries from old injuries would be another. Patients that have depression and patients that have [a] personality disorder, either overt or subclinical, [are others]. A patient, for example, who can be just very impatient can be a predisposing factor."

"Q. So generally what symptoms will specifically lead you to that diagnosis minimally?"

"A. Like I said, it is a very multi-faceted diagnosis. So, it's a little bit like [six] blind men trying to describe an elephant. The diagnosis is more accepted and recognized more commonly now than it was ten years ago. And that's because it is more common. There are some very subtle things that we're now recognizing that are part of it.

"It has been probably longest recognized in the upper extremity, in the hand and arm. But it has been manifested— we've known about it for hundreds of years—for example, in the [U.S.] Civil War when people had injuries. It has been written about in the old medical literature, and orthopedic surgeons have known about it for hundreds of years. I think we're getting better at understanding it in the last ten years than we've ever understood it before. Ten years ago, I distinctly remember [one] of my partners telling me I was not right in saying that there was RSD in the knee. And now it's commonly accepted."

"Q.   So lower extremities are following upper extremities as far as…"

"A. Lower extremities are [less] understood, but they can have RSD [symptoms like] an upper extremity. In fact, there [are] RSD-like syndromes in the back, neck and any part of the body that is not put in the right circumstances in a recovery or rehabilitation phase after an injury or [surgery]."

"Q. Has anybody ever misdiagnosed RSD?"

"A. It can be misdiagnosed, sure. It can have a lot of different manifestations. It can also mimic a lot of other things. It can also accompany other problems or diagnoses. It can accompany injuries, for example, that have a tumor.

"A patient can have an injury to the knee and a tumor in the knee, and either one of them or both of them can contribute to pain that's out of proportion to what we'd normally expect for those two particular problems. And [whether] the injury or [whether] the tumor is contributing to RSD sometimes can be very difficult to sort out because either one of them, or the combination of the two, can contribute to RSD. So, there [are] multi-factorial contributory causes to it, but fortunately most of the time, it's not that complicated to figure out."

"Q. Okay. I'm a little confused. Is the…"

"A.   Don't worry about that. Most patients, most physicians are confused about the diagnosis still at this point."

"Q. If I had to describe one very clear, most common characteristic, would it be pain out of proportion to the injury or the trauma?"

"A. That's certainly one of the most common."

"Q. Is there anything that would be that high up on the, anything else that's alarmingly, if you will…"

"A. Stiffness is another that's very common."

"Q.   Thank you. Is there a specific treatment that's used, once that diagnosis kicks in, to treat the RSD? A specific, I'm sorry, course of treatment?"

"A.   Yes. There [are] many levels of treatment for RSD. There [are] both good and bad simple as well as good and bad complex treatments for it. For example, the standard treatment for it is rest, appropriate stretching, physical therapy, limitation of activity and gradual progression of use when the patient is feeling better. Those are some of the basic things. In more advanced or resistant cases, sometimes things like sympathetic blocks, epidural blocks, regional blocks or anesthetic blocks locally can be used. But if the patient doesn't change how they are dealing with the problem, those blocks are almost always [only a] temporary benefit.

"If the patient is [ ] doing their best and doing the right things, sometimes the block can help the process a little bit. But the bottom line of getting patients with this particular problem better is assisting them, guiding them [and] teaching them because that's what works best."

"Q. What does the patient have to do to maximize the benefit of a block? What's the patient's part?"

"A. That's what I was just talking about. And what I mean by that is that the patient does need to learn how to rest, learn how to work on the stiffness in the appropriate ways and learn how to only gradually resume [use].

"One of the most common denominators of a chronic perpetuation of these kinds of complaints is the patient gets impatient. They try to go too fast to do things and never get well. And they try to figure out why they are always hurting."

"Q. Any kind of prescription medication that is used in the treatment?"

"A. There [are] lots of medications that are used. And again, if they are used in appropriate ways, they can be a good temporary benefit. But those patients can also be easily addicted to medications, unless they are guided and monitored like a hawk."

"Q. So the medication would be to treat the symptoms, the pain?"

"A. Well, when used appropriately, the medications would be used to help the patient do what I mentioned before, to be able to rest initially, temporarily [and] to be able to stretch. But if they don't taper off the medication soon, then they never learn how to deal with [the pain] appropriately.

"I think I'm going to keep a copy of this deposition, by the way, because you are asking some questions that I explain day in and day out to the patients, yet I have never [ ] written them down. But I've learned how to deal with it over the last 15 years, and I'm in the process of writing a book."

"Q. Okay. That was going to be one of my questions. Is there always a permanent disability from RSD?"

"A. No. [It can vary from] no residual problems to no use of the involved part. It varies between those extremes. But, fortunately, for 90 to 99 percent of the patients it is self-limiting, and it tends to improve."

"Q. Is it ever considered cured in a patient?"

"A. It's unusual, but yes."

"Q. So it's more as though it's in remission instead of cured?"

"A. When patients are really learning well how to take care of it, they can get over it. Yet, with all comers in my experience, probably 90 percent of them will improve significantly and dramatically. [Of those,] probably only 10 percent will be able to totally forget about it."

"Q. Okay. Now with Mr. Watson, who you examined, you were the first of about, I guess, four doctors who diagnosed this condition. That's why we're here today. What specifically about him and his condition led you to this diagnosis?"

"A. To do that, I literally would need to go through sentence by sentence, what the history was [and] sentence by sentence what the [physical] exam was in the records. I don't know if you want me to do that, but I look at all the factors combined. That's the best way I have of describing it.

"One of the things I see in the first paragraph, for example, is [that] the mechanism of the injury was a crush injury. That is another factor that is very common in reflex [sympathetic dystrophy] patients."

"Q. Anything else? I'd kind of like to get a little specific, if we can."

"A. That's only out of the first paragraph."

"Q. Do you want to take some time to review the file?"

"A. I have already done that. What I'm saying is, if you want me to go sentence by sentence, I'd be happy to do

136

that because there will probably be things like that in [ ] almost every paragraph as we go through [them]."

"Q. I assume not everybody who has a crush injury develops this?"

"A. That's correct."

"Q. If you have to go through it sentence by sentence—I'd just like to know. Sorry."

"A. Let me tell you this and then you can tell me whether that's answering your question or not. Probably 70 percent of the patients with a crush injury will have some degree of reflex sympathetic dystrophy, whether it's a hand crush injury or whether it's a foot crush injury. It's very, very common in those injuries.

"And 5 percent of all wrist fractures, whether they are minimal or severe, will have reflex sympathetic dystrophy. No matter how well we treat them or how well the patient tries, sometimes they misunderstand when we take the cast off. Sometimes they misunderstand what they are to do.

"Even though we tell them, they don't get it, and they hear what they want to hear. They go out and do what they want to do despite the instructions. I say, 'Okay, your cast is off, [and] your fracture is healed. Go out and get the stiffness out; move it, but don't use it.'

"Well, they hear what they want to hear, and they say, 'Well, he said move it,' and they start to use it. Even though I told them not to use it, they start to use it to move it. By doing that, they [exacerbate] stiffness. And they also start noticing, 'Well, that kind of hurts so I better kind of hold back a little bit.' Then they stop moving it and [ ] stop stretching it. That combination is the exact opposite of the direction that they are supposed to go, and it causes increased pain.

"So the pain that is out of proportion to what the findings are doesn't mean that the pain is not understandable. It's understandable from the standpoint that they are doing the wrong things and that's contributing to the pain. Very soon it can lead into a severe vicious cycle.

"Again, this is just as an example. Some of those wrist patients will have an atrophic arm that is useless within two or three months. That can happen even though they just had a wrist fracture. Even though it is a nondisplaced fracture. Even though they were casted for six weeks. Even though it looked just like another patient who had the same exact injury and is fine two or three weeks after the cast comes off.

"Okay. That's how different some of those patients that have RSD are from the normal. Now, going back to this patient and in the second paragraph under history of present illness, the patient saw Dr. Baker for three months [and] had physical therapy for four months. 'Patient states that the therapy did not help. In fact, [it] made him worse.' That's very typical of a reflex sympathy dystrophy patient.

"It used to be that physical therapy was one of the best helps and treatments for RSD. But that's unfortunately changing because of all the economic pressures on all medical providers. Rather than assisting therapists or their brace makers or their physicians, [there are more obstacles] with managed care and some of the constraints in industrial care. [Physical therapists] are forced to kind of look at the diagnosis, put them on a treadmill and let them do some of their own exercises. They don't listen to the patients enough. [They may] treat just what the diagnosis is instead of the individual.

"It's very easy to make these patients worse because the patient actually wants to get better. The therapist tells them, 'Okay, do this.' And the patient does it and they keep hurting. And they think, 'Well, the therapist told me to do it, but it still hurts.' And they think, 'Well, the therapist must know what they are doing,' and they keep trying. And they are still, when they go to therapy, going in the wrong direction. And that perpetuates the pain, that vicious cycle. So the patient recognizes, 'This hurts; it makes things worse so I will stop therapy and see what happens.' So again, that's very typical [for] this kind of patient."

"Q. Just to digress for a moment, how would you, if you had seen this patient right at the beginning, have handled that? Would you not have prescribed physical therapy?"

"A. Well, every physical therapy facility is a little different. In ours, we do try to listen to the patients a little bit more. But I have to tell you quite honestly even our therapists I have to watch like a hawk. I have to watch the patients like a hawk—just to make sure they are going in the right direction as I said—so they are not tending to do too much with the wrong things, [and] they are doing the right amounts with the right things.

"The other thing that also is in that second paragraph, for example, is that he was last seen by the doctor in February of 1998, who recommended an MRI scan of the right foot for nerve damage. That's another contributory factor. Not that I'm trying to fault the doctor, who is trying to understand what the patient is having, [and] is explaining it in his own way. Sometimes the patient may have understood that because they feel a sharp pain, 'it must be a nerve.' So again, he wants to hear what [the doctor] thinks. But sometimes that contributes to the confusion. And if he understands that it is stiffness, it is a problem that he can control by knowing what to do and what not to do. Then things like [the MRI scan] don't confuse the issue.

"For example, if I send an RSD patient for an MRI scan, they start assuming that 'Okay, he's doing a diagnostic test. He's going to actually find something.' So, they are terribly disappointed when I tell them, 'Well, the MRI scan shows a little degenerative change. But I don't think that's causing the pain.' Or if the MRI is normal, then they really get concerned because, 'He is telling me that it's normal. I'm having all this severe pain, and they really don't understand.'"

"Q. So if I'm hearing you correctly you are saying his being told that by the doctor could have added some psychological reaction or component?"

"A. No. Not so much that. It's just [that] sometimes it delays understanding the actual problem. Again, the patient thinks, 'Okay, he's doing something. He is ordering a test and hopefully it will show something.' And it doesn't matter, you know, whether it's this particular problem or another problem, but if we're doing tests on patients that are [ ] likely going to be negative, we may be trying to rule other problems out like a tumor [or] something else that might show up on an MRI scan.

"But if it's not helping us with directing the treatment, then sometimes, again, the patients tend to have false hopes saying, 'Okay, the MRI scan is really going to show us something, and then [ ] my pain is going to go away.' And so they are floored many times when they come back, and I tell them the MRI scan is normal. But if the physician and the patient keep that in perspective, then an MRI scan may not be a bad thing. But I certainly don't use it very often with an RSD patient.

"You started to ask what I would have done. And the most important thing that I have found over the years that helps these patients is—from the first time I see them—explain what they've got and what they can do and what they shouldn't do. And then, if they'll listen and if they will apply those things, like I said, 90 percent of the time they will start improving, and they will do significantly better."

[ ] "MS. SMITH: Did your client have an MRI scan?"

"MR. HERNANDEZ: No. They didn't say he had one. Just recommended."

"Q. BY MS. SMITH: So just this statement that the doctor would recommend that is somehow a background, part of why you came to that diagnosis? I mean I am not sure what you were saying. I'm sorry. I just didn't understand the connection of the fact that an MRI scan was talked about to your actually diagnosing the condition."

"A. What that means to me... I'm picking out things that are contributing to the patient's confusion. An MRI scan was recommended. For what purpose? What was he trying to look for? What was he trying to rule out? If [the MRI scan] was just because the patient had severe pain, that doesn't necessarily make any sense. But if he is actually looking for a tumor, okay, that's great. That's understandable. But if not, if he's just trying to figure out why the patient is having pain, but then never explains to the patient what to do or what not to do, then yes, that's a contributory factor."

"Q. Is the patient's confusion..."

"A. Yes. Not knowing what to do."

"Q. No direction. All right. Continuing okay. We were talking about the things that led you to this diagnosis with Mr. Watson. And we had just talked about the MRI, the recommendation of the MRI, and the fact that you felt that it could add to his confusion. What else could have suggested to you that he had this condition?"

"A. In the next paragraph, the first paragraph on page 2, he states that at the present time he has constant pain, except when he is off of his feet. Constant pain is not a good sign, especially if the injury is November 1996. He's still having constant pain. That seems to me, and I think to most orthopedic surgeons, that's kind of out of proportion to what we'd expect. And certainly, it's possible. It can happen. But that's part of what I meant before by things being out of proportion to what we'd expect."

"Q. Okay. Was there anything in the way of an objective finding, a test, anything we could look at and say, oh, yes?"

"A. An MRI scan?"

"Q. Anything like that, yes. That helped you arrive at that diagnosis as well?"

"A. Well, again, I explain this to patients as well as their families many, many times, but the history and the physical exam do tell us [ ] most diagnoses. A lot of people are kind of surprised about that, but we've done arthroscopy and back surgery long before we had MRI scans. And most of the time we didn't need them. We've [ ] become dependent upon them in abnormal ways.

"The history and the physical are still some of the most important parts of making [a] diagnosis. And I think most of the doctors in our [ ] medical schools at the time that I was going through were taught that 90 percent of the time you can figure out what the patient has by the history. Then the physical exam confirms it. Then tests such as x-rays or an MRI scan are contributing things that we need to look at. But the history and the physical [exam] is always important.

"That's why it's ludicrous to assume that some of the industrial [clinic] mills that are out there can buy a cookbook, treat some of these patients, understand them and get them better. That's why [the patients] don't [get better]. That's why [the clinics] can't [help these patients]. They are not listening to the patient. Someone is taking the history and somebody else is [doing the physical exam]. They are thinking of 50 other things while they are trying to examine them in two minutes.

"The patient needs to know that he has been listened to, and the patient needs to know that he has been examined. He needs to be told in no uncertain terms what he has wrong, so he knows what to do about it. And surprisingly they get better!"

"Q. Let's presume that you had no... you didn't have any conversation with Mr. Watson. Or actually what I'm trying to get at is—other than his own telling you personally of his complaints and his history—what other factors are markers, if you will?"

"A. Are you asking me to go on to the physical exam?"

"Q. Yes. If you have to do that, please do."

"A. Let's do it."

"Q. Are we missing anything?"

"A. From the history?"

"Q. Are we missing anything in the report that contributed to your diagnosis? I don't want to miss anything. I didn't realize..."

"A. Well, [in] the next paragraph on page 2, he's taking two different anti-inflammatory medications. He's confused as far as what he's supposed to be doing. That's not a big deal, but it still indicates that he is not sure what he's doing. Under review of systems, he describes needle-like sensations in the right foot. That's very typical of RSD. [The symptoms] were in a location that was different than the gout that he described. And the gout was very specific and doesn't seem to be related."

"Q. You knew I had that highlighted, didn't you?"

"A. No."

"Q. That's just a joke. Sorry."

"A. No, I didn't. In the last paragraph of the review of systems, the patient described a previous Workers' Comp

142

claim for which he was hospitalized in 1988 for his low back. He was off work for six months. That, again, just by itself suggests that he struggled to get over his low back. It could have been a significant injury. It could have been a minor injury, but that's a long time. He also saw a chiropractor. Those visits sometimes will perpetuate misinformation. And that is also a contributory factor. There are many chiropractors [who] do good things, but it's something that [can] contribute to the patient's misinformation.

"The patient states that he limps constantly at the present time because of his right foot and leg injury. That limping [ ] indicates that he is not using his legs appropriately. In other words, if you are really limping, you should be using crutches, a cane or something else to help. It not only increases the stress on your back when you limp all the time, but it also can spread the problems to the other lower extremity. It also contributes to poorly controlling the amount of weight bearing that actually is appropriate for the right leg.

"In other words, when they are limping, they are going from 10 percent to sometimes 90 percent weight bearing. And what helps the patients, as they are being treated, is to actually get them on ambulatory aids so they control how much weight bearing they are putting on [the foot] that's comfortable for them. So, if they are comfortable [with] 30 percent weight bearing, fine. But he doesn't know [or] understand that, and he has continued to do things such as the limping that contribute to the problem. Now, we're finally getting to the physical exam."

"Q. Great."

≈ *Chapter 15* ≈

Clues in the Physical Exam

The following is the conclusion of the deposition of February 17, 1999. I was answering questions posed by MS. SMITH about how I made a diagnosis for the patient.

"A. Under the physical exam, the puncture marks were well healed, which means there is no infection. There [are] no other findings that are a source of the pain.

"Again, these are all clues. There are two anterior (top of the)[48] foot lacerations, abrasions, which are well healed, nontender, no [altered] (abnormal) sensation. There is hyperactivity of the right dorsal [great toe extensor tendon] (the right big toe was cocked up), not on the left. The hyperactivity of the dorsal [tendons] of the foot is another clue (second to fifth clawed toes). It's very typical of patients with RSD. The patient's toe range of motion is slightly stiff at the [extremes of motion].

"Sometimes, some of these patients will have pressure [in] the foot. The toes are uninvolved. But the toes can get stiff and be part of the overall problem when the stiffness exists longer than it should. In other words, it's out of proportion. And not only the stiffness is out of proportion, but the pain [is] out of proportion. Next paragraph, the stiffness is fairly well described. So, I am not sure if you want me to [go into] detail [on] that anymore."

"Q. Are those just the range-of-motion tests that are indicating that?"

"A. Yes."

"Q. So those tests are indicating a loss of motion?"

"A. Yes. And the other interesting thing [ ] that is a factor leaning towards RSD is that the stiffness is generalized. It's in all directions. It's in all the toes. If you break your foot and you've got a little stiffness in one direction, that's understandable for a little while after the injury. But eventually you're going to stretch that out. But patients with

---

[48] For this chapter only, a basic explanation of medical and Workers' Compensation terminology is added in ( ). In all other chapters, medical terms are in ( ).

RSD allow the stiffness to accumulate everywhere and in all directions."

"Q. Okay."

"A. The following paragraphs after that, 'Color and temperature of the lower extremities [are] normal and equal.' That's a good sign because if the color is different or the temperature is significantly different, where I can [ ] feel a difference, that just means that the RSD is worse. 'No joint effusion.' Again, I'm looking for other things that may be factors. Or it helps me to understand the severity of his problem. 'There is minimal generalized [induration] of the right foot.' That's consistent with the stiffness."

"Q. What's [induration]?"

"A. [Induration] is generalized firm swelling that tends to hang around when stiffness hangs around longer than it should. The next paragraph talks about the minimal antalgic gait on the right (limp). We've already talked about that. Under measurements, there is a little decrease in the thigh size and a little increase in the foot size on the right. Again, [ ] they are not dramatic differences, but they are very consistent with the problem as described. The muscles of the right thigh and the right calf sometimes [ ] are not used as much as they should be, so they can get a little smaller. Yet the swelling in the right foot is persistent. So the right foot is a little bit bigger than the left. It makes sense."

"Q. This could develop over time, the difference in the thigh measurement?"

"A. Yes. We're all a little asymmetric, so that could also be normal. It is not uncommon in right-handed individuals, that the right thigh is a little bit bigger than the left even though we're talking about hand dependency or hand dominance. [ ] That's the most common [pattern]. But again, there are always variations of that. But the key there is that the findings are consistent with what the diagnosis was. In the paragraphs after that, I described the x-ray changes, and I described, 'Mild disuse osteoporosis of the right foot.' It has a very suggestive pattern [with subtle tiny bony holes]. That can happen after a normal fracture, normal casting, normal recovery. But not this long after an injury."

"Q. In reference to those x-rays, would there be any significance to the fact that prior x-rays might not have shown that?"

"A. It's not uncommon for RSD to continue to develop after an injury. In other words, it doesn't always have to start within a month or two after the injury. It can start three months down the road. The bony changes of osteoporosis and the specific kind of osteoporosis that I described can, again, change down the road. It kind of depends on what the patient is doing and how fast they work themselves into that vicious cycle that I described before.

"We can have patients with RSD without bony changes. But when they do have bony changes, that just means it's more ingrained. And if it's affecting the bone to that degree, it just means it's probably affecting all the tissue[s] at least to some degree. That's different than severity. [All of the tissues being involved] describes the pervasive [nature] of the problem."

"Q. He did, in fact, have x-rays. You x-rayed him July of '98. He had x-rays before that in January of '98 by Dr. Davis. I wonder if you had an opportunity to review those x-rays or the report of Dr. Davis."

"A. I didn't have a chance to review the x-rays. Under review of outside records beginning on page 4, I do see [that] I reviewed a letter by Dr. Davis from January of '98."

"Q. I think that was his medical report. And he did at that time, he took x-rays. Do you have the report there?"

"A. I don't have the report here with me. When I reviewed that, I described what I [saw] as important."

"Q. Well, if I may indulge myself, x-ray examination of AP and lateral with obliques was normal. There was no evidence of acute fracture, no evidence of joint line displacement. X-ray examination, AP and lateral, of the right foot revealed no evidence of acute fractures, overall alignment [is satisfactory]. There was a small spur off the distal fibular aspect of the first metatarsal. Is that consistent with what you found in your x-rays?"

"A. Well, it's certainly consistent with it, as far as the bone spur that they described. When we described the x-ray, and I mean both myself as well as Dr. Ta who is the radiologist that interpreted our films, we described degenerative disease (arthritis) of the first [metatarsal] both proximal and distal (midfoot and big toe joints). And Dr. Ta did not mention the disuse osteoporosis, but that's not uncommon for a radiologist. Many times, they don't notice it or don't mention it. But as an orthopedic surgeon, it's my job to notice things like that."

"Q. And then there was an X-ray done by Dr. Wong in December of 1997. That would have been 13 months after his injury. And I guess that one was right ankle (sic). There is no evidence of fracture, dislocation or other bony injury. Joint spaces are well maintained. There is no arthritic spurring. There is no ectopic calcification. There is no evidence of a soft-tissue mass. And then right foot [3 view] x-rays reveal no evidence of fracture, dislocation or other bony injury. Joint spaces are well maintained. There is no arthritic spurring. There is no disuse osteopenia if I'm pronouncing that correctly. Is that consistent with your findings?"

"A. What's the date of the x-ray?"

"Q. The x-rays were taken in December of 1997."

"A. All I know is each radiologist describes things sometimes slightly differently and puts emphasis on things slightly differently. And what I'd have to say with that report, basically he's describing a normal x-ray of the foot, as far as I heard from what you read. He didn't describe any abnormality. And yet, there were significant abnormalities.

"Now, maybe significant abnormalities developed since December of 1997. However, I think more likely is that he just felt that those things were not significant, or he just didn't notice them. But certainly, in this age of managed care, which I like to call 'mangled care' by the way, it's very common for a radiologist to gloss over things that are minor. I can understand why they do that because [the findings] are minor and are not all that significant.

"The bone spurring that I described is not significant, as far as the patient's RSD, which is the most important part of his symptoms. So as far as the patient's symptoms, the arthritis that I described, and our radiologist described, is not significant.

"What is significant from our x-rays is that the findings were not real terrible. Yes, he did have some degenerative disease. I can't tell you whether that degenerative disease is worse without being able to physically look at both sets of films myself and then compare them. And then I can tell you. Looking at those old x-ray reports doesn't tell me whether those films show a significant difference or not [ ].

"So, if I'm treating a private or industrial patient, they may ask me, 'Well, is my foot different on x-ray from now to then?' The only way for me to do that is to have the films and directly compare them."

"Q. If you actually did review the films and there was no evidence of what you found and you agreed with what the individual doctors have talked about, what would be relevant in the overall picture?"

"A. Well, it does not change what I found in July."

"Q. Right."

"A. It would give us a perspective as far as what had happened to the patient's foot between December 1997 and July of 1998. In other words, maybe his crush injury was significant enough that some of the joints were damaged enough that they did develop arthritic changes in a very short period of time. That would be unusual but [ ] possible.

"The other thing that we noticed was the osteoporosis. It's possible to develop the disuse osteoporosis late in the course of reflex sympathetic dystrophy. It just depends on how the patient is dealing with his pain and how he is using his leg."

"Q. I see. Okay. We can move an (sic) ahead. Is there anything else?"

"A. Did you want me to go through the review of records? I'll skip that if you agree to that."

148

"Q. I just wanted you to give me the factors that contributed to your diagnosis. If you do need to go through the review of records, if that's the quickest way we can do it, so be it. Is that necessary for you to be able to answer that question?"

"A. Well, I'll give you an example. I would rather leave it at that if that's okay. Because, for example, in the first paragraph of page 6, Dr. Gomez saw the patient for orthopedic consultation because of the patient's inability to return to work and persisting problems. He was skeptical and concerned because the patient appeared to embellish his symptoms by saying repeatedly that he didn't think he could do this type of work and that he had been off work for two years with a previous back strain [which was] nonsurgical. Initially Dr. Gomez made the patient TTD (temporarily totally disabled).

"The thing that I got out of that was [ ] that the doctor was at least thinking that the patient was embellishing his symptoms. And maybe he told him that, maybe he didn't. But always when we're thinking of patients malingering or embellishing, one of the things that mimics that is RSD.

"So it's not uncommon with RSD patients to have multiple previous physicians concerned about patient malingering or concerned about the patient not doing what they are supposed to be doing or concerned about exaggerating or concerned about embellishing. That is, again, a very typical pattern. Let me say one other thing just to kind of round this out a little bit. I fully well recognize there are patients [who] malinger. There are patients [who] exaggerate, and there are patients who are [ ] liars.

"That is usually not the case with reflex sympathetic dystrophy patients. There probably is a small percentage of those patients [who] use their symptoms because they know how to control them, make them better [and] make them worse. [They] use [them] for inappropriate purposes."

"Q. Okay. Do you think we've covered the components of your diagnosis?"

"A. Yes. I hope I didn't bore you."

"Q. No. It's interesting. I'm going to save the deposition too. Just on that point, one of the hardest problems we have in our business and I'm sure you have is assessing the credibility of a patient. And I'm wondering how you... I mean could Mr. Watson have been simply lying to you about his symptoms?"

"A. No."

"Q. And what kinds of things do you take into account when you talk to a patient that would lead you to believe whether or not he's legitimate or he's embellishing or lying?"

"A. Well, again, [there are] a lot of factors along the way in the history [and] physical exam as well as the records. Those all help me to think of that. The first part of figuring out whether somebody is lying or malingering is to think of it and then test that [ ] as a hypothesis based on what the facts are. And if there is evidence of him telling me that he limps, yet he doesn't at times, that means one of two things. Either he limps part time or not.

"And so sometimes understanding what patients mean when they say they are limping, implies that we have to look into it a little bit more. We have to understand, 'Okay, is it a limp where you are limping all the time, or is it part time?'

"If somebody is telling me that they are limping constantly and severely and then they go outside my office and they are not limping, then they are lying; they are malingering. And that's not RSD. It has nothing to do with RSD. Those patients don't belong in the Workers' Compensation system.

"Patients with RSD have a real problem and most of the time, they just don't understand how to deal with it and how to improve it. And once they are taught and shown, many times they are some of the most [grateful] patients I have. They are [also] very difficult to deal with. Because they are so set in their ways [in] doing things the wrong way, they can be very difficult patients to treat."

"Q. So you felt that Mr. Watson was pretty straightforward with you?"

"A. Yes."

"Q. I don't know if you noted this, but one of the doctors that saw him commented that he was using a cane. Did he ever discuss his use of a cane with you?"

"A. I don't recall. If it's not in the report, I don't have any independent recollection of what he told me at this point."

"Q. This particular doctor, Dr. Wong, also observed him using the cane and indicated that he used the cane on his right side with his right hand, which would have been inconsistent with the complaints to his right foot. Do you have any comments about that?"

"A. Yes. That's another example of patients not understanding how to use the cane appropriately. That can occur in patients who are malingering, using the cane on the wrong side. But that one fact by itself doesn't prove whether it's RSD or malingering. And not understanding and disuse—which is inappropriate use of an extremity or an appliance—don't differentiate between the two."

"Q. So that could simply more likely be a matter of his just not understanding how to use the cane if, in fact, he was using the cane?"

"A. It also means he probably, at least at that point, needed more than a cane and that's why he didn't feel steady using the cane on the left side. So he was trying to use it on the right side [and] using it with too much force in his right hand. And it just doesn't work that way. Canes don't work very well when they are used inappropriately. But patients with RSD can get into trouble with crutches too if they are not using the crutches appropriately. And that's why I said before that these patients are very difficult to treat.

"But when we teach them and guide them and then they do learn and they come back and they are showing us that they are learning and they are telling us that they are feeling better, that even proves the diagnosis [ ] further. A patient [ ] knowing all that, which they don't, but even if a patient knew all that, they would have a terrible time trying to reproduce that and malinger."

"Q. Okay. Moving along. You found that Mr. Watson had some permanent disability and you precluded him from prolonged sitting, standing, walking, and from heavy work. What did you mean by the use of the word prolonged?"

"A. Prolonged is a general term. I realize that. It doesn't describe things in terms of minutes. It doesn't describe things in terms of how many hours the patient can do it. I use it because it's a way of describing it to the patient, as well as any future employers. Hopefully they understand that they need to not do things for any prolonged period. Now, that could mean a few minutes or a few hours depending on what activity specifically we are talking about. But basically, the long and short of the instruction is that they should not be doing anything for a prolonged period of time, enough to cause pain.

"So, for example, with sitting, if he sits for a prolonged period of time and because of that his foot is overly sensitive when he first starts to put weight on it, that wouldn't be surprising in a reflex sympathetic dystrophy patient. They need to stimulate it enough in small amounts in the right ways so that it's not hours and hours between the times they are putting a little weight on it. [ ] It becomes more sensitive if they do [it infrequently]."

"Q. So in his case, prolonged sitting would mean to you what? Two hours? 30 minutes?"

"A. I can't put any specific time on it. It's a general guideline, and I literally can't tell you whether it's minutes or hours. [ ] If you want me to estimate it, I can. But it is really unproductive to do that. It's better to tell the patient what the principal is and let them learn how to apply it because that's [ ] how they start to get better.

"And sometimes [ ] if a patient still doesn't understand and they come back and they show me or they tell me that they are sitting for two hours because they are limiting their sitting, yet they are watching a TV program or a movie and they can't understand why they are still hurting when they are getting up after sitting for two hours, then I have to tell them 'Well, that's too long. That's what your body is telling you, and that's what your leg is telling you. You do have to make it shorter than that, and you do have to warm it up while you are sitting by moving around and changing positions.'"

"Q. So that particular preclusion as to sitting, we're trying to prevent pain? I mean the preclusion is to prevent pain or reinjury?"

"A. It is just what he has to do to keep from adding to his disability."

"Q. And is that the same with the prolonged standing restriction?"

"A. Yes."

"Q. And there is no, you couldn't give us a time frame? Unfortunately the Workers' Comp system wants to know what you mean by prolonged. And I don't want you to tell me something if it's not the case. But a guideline would be helpful."

"A. In back injuries, as you well know, a heavy work restriction has [specific] capacities that are associated with it. So hopefully the Workers' Compensation system in all their wisdom will figure out work capacities eventually for things like that. I think to some extent they already have because otherwise these kinds of things wouldn't be ratable. But they are ratable. Okay, the system kind of puts a number on it. That number may apply to the average, which is okay. That is a good way of describing it, but it doesn't mean anything else.

"If a patient comes in and I know that he can't sit for a long time, he can't stand for a long time, he can't walk for a long time, he can't do heavy work, am I going to hire him? Well, he might have a tough time finding a job. But if he's always uncomfortable, having pain, he's going to have a hard time finding a job anyway.

"On the other hand, once he has his symptoms under control, and he knows how to deal with it, and he [stays] within those restrictions, he could do a lot of things. There [are] a lot of things he could do, where he could make a lot more money than I do."

"Q. Right. That's probably true. So all the restrictions you have given him are basically to prevent his condition from worsening? If he would abide by those restrictions, that's the desired effect?"

"A. They are all designed to help prevent additional disability."

"Q. A couple more things. On page 7 of your report, about the third paragraph down, you have discussed... quoting from the report, 'significant improvement is possible if the provider and the patient treat his right lower extremity appropriately.' Can you elaborate on that?"

"A. Sure. It's [ ] important for both the provider and the patient to do what I've outlined before in this deposition. For example, there is no difference between the patient that gets RSD and doesn't get RSD.

"Like I explained before with a patient with a wrist fracture. They can have the same fracture, a nondisplaced wrist fracture, and one gets RSD and the other doesn't. But if the patient understands, [ ] tries to learn and actually does learn how to apply the knowledge that he's given from the provider, fortunately most of the time it works just fine.

"If the provider doesn't know what to tell him and confuses him, fortunately most patients do the right things. And that's why 95 percent of the wrist fractures get better anyway [ ] even if some physicians tell them to do the wrong things. Patients are smart enough that they don't like to hurt, and most patients do it right. They recover just fine.

"But if that combination of problems occurs where the provider is confusing them or telling them to do the wrong things and the patient buys into that and does the wrong things—or the other way around, if the provider tells them to do the right things and the patient continues to do things inappropriately—it prolongs the problem until [something] changes."

"Q. Well, in light of what you said here, should he be having treatment now? Should he be seeing some type of specialist and having some sort of ongoing treatment to significantly improve?"

"A. I believe what I said in my report is still what I am thinking now, and that is that... I'm not finding it. I think I addressed that when I described that the patient should have provisions for further care on demand." [ ]

"Q. BY MS. SMITH: 'Treatment is not necessary at the present time, however, should be provided on a demand basis.' Well, what I'm wondering is just in light of your comment that significant improvement is possible if the provider and patient treat his right lower extremity appropriately. Could he recover or reduce his symptoms significantly?"

"A. Sure."

"Q. Would he still be permanent and stationary then?"

"A. Well, permanent and stationary (P&S) is an interesting concept because it depends on when the patient improves [to a] maximum, medically (a point of 'maximal medical improvement' in California Workers' Compensation). So, that presumes that the patient is going on with their life and there is nothing else different that they want to do or accept.

"And the same thing with the provider. If the provider can't figure out anything else to tell them, they've done basically what they can think of, then yes, that patient is probably permanent and stationary. If the patient is motivated to change, some of these patients over the years can improve.

"We all know patients that are made permanent and stationary with and without a diagnosis of RSD. [After] they are made P&S, within five years, they can be significantly better.

"It happens in patients with RSD and it also happens with many other diagnoses. It just kind of depends on how the patient continues to handle that body part in relationship to their activity level. That's kind of a simplified approach to it, but it is generally true."

"Q. BY MS. SMITH: Just a couple more things. Generally, with the type of situation that Mr. Watson has, what about exercise, an exercise regimen, would that hurt him? Help him? Would he be able to do it?"

"A. As I was explaining before with physical therapy, it's very easy to do too much. It's also very easy to not do enough. And that's part of what the treating physician needs to be able to do in these types of syndromes. And it is a chronic pain syndrome that he needs help with. And that's why he is P&S [ ] because when he gets tired enough [of] the pain and wants to do something about it, then he is going to be more willing and ready to learn (California Workers' Compensation allows for 'provisions for future medical care')."

"Q. All right. You had mentioned before that Mr. Watson had a history of a back injury with a prolonged recovery. These records apparently are not available. Would the availability of these records... would you want to review them? Could there be something in those records that could change your mind about his current condition?"

"A. I wouldn't think so."

"Q. If it turned out that he did actually have a back injury that reasonably required that length of time to recover— I can't tell you exactly what, maybe a herniated disc, but something that would require that amount of time for an average or normal person—would that change your opinion?"

"A. No."

"Q. And you also had discussed the fact that he went to his family doctor for some treatment. Would reviewing those records at all be helpful to you?"

"A. No."

"MS. SMITH: That's it for me."

"MR. HERNANDEZ: I have no questions."

"Q. BY MS. SMITH: One more. You mentioned you are in the process of writing a book on RSD. Have you written papers as well?"

"A. I have written many things, but it has been a long time since I have written anything for the medical community. In fact, what I'm writing is for lay people. [ ]"

"Q. And you have patients now that have this syndrome that you are treating?"

"A. Yes."

"Q. Can you estimate the percentage of your patients?"

"A. That have reflex sympathetic dystrophy?"

"Q. Yes. That are under treatment now."

"A. Most of the ones that I get are like this where they've been treated elsewhere, and it's probably on the order of 5 to 10 percent. Again, it kind of depends on the severity that we're talking about. Full-blown RSD, where it's obvious to all orthopedic surgeons, I don't think I have any of those right now, fortunately."

"Q. That's good."

"A. The last one I can remember that had significant loss of function of the upper extremity was a year ago, and he ended up doing actually pretty well. And a year or two before that was another one that was very, very severe. And I could not convince him to do the right things. He continued to want to do the wrong things. He ended up going [elsewhere] through pain clinics, dorsal column stimulators [and] all kinds of stuff that made him worse and added to the problem."

"Q. Okay."

"A. Can't help everybody."

"Q. No. I guess you can't."

"MS. SMITH: Help me with the stipulations because I never remember them."

"MR. HERNANDEZ: Doctor, would you like to waive signature or like to review it?"

"THE WITNESS: [ ] I just need a copy of it."

"MR. HERNANDEZ: So original to defendants, copy to doctor, copy to our office. Waive the court reporter of her duties under the appropriate Code of Civil Procedure. So stipulated."

"MS. SMITH: So stipulated."

"(Deposition adjourned at 11:43 AM. Witness waived signature.)"

Chapter 16

The Pain Resolution Clinic Experiment

In January 1997, I wondered if I could help chronic pain patients by talking with them in a classroom setting. To keep it positive, I called it a Pain Resolution Clinic. Helping one patient at a time in my office with traditional evaluation and treatment was working well. However, it required a significant amount of time for each patient with an initial evaluation and follow-up visits. So, I planned small, short sessions with up to five orthopedic patients with chronic pain. Each clinic session would be 30 minutes.

I decided that any orthopedic patients with chronic pain would be eligible to participate in the clinic sessions if their worst pain was not in the head, front of the chest, abdomen or groin. For example, if they had neck pain but their worst pain was in the head, they needed to see a neurologist. I was curious if patients, their families or insurance carriers were willing to pay the ten-dollar fee to attend a session. Up to two family members could attend for five dollars each. Because the clinic was something for me to learn from, I wanted to keep the fee nominal.

After setting up the time and place, I asked my office staff to create a flyer (Picture 1) and a signup sheet for use in our office reception area. I did not use any other marketing because I wanted to keep clinic sessions small. To help my partners know what to tell their patients, I told them that I would not accept a clinic participant later as a patient. Because chronic pain patients present many trials, I did not want to accumulate more in my practice. I already had plenty of chronic pain patients. For many of them, treatment by a doctor specializing in pain management had been unsuccessful with no improvement after injections had worn off. A few needed surgery, but most simply needed to be pointed in the right direction.

In each clinic session, I wanted to have participants with pain in different body areas. Then, the focus could be on coping skills and habit pattern changes rather than anatomy or procedures for a specific body area. Another area of focus was

158

for them to understand their diagnosis and the mechanism of their pain. The registration information collected for each session participant included their name, age, phone, worst body part, diagnosis, treating orthopedic surgeon, clinic session number and payment method. We noted any family members who were coming and asked for full payment in advance.

Community Medical Group of Riverside, Inc.

NOW OFFERS

A NEW PROGRAM

PAIN RESOLUTION CLINIC

When: Workshops Every Tuesday
Session I: 4:00 - 4:30 PM
Session II: 4:30 - 5:00 PM

Where: Health Education Room
Community Medical Group

Director: David E. Smalley, MD
Orthopaedic Surgeon

Objective:
An active workshop designed to assist those who suffer from chronic pain. The program will provide a comprehensive, practical, positive treatment plan to help patients learn how to control pain by recovering pain-free muscle function.

Who Should Attend:
Anyone experiencing pain that does not go away or get better. Participants must be currently treating, or recently released from treatment, with an orthopaedic surgeon. The program is designed to compliment, not replace, current treatment.

Cost for Each Session:
$10 for each participant
$ 5 for each accompanying family member

Sign-Up Procedure:
Arrangements for Clinic participation may be made with the front-desk receptionist. Payment must be made prior to each program. Sessions are only open to those who register.

4444 Magnolia Avenue   •   Riverside, CA 92501   •   909/682-5661   •   909/686-3758 Fax
(Corner of Magnolia Avenue and 14th Street)

Picture 1, Pain Resolution Clinic flyer

In the clinic sessions, I encouraged the participants to listen to understand and not to take notes until afterwards. At the end of each session, I gave them a reference card with some principles to remember after they left the session (Pictures 2 and 3). At the bottom of the reference card was a detachable postcard that class members could fill out as a survey and return it with comments. The reference card was the size of a bookmark. The back of the reference card had space for participants to make notes and write specific goals. The reference card they created would therefore be different for each session they attended.

COMMUNITY MEDICAL GROUP OF RIVERSIDE, iNC.
4444 Magnolia Avenue • Riverside, CA 92501 • (909) 682-5661 • (909) 686-3758 Fax

COMMUNITY PAIN RESOLUTION CLINIC WORKSHOPS

I will learn what I can do without pain,
even if it is very little.

No pain, no gain does not mean to push through pain;
it means to learn from pain.

Workshops are on Tuesdays at 4:00 pm and 4:30 pm
Call: (909) 682-5661 for more information

(Detach and return the postcard below)

Stamp

COMMUNITY PAIN RESOLUTION CLINIC
Community Medical Group of Riverside, Inc.
4444 Magnolia Avenue
Riverside, CA 92501

Picture 2, Front of reference card (top) and survey (bottom)

We called each clinic session a workshop because active movement and position changes were encouraged. Comfortable exam tables and pillows were available in the room, so patients could recline completely. Each session, I asked class members to change positions or, "do something at least every 10 minutes to improve or resolve pain, or do it before you have pain." At the start of each follow-up session, I asked participants to say what they had learned about pain.

Date _____

I have learned to _____

I have learned not to _____

I have more hope to _____

I will control _____

I will ask my orthopaedic surgeon _____

I will ask my physical therapist _____

_____

- -

PLEASE TELL US WHAT YOU THINK AND KEEP THE ABOVE BOOKMARK AND REFERENCE CARD

How many workshop sessions have you attended? _____

What could we do better? _____

Is there something that doesn't make sense? _____

Are you still dependent upon something you don't want to be? _____

Do you believe your diagnosis? _____

Do you understand your diagnosis? _____

Do your symptoms make sense yet? _____

Other comments to help us or you _____

Picture 3, Back of reference card (top) and survey (bottom)

The session general outline was first, to start the class participants moving, including changing between standing, sitting or lying down positions. Second, I gave a description of normal healing time for chronic pain. Third, I offered easy to understand descriptions of common diagnoses. And fourth, I discussed high pain tolerance. Next, I discussed symptom area size and the meaning of pain. I applied principles to different musculoskeletal parts of the body and gave assurance that, "If you are right, it will feel good."

Then, I provided hope for pain resolution. Exceptions are symptoms from some unremitting cancers and diseases, which can get worse. Good temporary tools such as medications and physical therapy versus permanent helps such as stretching and surgery were described. Misuse of good temporary tools such as ice and heat were discussed. I described low-percentage helps such as vitamins, diet, losing weight and repeated injections. Weight loss can be good but not in the short term. I described common sources of misinformation, including "war stories" or embellishments where "my story is better than yours," advice from a relative, a friend and various providers.

I asked participants to notice during the session if less pain or resolution of pain occurred with gentle motions. I also asked them to measure the longest period of time without pain. If time remained in the session, I reviewed methods to relax muscle groups including rest and stretching with modifications. I described other specific dos and don'ts. They included not holding or bouncing a stretch. They included using light, gradual strengthening but only after 2 to 3 weeks of no pain.

Recognition of all early warning signs, such as tingling, instead of waiting until any late warning signs, such as burning, was encouraged. In the last few minutes of each workshop session, I encouraged questions from each participant. I wanted to give them a tool such as a position change or a stretch to try when dealing with their worst symptoms. At the end of each session, I handed out the reference card with the survey.

My first session goals were as follows: 1) Teach what chronic pain is. 2) Help participants understand the diagnosis. 3) Give hope to resolve pain or to lessen pain and live with it well.

The second session goals were as follows: 1) Help participants recognize short periods of no pain or less pain. 2) Help participants appreciate what they can do without pain. 3) Help them to not want to ignore pain and to want to learn.

There were additional third session goals: 1) Teach participants how to apply principles and ask specific questions.

2) Encourage them to find more than one stretch that helps their pain. 3) Teach proper use of temporary helps such as heat, cold and massage.

My goals for the fourth session were fine-tuning: 1) Help participants recognize little areas of progress. 2) Ask them to tell others that they know how to control activity and then do it. 3) If it is true, ask them to tell others that they understand what is wrong and what to do about it, and do it.

I outlined goals for each participant: 1) Learn to ask good questions of good sources and learn from answers they feel good about. 2) Be consistent and less impatient. 3) Test the diagnosis, then as progress is made believe the diagnosis. 4) Listen to the symptoms of their body early. 5) Become medication free if their doctor agrees. 6) Let their therapist know if something in therapy hurts and learn from it. 7) Never push through pain and never give up. 8) Limit activity, especially heavy or prolonged activity. 9) Learn what they can do without pain even if it is very little. 10) Remember, "no pain, no gain," does not mean to push through pain. It means to learn from the pain.

The first clinic session was in March 1997. There were 4 participants with a variety of orthopedic conditions in different areas of the body. I thought the class went well, but letting the surveys go home and expecting the participants to mail the surveys back was a mistake. I needed the feedback. However, none of the surveys came back. For the following workshop sessions, I asked the participants to fill out the survey before they left. I asked them to ask questions on the survey if they desired. That resulted in an overall 89 percent return rate of participant surveys for subsequent sessions (16/18).

At the beginning of each session, I requested, "No note taking or tape recording is allowed during the session. At the end of this workshop session you can make your own notes on the reference card handout that you will be given." Then, I gave a disclaimer, "These sessions are not an attempt to diagnose your pain. If pain continues or worsens, you should call your current treating orthopedic surgeon, not me, who will listen to your symptoms and re-examine you." I got to know each participant's name, involved body part, diagnosis, worst pain, time without pain, first onset of the pain and number of workshop sessions each had attended. The average duration of pain of the participants attending all sessions was 18 years with a range of 1 to 40 years.

The second session was 2 weeks later, and 4 participants attended. During the second class, the first thing I learned was that I was doing a lot of work. My enthusiasm had faded slightly. It felt like the workshop participants were in a passenger van with the transmission in neutral on a level surface with me trying to pull them forward with a rope. The resistance was not overwhelming, but by the end of the 30-minute class, I was exhausted. Nevertheless, I was excited because I had in my hands all 4 surveys from the second workshop session. All were completely filled out!

The results of the first 4 surveys were as follows:

Number of workshop sessions attended? "2; 1; 2; 2."

What could we do better? "Need more detail about injuries; More examples of exercise; Classes are good; More practice with exercise."

Is there something that doesn't make sense? "Explain why muscles burn; Explain how I will be able to make progress with spinal canal narrowing; No; No."

Are you still dependent upon something you don't want to be? "Pain pills; ?; Yes; ?."

Do you believe your diagnosis? "Yes; Yes; Yes; Yes."

Do you understand your diagnosis? "Yes; Yes; Yes; Partly."

Do your symptoms make sense yet? "No; Yes; Yes except hip pain; Yes."

Other comments to help us or you? "—; Need movement demos; —; More practice on personal exercises."

The participants had given constructive comments, relevant observations and posed excellent questions. The questions returned with the surveys were easy to answer. Muscle burning is from metabolism byproducts that build up in muscles with use or with pressure that inhibits blood flow out of the muscle. The answer for spinal canal narrowing depends on the degree of narrowing. If the narrowing is mild or moderate, the nerves can adapt to it with time and symptoms can resolve. If the narrowing is severe, it takes many years of arthritis for it to develop to that degree. In that case, surgery could be a good answer if symptoms are persistent and the findings are consistent with the symptoms.

In the 7 workshop sessions I held, a total of 22 session participants attended. In addition, 2 family members attended. There were only 4 participants who failed to show. My enthusiasm was continuing to fade by the seventh session. It felt like I was still pulling the passenger van along and the participants were enjoying the ride and entertainment. They only had a mild interest in where we were going because they did not want to be too hopeful and then be disappointed.

A total of 13 different participants attended, 3 males and 10 females. They completed 16 surveys. Four of the 13 participants attended 9 follow-up sessions (3, 3, 2 and 1).

Results of the last 12 surveys are as follows:

Number of workshop sessions attended? "3; 2; 3; 4; 4; 3; 1; 1; 1; 1; 1; 1."

What could we do better? "Need more demonstration of exercises; Need notes of examples; ?; ?; Need to learn about origins of the pain; Need more detail in muscle and nerve reactions; Nothing; Individual ways to relieve and set mind in rest (sic); —; Make the session longer; Make it a 1-hour class; Need more time on how to use the exercise for the hurt area and hands on."

Is there something that doesn't make sense? "No; No; A lot but mostly makes sense; Not really; No; No; No; Hurry up, slow is better; —; No; No; —."

Are you still dependent upon something you don't want to be? "Elavil 15 mg every day; No; Yes; Yes but not guilty about it; No; Fear of pain with movement; Yes; Ansaid (an NSAID); —; No; No; Meds when the pain is real bad."

Do you believe your diagnosis? "Yes; Yes; To a point; To a point; Yes; Yes; Yes; Yes; Yes; Yes; Yes; Yes."

Do you understand your diagnosis? "Yes; Yes; To a point; To a point; At times; Yes; Yes; Am understanding it better; Yes; Yes; Yes; Yes."

Do your symptoms make sense yet? "Yes; Yes; To a point; To a point; Yes; Yes; Yes; Yes; Yes; At times; Yes; Yes."

Other comments to help us or you? "—; —; —; Do not know what I need that I am not getting; More explanation about pain origin than muscles and nerves; Need a session on mechanics of the skeleton, muscle and nerve interactions; —; To understand when you try something and what happens when you do; —; The class was well done; —; Very nice doctor."

Interestingly, one participant, wrote that they had attended 4 sessions though it was only 3. Then, on the fourth survey they wrote that they had attended "all but 1" though they had by that time attended all 4 sessions. For this participant only, I corrected the results of their survey. The lack of accuracy and their assumption that they missed a session may be from a learning disability or other issues. For many patients who are struggling with chronic pain, learning disabilities can be a factor. Though they may take more time, it does not mean they cannot learn.

I will answer the participant who wrote, "Do not know what I need that I am not getting." They need to pay attention to and learn from the pain. It is easier than they are thinking. Our body will usually try to tell us what it needs. Under normal circumstances, our body regulates many things automatically such as salt excretion and water output. With other problems such as overeating and fatigue, our body will tell us if we are going in the wrong direction. The body will not, however, control those things for us. Are we listening and learning? Do we have bad habits that hold us back from healing? Are we misled by ads or distracted by fads?

The survey responses reminded me again, as I pondered them, that I am fallible like anyone else. But we have answers to many questions that many patients need to ask. Patients can also learn to ask better questions to achieve a sense of direction and sustain hope. I noticed that none of the clinic participants used the exam tables or pillows for horizontal positions before, during or after the sessions. That surprised me, and for them it was a lost opportunity. We control more variables contributing to pain than we realize.

Chronic pain may resolve quickly when we rest and use position changes early. Pain stays resolved more quickly when we add limited activity without pain or other warning signs. Pain resolves more slowly or not at all when limited activity aggravates pain, swelling or other warning signs. Pain resolves more slowly when patients are afraid to move or to warm up or when they overuse a position, even when resting. Pain resolution comes to a halt if we stretch too far or too fast. When we feel no pain, overdoing things is easy. Resuming activity too early is a common mistake. Chronic pain needs to be gone for 2 to 3 weeks before starting light strengthening or easy activity.

The Pain Resolution Clinic experiment was humbling, but it answered my question, "Could it help patients with chronic pain?" The answer was yes, to a degree. It seemed helpful for most participants, and pain resolution is a nice goal to shoot for. I suspect that the clinic class setting may have obtained a 50 percent good to excellent result. It was not as effective as the one-on-one care in my office that gave a 90 percent good to excellent end result.

My hope is that the concepts in this book will give a 40 percent good to excellent end result. That would be a little higher than a placebo effect. If so, the potential number of persons improved could be many times greater than the number of patients in my years of office and surgical practice. A book will, however, never take the place of diligent, compassionate, individual orthopedic medical and surgical care.

Chapter 17

Olympic Mentality

The 2004 Summer Olympics were in Athens, Greece. The Winter Olympics were in Torino, Italy in 2006. They are always exciting to watch. The Olympics were in Beijing, China in 2008, in Vancouver, British Columbia in 2010 and in London, England in 2012. I noticed my patients attended their appointments after watching Olympic events on television with the attitude that they needed to be tough. They wanted to ignore or push through pain. That counterproductive Olympic mentality was prevalent in my patients, who would push too hard then crash and burn. But that mindset does not reflect how most Olympic athletes got to where they are. If an athlete pushes through pain during training, they are an accident waiting to happen. Others are ready, willing and able to replace them. Underappreciated risk during training and recovery is real and common.

If an athlete takes good care of an injury over the course of their recovery, it does not make an exciting news story. In June 2012, Miami Heat forward Chris Bosh decided to bow out the Summer Olympics on the USA Basketball team. He was concerned about participating because of a recurrent abdominal muscle strain. His agent Henry Thomas was right when he observed that Bosh could develop a chronic injury. The pain and discomfort were still there, and the worry was real without rest and appropriate recovery.[49]

Time for recovery is an expensive commodity, but extra time is a priceless gift. American Olympic downhill skier Lindsey Vonn experienced that in the 2010 Winter Olympic Games. She was training in the first week of February 2010 before the Vancouver Olympics. During the training, Lindsey sustained a severely bruised right shin. She told reporters a week later that the shin was still hurting and was the most painful injury she had ever had. She admitted

---

[49] ESPN, "Chris Bosh will sit out Olympics," Associated Press, June 30, 2012, www.espn.com/olympics/summer/2012/basketball/story/_/id/8112341/olympics-2012-chris-bosh-olympics-rehab-injury, accessed May 9, 2018.

that she might not be able to ski her five events.[50]   With subsequent snow storms, Olympic events were delayed several days. For Lindsey, the delay was an enormous help to allow for some healing of her shin.

A reporter described Lindsey trying some unorthodox treatments. She also took anti-inflammatory medication. But Lindsey said that she had not tried other pain medication and was willing to try other things. The reporter then commented that like other ski racers, Vonn has had many injuries and it would not "be anything new for her to try to shut one out while speeding down a slope."[51]

Maria Riesch, a friend and rival of Lindsey Vonn, after another day minimized the injury. Riesch commented that elite ski racers ignore the pain and may take painkillers. She thought that the media was embellishing the injury and said that Lindsey is always difficult to beat.[52]

Three days later, Lindsey's husband and coach at the time, Thomas Vonn, said that she needed the time off from skiing. He also said that she likely would not compete without the delays in the races. He continued, saying that she was still taking pain pills for the aching leg.[53] With more delays, a day later Lindsey Vonn said that the delays were a critical help for her to be able to recover.[54]

After two more days, on February 17, 2010, Lindsey Vonn became the first American to win an Olympic gold medal in the women's downhill. In a video interview, she told NBC's Todd Brooker that she had to try to get everything in her right shin healthy again as soon as she could. In describing her shin injury, she said that it was, "so painful to ski, especially on this course… It was so tough, just to make it down."[55]

---

[50] NBC Universal, February 10, 2010.
[51] ESPN, "Shin bruise has Vonn concerned," Associated Press, February 10, 2010, www.espn.com/olympics/winter/2010/alpineskiing/news/story?id=4902100, accessed May 9, 2018.
[52] Agence France-Presse (AFP), February 11, 2010.
[53] Associated Press, February 14, 2010.
[54] Associated Press, February 15, 2010.
[55] NBC, Lindsey Vonn interview by Todd Brooker, February 17, 2010.

The Miracle of Pain

Yes, Lindsey ignored the pain when she had to compete. That was, however, after considerable time and multiple little steps that were necessary for her recovery. Before competing, she did not ignore the pain while taking care of it and recovering. She did not ignore the pain as she gradually resumed training and when she made the decision whether to compete or not. On February 10, 2010, she was right when she explained a week before she competed, "I have to play it by ear."[56] That common expression was a perfect explanation. Each one of the steps for recovery cannot be minimized without an elevated risk of reinjury. During the recovery, she was calculating how much risk she was willing to take as the pain subsided.

Another American athlete in the Vancouver Winter Olympics was Evan Lysacek. He became the Men's Figure Skating gold medal Olympic champion on February 18, 2010. Before the Olympics, he had done the quad jump many times. However, he broke his left foot in 2009, and he had pain in the left foot again in January 2010 after the U.S. Championships. With the help of his coach Frank Carroll, he decided to change his program and not include the quad jump. His brilliant performance was like smooth, flawless velvet. Afterwards, silver medalist Yevgeny Plushenko criticized him, but Lysacek was a gracious champion. He knew his limits and did not want to significantly increase his risk prior to and during the Olympic Games. It worked for him and the judges rewarded him with a gold medal to the dismay of Plushenko.[57]

In the 2008 Summer Olympic Games in Beijing, Samuel Wanjiru was a marathon runner from Kenya. He kept a blistering pace along with several other leaders. As I listened to the NBC commentators on TV, they expected all the leaders to fade. At his tender age of 21, Samuel knew his limits better

---

[56] MPR News, Associated Press, February 10, 2010, "Vonn says injury may keep her out of Olympics," www.mprnews.org/story/2010/02/10/vonn-injury, accessed May 9, 2018.

[57] CBS News, Associated Press, February 19, 2010, "American Takes Figure Skating Gold," www.cbsnews.com/news/american-takes-figure-skating-gold/, accessed May 9, 2018.

than the commentators did. He finished with a gold medal and a new Olympic record time of 2 hours, 6 minutes and 32 seconds. He was 44 seconds in front of his nearest competitor. Wanjiru broke the previous Olympic marathon record set in the 1984 Los Angeles Games by almost 3 minutes. This was only his third marathon. He broke the world record for the half-marathon twice in 2007.[58] What is most important about his rise to fame is the short distance interval training that led up to his marathons and kept him away from injury. Before his half-marathons, he was a track runner. In 2002, he attracted attention with an age 15 world record of 28 minutes and 36.08 seconds for 10,000 meters, which is only a little more than 6.2 miles.[59]

Marathon runners at many diverse levels train with short intervals. They may run 5 to 10 miles per day, occasionally 15 miles. They use interval training and do not run 26.2 miles for practice. By keeping the distances short, they build endurance and stay injury free more easily. Short, varied distances build endurance in a distinct way. They run longer distances less often and at a relaxed pace. Marathon beginners with running experience can train with 15 to 45 miles per week.[60] The number of miles per day or miles per week, however, is less important. Sometimes less is more fun and better than personal best times![61]

For world class marathoners, a weekly mileage of 40 to 130 miles may be imperative. But a relaxed pace and staying injury free is also important. Training less than the threshold of injury is always better. When pain free after recovering from injury, increase training frequency, distances or running

---

[58] NBC Universal, Associated Press, August 23, 2008, 4:31 PM ET, www.2008.nbcolympics.com/trackandfield/news/newsid=252832.html#kenyas+wanjiru+wins+mens+marathon, accessed May 1, 2014 no longer available.
[59] World Marathon Majors, www.worldmarathonmajors.com/US/athletes/athlete/169/, accessed July 21, 2010 no longer available.
[60] Runner's World, "Beginners Marathon, 16-week training plan," www.runnersworld.com/training-plans/printable-pdf-plans, accessed May 9, 2018.
[61] Runner's World, "The Benefits of Running Less," by Jenny Hadfield, November 12, 2013, www.runnersworld.com/ask-coach-jenny/the-benefits-of-running-less, accessed May 9, 2018.

pace slowly and not at the same time. Likewise, the same is true for building a marathon running program. That means that you must time your running pace often. If you know your pace, then you can change it as needed. Run 3 to 6 days per week. The other days are for recovery. Using recovery weeks is also okay. Tapering down before a race or a long run is an excellent idea. When injury does occur, decisions about changing or stopping training runs are tough. Decisions whether to compete or not are especially difficult.

Before the Torino Winter Olympics in 2006, there was a lot of news media coverage for figure skater Michelle Kwan. It centered on whether she would compete or not. Right before the Olympic Games, she had a new groin injury. After their anxious coverage, the media could not avoid covering her announcement. She withdrew from competition. For the media, her decision was a letdown. Michelle took herself out early enough to allow her replacement, Emily Hughes, enough time to travel to the venue in Italy. Emily is the younger sister of Sarah Hughes, who won the Figure Skating singles gold medal in the 2002 Salt Lake Winter Olympics.

Michelle decided that the risks of not performing well, or hurting herself worse, were too high. I loved what she did for herself and her sport. She set a perfect example by taking care of herself and helping others. Those decisions are difficult personal choices that only the athlete, their doctor, their coach and their certified athletic trainer can make. The news media analysts and all the rest of us should just listen to understand. After her decision in 2006, Michelle related that she had always had a dream to win an Olympic gold medal, but she learned that the Olympic spirit and the sport itself are more important. She had to make a tough decision and felt that it was right. After hearing from the U.S. team doctor, Michelle explained, "You don't have to hear it from somebody else to know you're in pain..."[62]

---

[62] NBC Universal, Associated Press, February 13, 2006, nbcsports.msnbc.com/id/11302192/ns/sports-winter_olympics/#, accessed September 14, 2011 no longer available.

Though Michelle Kwan never won a gold medal in the Olympic Games, she was a great Olympic athlete. She won an Olympic silver medal in Nagano, Japan in 1998 and an Olympic bronze medal in Salt Lake City in 2002. She won five World Titles and nine US Championships and is a hero to many people. Michelle Kwan had years of prominence in American and international women's figure skating. She always exemplified true sportsmanship. Many young skaters are inspired by Michelle Kwan and want to be like her. She set a wonderful example by paying attention to her pain and injury. Because of her, there are probably fewer injuries in women's figure skating at multiple levels.

When described accurately, I love it when athletes overcome the obstacles of an injury to be able to compete again. It is not flashy when reported appropriately. It does not sell as well because describing it is usually harder. It takes a little longer to explain for others to take away correct ideas and principles. Without the correct detail, we can come away with a false impression that the recovered athlete is lucky, unusually tough or a miracle occurred. I believe that amazing miracles occasionally happen. For most of us, however, our Creator, the God of Heaven and Earth, expects us to learn and grow through the experiences and trials we face.

Paying attention to detail, respect for an injured part, patience and perseverance are all vital elements of recovery. Also important is the gradual building of endurance without pain. Patients will get farther with their recovery with less risk if they follow those simple steps. As a patient feels success with relief of pain, the temptation to add exercises and suddenly increase them can derail improvement. The truth about recovery from athletic injuries helps patients, both athletes and non-athletes, have correct ideas and realistic expectations. We can then test those credible ideas and apply them in small steps.

What happens when athletes have an injury and do not listen to what their body is telling them? Do they get away with it as some sensational news stories want us to believe? Sometimes the noise and pressure of continuing in the Olympic

Games can reach a feverish pitch. In 2003, Tom Pappas was included among great American decathlon athletes when he won the world decathlon in Paris. He had surpassed the world record holder Roman Šebrle from the Czech Republic. Since Dan O'Brien won a Gold medal at the 1996 Atlanta Olympics, Pappas was the first American to win a major decathlon.[63] No pressure? The pressure was tremendous.

Many envisioned American decathlete, Tom Pappas, with a triumphal return to the land of his heritage. At the 2004 Summer Olympics in Athens, Greece, they expected him to be in contention for an Olympic medal. His family came to Athens to watch, paid for by a Greek bank. Monday was the first day of his events. After competing in the high jump and the long jump, he reported that he had a lack of confidence. Later the same day, he described only some aches and pains. The next day, after treatments for stiffness, his left foot felt better. Nevertheless, on the practice track after a hurdle repetition, his foot started hurting. After the discus, the foot pain continued, and it was not getting any better. He was trying to ignore the pain and run more on the outside of his foot. After getting the foot retaped and trying a few strides, the pain was still there.

The worst injury to his left foot happened next when he ran down the runway with his first pole vault attempt at a height of 15 feet and 1 inch. He ran through the jump. Afterwards, he withdrew from competition and confessed that his left foot got even worse on his first pole vault attempt. The medical diagnosis was an acute foot strain. Afterwards, Tom acknowledged grand expectations, but he said, "more than anything I'm worried about my foot." Although compensating for the pain by running on the outside of his foot may not have been the best idea, at the time he felt that he should try.[64]

---

[63] CBC/Radio Canada, CBC Sports, August 27, 2003, "American Pappas wins decathlon gold," www.cbc.ca/sports/american-pappas-wins-decathlon-gold-1.362905, accessed May 9, 2018.

[64] SportsLine.com wire reports, Associated Press, August 24, 2004, www.cbssports.com/olympics/story/7609819, accessed July 21, 2010 no longer available.

Whether to continue or not is a difficult decision even when you have a medical doctor, coach and an athletic trainer to consult with. In the past few decades, a doctor telling someone, especially an athlete, to rest and pay attention to the pain has become heresy to many people. Speaking of pain as something to ignore, work through or "tough through" is flattering and sells news reports as well. How well did that work for Tom Pappas? When he made the pain worse, no wonder Tom was more concerned about his foot than anything he could think of in the future.

An aspiring athlete trying to ignore pain and push through it will accumulate injuries. If they ignore a first injury, the second injury happens more easily. Athletes who have accumulated three different injured areas, even if minor, will likely be out of contention. To get over three injuries is much more difficult than getting over one. It also takes longer to get over three injuries than more carefully dealing with the first injury. Many athletes are ready and willing to replace injured athletes who do not recover or who only partially recover.

We all tend to look up to individual and team athletes who have endured what it takes to get to the Summer or Winter Olympic Games. Yes, pain happens along the way. For athletes, however, who succeed with any staying power, they deal with the pain appropriately. They learn from it, resolve it and do not ignore it.

Chapter 18

Endurance from Breaking Things Up

Early in his college career, baseball player Chad Brooks had an early season throwing arm injury to his elbow. He did not need surgery, but recovering was going to take some time and patience for him to get back to throwing. When returning to a sport mid-season, there is always a pressure to return to play too early. Returning safely by breaking things up takes extra time and patience, so it is difficult to want to use. However, the results can be dramatic. Breaking up activity to recover fully from any injury in a reasonable time sounds easy, but it is not.

After the pain in Chad's throwing arm was gone, he started practicing short throws and then longer distances, but not in team practices. After 7 days, his throwing and endurance was improving. If he had returned to full games, he would have easily flared up his injury. I asked him to tell his coach that he could return to games earlier if he was used for a few innings instead of a whole game. Chad never looked back. He played full games within a few more weeks. He had a very successful career in college and then professional baseball.

Breaking up activity to prevent an injury is much harder than doing it to treat an injury. For many years in baseball at all levels, there was great resistance to the simple concept of breaking up pitching assignments. Baseball pitching for half a game or only a few innings was less desirable and less impressive than pitching a complete game. The rationale was that it took some time for a pitcher to warm up and, "get in the groove." That is true to some extent. Plus, for a starting pitcher to throw a complete game and tough it out to the end was a macho thing, a matter of pride. A complete game (CG) is a statistic that helped determine a pitcher's value to his team and, if he is a professional, his salary. The question was, "Could the pitcher hold on to finish the game?"

At all levels, however, most starting pitchers will rarely be at their best in the ninth inning. They will usually get into trouble before that. A closing pitcher is often a winning baseball team's best relief pitcher. He is assigned the role of getting the save or the last few outs of a game. Fortunately, for the health of the throwing shoulder of most baseball pitchers, complete games since the 1980s have continued to become less common. The use of relief pitchers and closers in professional baseball has become more common.[65]

Oakland Athletics' manager Tony La Russa advanced the concept of a closer. His incredible closer Dennis Eckersley recorded 4 saves in 4 games when they swept the Red Sox in the 1988 American League Championship Series. Oakland also had power hitter José Canseco. The Oakland A's team was respected and feared. For Game 1 of the 1988 World Series, they came to Los Angeles to play the underdog Los Angeles Dodgers.

Having admired Vin Scully and the Dodgers since they were in Brooklyn, New York, I called a local ticket agent. The agent surprised me when he told me that they had four $75 seats still available for Game 1 above first base. I had patients to see in my office, but the ticket agency did not want to hold the tickets. So, I called my wife and asked her to pick up the tickets. When she arrived less than 15 minutes later, only two of the four tickets were still there. We felt fortunate to have those two tickets. Before game time on October 15, 1988, my wife and I walked into Dodger Stadium. It was surprising how close we were to the field in Aisle 1, Row N between home plate and first base. Renovation of the stadium seating and numbering has occurred since then. We saw media personnel and their equipment just to the left of us.

Oakland did their usual damage early with Canseco hitting a grand slam home run in the second inning. In the bottom of the ninth inning, the Dodgers were behind 3 to 4 and Eckersley was the closing pitcher. At the last minute, with 2 outs and Mike Davis on first base, manager Tommy Lasorda surprised everyone. Instead of another Dodger already in the on-deck circle to pinch-hit for the pitcher, he brought out number 23, Kirk Gibson, limping on two bad legs. He had not

---

[65] Wikipedia, "Complete game," en.wikipedia.org/wiki/Complete_game, accessed May 9, 2018.

even dressed for the game until the last inning. Gibson had been a spark plug for the Dodger offense nearly all season.

With 2 balls and 2 strikes on Gibson, Davis stole second base. It went to a full count with 3 balls and 2 strikes. Fortunately, we were not with the small number who we saw leaving the stadium. What we saw next was barely believable. With a crack of the bat, we saw a high fly ball go deep into right field over the fence and well up into the stands. Gibson's two-run home run brought in the tying and winning runs. In our stadium seats, we did not hear the call by Vin Scully on television. Later, when I watched the video replay, he was speechless for 67 seconds after the game ending home run. Yes, sometimes good things can seem unlikely. Then, with his usual class, Scully said that the impossible had happened.[66]

The atmosphere at Dodger Stadium after the game was electric. We and everyone else stood there and cheered for what seemed like a half hour. Oakland never fully recovered after that first game. The Dodgers went on to win the 1988 World Series Championship in 5 games. That first game in the October 1988 World Series remains a classic for many fans and sports announcers. Though the closing pitcher, Dennis Eckersley, gave up the dramatic game winning home run for Game 1 of the World Series, he had contributed to the use of the term "walk-off" home run earlier in 1988.[67] He continued to be a consistent, incredible competitor. The next year, Eckersley and the Oakland A's swept the San Francisco Giants to win the 1989 World Series in only 4 games.

When Eckersley as a professional athlete is breaking up throwing, talking a patient into breaking up their activity is easier. When we are recovering from a musculoskeletal problem, breaking up activity can be tremendously helpful. It keeps recovery going to finish in a reasonable time frame. Because simple things such as sitting, walking, running or biking are prolonged positions, they are important to break up

[66] YouTube.com, MLB Classics, "1988 World Series, Game 1: A's @ Dodgers," www.youtube.com/watch?v=b1_0373UNDc, accessed May 9, 2018.
[67] Wikipedia, "Walk-off home run," en.wikipedia.org/wiki/Walk-off_home_run, History and Usage of the Term, accessed May 9, 2018.

when recovering. Common pitfalls that keep us from recovering are sitting too long and walking too far. We are a society of sitting. We tend to sit too long with computers, TV, movies, driving and airplane flights. Direct consequences can be pain, stiffness, spinal disc degeneration, hemorrhoids, constipation, leg clots, leg swelling or varicose veins. We need to remind ourselves to get up and move around. On an airplane flight, request an aisle seat. If you have a window seat, do not hesitate to get up from it several times. Learn to break up prolonged positions.

Endurance is a form of strength that allows a person to maintain a position or an activity for a certain length of time. The activity can be at a high or low level. After an injury of the low back, sitting endurance is usually very limited. When those patients complain that they cannot sit, they often describe flaring up their pain easily with the use of a computer or going to a movie. The solution seems to be to tell them to not sit that long. However, their sitting is often limited to 10 minutes or less before flaring up their back or associated leg pain. Patients can make a mental note of what their sitting time limit is and cut it in half. When I can convince them to sit for half the time it takes to cause pain and they do it often, their sitting endurance will slowly improve.

We tend to push our limits until it hurts and then remember, "Oh yah, that hurts." If we do not learn and change, we will not improve. Sitting through a 2-hour movie until it hurts or ignoring the pain during the movie is not the answer to improve endurance for sitting. Even when we try to sit in shorter amounts, the most common pitfall is not keeping it short enough. That not only aggravates the pain, it makes sitting endurance worse. It causes low back muscle irritability, tightness and pressure. That can affect the low back nerves, causing nerve irritation with radiating leg pain or numbness.

Occasionally, patients tell me that they, "cannot sit at all," referring to their pain. We too easily go from doing something too much to not doing it at all. Staying at either extreme, whether it is no sitting or sitting until it hurts, will continue to generate problems and pain. Being afraid to do something at all, diminishes our capacity to do it in the future. When we ignore little things that we can do without pain, we lose an opportunity to improve them. Occasionally, patients cannot get to a sitting position without aggravating their back pain. Warming up to it before changing positions is important.

If the pain occurs right after sitting, gently squirm and stretch the hips, knees and ankles to keep muscles from tightening up. Do not stay there. Change positions again. Then after an hour, warm up before and after sitting, so there is less pain or no pain. With experience, I learned to be more specific for patients. I often had to encourage cutting sitting time in half a second time. Getting patients to try 1 to 2-minute intervals at a time, 3 or more times per day, is hard. A good starting point is where no increase in the pain occurs. Stirring up less pain is okay, but getting to no pain may require further adjustments to the duration. Short durations without pain are important interval training methods for all activity levels, from couch potato to marathon runner.

After we tolerate a short sitting interval well for several days, increasing the frequency, not duration, is the safest way to stay away from pain and to build endurance. Therefore, an example of progression is 4 times per day, then 6 times per day and then 10 times per day. The last step is to do it every hour or about 15 times per day. Doubling the frequency is not a good idea. Once further progression of sitting frequency becomes impractical, then we decrease the frequency back to 3 times per day and increase the duration from 2 to 3 minutes. The same steps of increasing frequency are then repeated. The duration is later increased with multiple steps to 4 minutes, 6 minutes, 10 minutes, 15 minutes and so on. Doubling duration is also not a good idea. Increasing frequency and duration at the same time is never a good idea! Increasing either of them every day is also an easy way to get into trouble.

Any position or activity with a reoccurrence of pain during interval training for endurance necessitates a decrease in the duration first. Cutting the duration in half is usually the best approach. The need to cut it in half again, down to 25 percent, is common. The tendency for most of us is to not cut back enough and it allows the symptoms to continue. Decreasing the frequency is not enough to help quickly. On the other hand, when we slow down the duration quickly enough, the resolution of the recurrent pain is usually much faster than we think.

A patient having persisting pain after an injury will often say, "Every time I do something it hurts." It is as if they think that the effort of doing something should be good enough to solve the pain. Patients are often not aware that they are causing reinjury every time it hurts. They justify their pain by saying, "I'm just trying to get better." Merely doing something, is never enough for rehabilitation and full recovery. "Doing nothing" will also never work.

We should not be afraid to try, and we must find the right level, frequency and duration for each activity or position. It should not hurt at the time or afterwards. When we are better and not having pain, we tend to progress everything too quickly. When strength and endurance are improving, we must assess risk levels when returning to a sport or an activity. We need to decide what activity is most important for us to return to first, and then break it up into smaller tasks. As progress continues, we can then realistically find what we can get back to and when, without causing reinjury.

If we win a new Ferrari on a TV game show, we might be tempted to drive it on a mountain road. If we drive fast and are always on the edge of the road, risks of damage, injury and death are higher. On the other hand, we could drive it more slowly and err on the side of caution. Though not as exciting, we will much more likely enjoy the mountain road and return safely. Since reinjury is a concern during all recovery levels, erring on the side of caution is always better.

Every sport has a different level of risk when an athlete returns after an injury. Occasionally I heard a high school athlete with an injury in basketball say that their football coach was "going to kill" them. They may have had more promise in football. Then a few have also asked another question, "Should I go out for track?" Those are very confused goals, each with differing risks. More importantly, an athlete needs to decide what they like the most and what they want in the long term. Some athletes know the answers right away, and some do not. A doctor cannot give them those answers. Their coach, family or friends can help them, but those choices require the athlete's own individual motivation.

If long-term goals are known, short-term goals can be more specific during the path of recovery. The risk of returning to track is less than returning to basketball or football. For each track event, however, there are diverse levels of risk. Each contact sport and each position in a sport have different levels of risk. The risks with volleyball are less than football or basketball, but volleyball is also a contact sport. Jumping at the net and diving for digs includes contact with other players. Like basketball, sustaining an injury when landing on someone else's foot is easy to do.

Activities like walking, running or swimming that are more predictable than contact sports have less risk. Running is a necessary part of many sports. Therefore, resuming running is one of several basic steps for most rehabilitations back to a sport. Further steps for increasing running are balance, speed, duration, intensity, inclines and different surfaces. Running forward, backward and cutting to each side are then important for some sports. The timing for a return to a sport will depend on the body part and the toughening that is needed. In addition to strength, a maturation of the healing must occur.

A patient who is not an athlete will go through similar steps though at a different level. All patients go through many steps to achieve full recovery. Early rehabilitation may be as simple as very short walks. Our choices of what to do along the recovery route make huge differences in whether we progress or continue to have setbacks. Though "doing something" is not good enough for full recovery, learning from it is better than doing nothing. To help break things up for patients who are walking or biking, we can encourage them to leave early and then, "stop and smell the roses." Breaking up distances is hard to want to do because we know that getting where we want to go will always take longer. Breaking tasks up means that they will also take more time to complete. The benefits, however, are significant and useful for recovery. Limited activity that is consistently without pain is constructive. It builds ability and endurance.

During walking intervals, if any pain reappears, we must slow or stop the exercise level. We can resume lesser amounts again after the pain is gone and when there is also full flexibility without pain. Very limited strengthening exercises may help resolve stiffness and should also be without pain. A starting point for building walking endurance may be intervals of only 10 feet, 3 times per day. We can increase frequency gradually over several days to 10 times per day. After being comfortable with 10 times per day for several days, the interval length could increase up to 15 feet and the frequency should decrease back to 3 times per day. Again, over a period of days, the frequency could increase to 10 times per day. Once a person is comfortable with that, the same pattern would continue. Do not increase every day. When doing well, letting it stay good for a few days at the same level is okay!

Weight lifting principles for building power, another type of strength, are like interval training patterns for building endurance. Weight lifters use a weight light enough to allow 8 comfortable exercise repetitions. With 3 to 4 sessions in a week, the weight lifter increases to 10 and then 12 repetitions. When comfortable at 12 repetitions, the next step is to increase the weight and return to 8 repetitions. The days off weight training allow recovery and decrease the risk of accumulating stiffness or injury. Short cutting a step increases the risks.

For patients who are struggling with recovery, specific concepts for building endurance give substance and interest to the task of breaking things up. For many types of pain and musculoskeletal injuries, patients need to learn these concepts at many levels when trying to recover fully. When teaching patients, I looked for an example of building endurance that would give them hope that the little things that they were trying would work.

The best example of building endurance was marathon running. If marathon runners are always pushing their interval training limits, it is easy to have pain and accumulate injuries.

The Miracle of Pain

Pain is one of many guides that we use to adjust a training schedule. Other signs are fatigue, soreness, stiffness, swelling, numbness and weakness. When dealing with a warning sign, decreasing the amount of running is hard for runners to accept, but it is sometimes necessary. If they have waited too long to get help, some patients have already stopped running on their own.

Between 1988 and July 2010, then 57-year-old John Bozung, a fellow Californian, completed 300 marathons. He won only one marathon during that time. His friends call him "Marathon Man." He has world class endurance for marathons and ultramarathons. In June 2016 he completed his 400th. John says, "Because my body is used to going the distance, I don't hurt after a race." He always finishes a race, and his interval training was good before the marathons. A friend says, "He is an anomaly in that he can go out every month and do a marathon without much training in between."[68]

Distance runners apply training concepts to the variables of running distance, pace, repeats and recovery. Pace is the time it takes to go a specific interval distance such as a 6-minute mile. Repeats or repetitions are the number of times the runner goes the interval distance, sometimes 4 to 8 repeats in a single work-out session. Repeat recovery and work-out recovery is the time it takes for a cool-down or a rest before the next repetition or the next work-out. Applying these concepts to other specific activities allows each of us to see how to break things up and build endurance for that activity. Increasing training distances, pace and repeats at the same time is not a good idea and does not allow recovery.

Professional baseball pitching ace Justin Verlander showed extraordinary speed and endurance early in his professional career. He played for the Detroit Tigers for years beginning in 2005. In the 2017 season, he pitched for the World Series champions, the Houston Astros. The research director for the American Sports Medicine Institute in

---

[68] BYU Magazine, Winter 2011, "Marathon Man," magazine.byu.edu/article/marathon-man/, accessed May 9, 2018.

Birmingham, Alabama, Glenn Fleisig, Ph.D., commented that repetition for the shoulders and elbows of baseball pitchers leads to microscopic tears of ligaments and tendons. Speaking of Verlander, he explained that we can limit damage by better mechanics and physical training. And he said further that the body can heal itself with easy exercise, good nutrition, adequate hydration and frequent rest.[69]

Building endurance for low levels of activity such as sitting, standing and walking is simply not as exciting as throwing a baseball or running. Most people are not going to want to hear about our improving sitting endurance. However, patients who are improving their endurance for sitting from very short durations should get excited about it! They cannot expect others to understand or to share their excitement.

Physical rehabilitation is necessary, but sometimes limited exercise needs to start from frustratingly low levels. We usually need to start at a level that is lower than we think. Interval training concepts are tedious. The detail to keep track of them is huge and does not eliminate all risk. Increasing frequency first is safer than increasing duration, distance or weight. When no pain persists, breaking things up allows a safer progression in developing various forms of strength, including load, power, speed and endurance. Usually the last strength component to return is endurance.

After recovering from pain, common sense and judgment is necessary as activity increases towards a full recovery. Since we are human and make mistakes, caution minimizes the level of risk. The efforts we must use for endurance and all forms of strength are learning, patience, commitment, diligence and persistence.

---

[69] USA Today, "The Koufax of his era?" Section C cover story by Paul White continued on page 2C, "Pitches, innings pile up," July 8, 2011.

Chapter 19

"How Long Is It Going to Take, Doc?"

For most injuries, recovery should be a few days. For significant injuries, it could be a few weeks or more. For many fractures, bone healing should be in 6 weeks and motion and basic strength recovery in another 6 weeks. For major injuries, recovery may be a number of months. Ligaments, tendons and large bone structures require even longer recovery times to heal and mature, many of which take a year.

Many large ligament injuries take a year for complete healing and maturation, including the following: 1) a complete tear of the knee medial collateral ligament (MCL), treated in a brace nonoperatively, 2) a surgically repaired patellar ligament below the kneecap (patella), 3) a knee anterior cruciate ligament (ACL) reconstructed with a ligament or tendon graft from the patient (autograft). Each ligament completes basic healing within 2 to 3 months. However, the newly healed ligament is immature and easy to tear for up to 6 months. It takes a year for the fibers to mature and regain their natural maximum tensile strength. During that time, because the new ligament is a structural weak link, the risk of a re-tear is higher than normal. For an ACL cadaver graft (allograft), the risk of a re-tear of the ligament is higher and remains longer.

The time for healing and maturation of many tendons is the same as ligaments. Examples are the Achilles tendon, the shoulder rotator cuff tendon, the biceps tendon at the front of the elbow and the quadriceps tendon above the kneecap. If we cut the time for activity restriction shorter than a year, the risk of rerupture increases. Some surgeons and patients push for shorter recovery times. Not giving the fibers in a torn tendon or ligament enough time with limited controlled stress to fully heal and mature will overload them and cause tendon fibers to degenerate. Then, recurrent symptoms or an increased rate of rerupture may occur even after a year.

For a second tear, or a reruptured ligament or tendon, the healing and mechanical integrity are always not as good as healing the first time. It is, again, better to err on the side of caution. For ligaments or tendons that are only partially torn or

186

degenerated, time and restricted activity will allow most of them to heal without surgery. Though the degeneration may have caused a large knot or mass, it often does not need surgery for a full recovery.

If recovery is not happening in reasonable time frames, start looking for factors that are holding a patient back. Usually a physician is not holding the healing back, unless they tell patients to do too much. Patients are often holding themselves back with choices they make. We are asking for problems if a doctor tells us not to bear weight, but we do it anyway thinking that we, "heal faster than anyone." Those patients may have an attitude of "no fear," and we cannot hold them back. "Fear not" is a better attitude because it respects what the body needs. Patients with that attitude hope for healing in the near future despite imperfections.

Other patients may have a fear of doing good things. When a physician tells a patient to start weight bearing on a healing ankle fracture, a common pitfall is to delay it. The patient may think that by being more careful, the healing will speed up. It will not; the bone healing can slow down. For most fractures, weight bearing at the right time with the right amount helps healing. On the other hand, weight bearing can slow bony healing for some fractures. Broken bone, ligament and tendon injuries need the right type of limited stresses to heal well. Because we see many different subtleties of injuries and fractures, listen to an orthopedic surgeon.

If something does not seem to be going right, ask. The more specific the question about what the patient is trying to do or trying not to do, the better a physician will be able to answer it. Motion can be an excellent limited stress to help healing. Motion of a finger joint in the right directions helps control swelling and helps sprained ligaments heal better and stronger. The index finger big knuckle joint has motion from the neutral straight position to about 15 degrees extension. Full flexion from neutral of the same joint is about 95 degrees. Side to side motions are not helpful for healing.

Many joints have multiple range-of-motion directions. A shoulder joint, for example, has 6 directions of motion.

Beginning from a neutral position with the hand at the side (the anatomic position), full forward motion is about 180 degrees (flexion). The other 5 shoulder motions are moving backwards (extension), reaching out and up (abduction), in and across the chest (adduction), turning the whole arm out (external rotation) and turning it in (internal rotation). With so much range of motion in so many directions, it is no wonder the shoulder is susceptible to being unstable with trauma or misuse (disuse). For an injury that does not need immobilization, limited movement helps pain and keeps stiffness from occurring. It encourages healing with more arterial and venous blood flow.

Two basic types of motion are active and passive. Active range of motion occurs when the muscles surrounding the joint are causing the movement. Active motion helps improve muscle tone and provides limited strengthening. Resisted active movement in varying degrees offers greater strengthening. Active-assisted motion occurs with limited help and provides much less strengthening than active motion. This movement type is between active and passive.

Passive range of motion occurs when anything else is moving the joint, such as gravity, the opposite hand or a mechanical device. Passive movement is a form of stretching and is easiest on a muscle, joint or tendon. It does not involve strengthening. With early passive motion in recovering from injury or surgery, a re-adjustment of muscle tone and joint tension occurs that can be extremely helpful.

Orthopedic surgeons are acutely aware that pain and the loss of active or passive range of motion are signs of a tight cast. There are also earlier signs such as tingling, numbness, stiffness and discomfort. A tight cast can cause early muscle and soft-tissue damage (muscle compartment syndrome and cast syndrome). It will prolong recovery and can cause long-term muscle shortening (contracture), muscle shrinkage (atrophy) and nerve damage (peripheral neuropathy). For a patient who has early symptoms of a tight cast, passive range of motion of the fingers or toes and elevation can resolve the symptoms. If not, we must split the cast on both sides (bivalve the cast), or we can remove it. After passive range of motion is re-established, we can add active range of motion. Active motion will then later gradually take over.

Since a study in 1980, by Dr. Robert Salter in Toronto, Canada, we understand the value of passive range of motion much better. He reported moving rabbit knee joints with continuous passive motion, compared to intermittent active motion. The results showed that passive motion helped the healing of joint surfaces. He also compared immobilization with passive motion. Passive motion was better for healing adequacy and speed.[70] He later studied human knee ligaments and other human joints. Passive motion again improved healing and recovery.[71]

Soon after the publication of those two studies, many biomedical companies built devices that provided the knee and many other joints with continuous passive motion (CPM). The CPM machines have been a tremendous help for patients recovering from total knee replacements as well as knee surgery for severe ligament injuries or joint fractures.

Because of human nature and because passive range of motion is easier, the most common mistake we make, as patients, is to stretch too far, too fast and too infrequently. This can be true when we are trying to do passive range of motion on our own or even in the presence of a physical therapist. A good physical therapist will therefore instruct patients not to stretch farther or faster than they are comfortable with. For muscle movement and joint range of motion, the opposite of going too far or too fast is to use short

---

[70] Robert B. Salter, M.D., David F. Simmonds, M.D., Barry W. Malcolm, M.D., Edward J. Rumble, M.D., Douglas MacMichael, M.D., et al., "The Biological Effect of Continuous Passive Motion on the Healing of Full-thickness Defects in Articular Cartilage. An Experimental Investigation in the Rabbit," The Journal of Bone and Joint Surgery, December 1980, Volume 62-A, Number 8, pages 1232–1251, journals.lww.com/jbjsjournal/Abstract/1980/62080/The_biological_effect_of_contin uous_passive_motion.2.aspx, accessed May 9, 2018.
[71] Robert B. Salter, M.D., Henry W. Hamilton, John H. Wedge, M.D., Marvin Tile, M.D., Ian P. Torode, et al., "Clinical Application of Basic Research on Continuous Passive Motion for Disorders and Injuries of Synovial Joints: A Preliminary Report of a Feasibility Study," Journal of Orthopedic Research, 1983, Volume 1, Issue 3, pages 325–342, onlinelibrary.wiley.com/doi/10.1002/jor.1100010313/pdf, accessed May 9, 2018.

motions or warm-ups and to go slowly. We may do this more often than most patients understand.

With the simplest range-of-motion exercises, at least every hour is a minimum. Then, gradually over a period of hours or days, if it feels good, it can be done more frequently. When the exercise consistently feels good, we can do it every few minutes if needed to resolve stiffness or every few seconds to control muscle spasm. If a stretch or an exercise hurts repeatedly, even a little, the pain will increase and will stop the patient from doing it.

We should avoid stretching that causes pain for almost all repetitions. Where the pain starts in a range of motion is good for the patient to know. After that is known, going 50 percent of that amount is useful with 3 to 5 repetitions to warm up. After the warm-up, if the fifth or sixth repetition goes to the point where it would have hurt but now it does not hurt, the patient has accomplished something. If warm-ups are done gently and often enough, the patient will be able to resolve the stiffness. Short motions are, therefore, best to start with. We should do them slowly and gradually more often. Then later, we can increase the amount of range of motion.

Muscle stretching is movement in a direction that lengthens the muscle and is often passive joint motion. In the other direction, contraction of a muscle shortens the muscle and causes a joint to move actively. Involuntary contraction of a muscle is muscle spasm. In early recovery phases, the stretching direction is the most important to work on. If the muscle is tight, however, stretching is also easy to overdo and can easily cause greater injury.

We often use a runner's stretch to stretch a tight calf muscle (gastrocnemius). We can do it by leaning forward and pushing against a wall or a solid piece of furniture, putting the involved leg behind us (Picture 4). That motion allows the foot on the same side to stretch passively upward using body weight to help the stretch. With persisting pain, using slower or easier techniques to allow movement without pain is important. If pain persists, stop. There is a strain or irritability in the muscle causing pain, which causes more injury. So, we should stop if we cannot do the passive or active movement without pain. We should not do it because it will keep irritating or hurting the muscle.

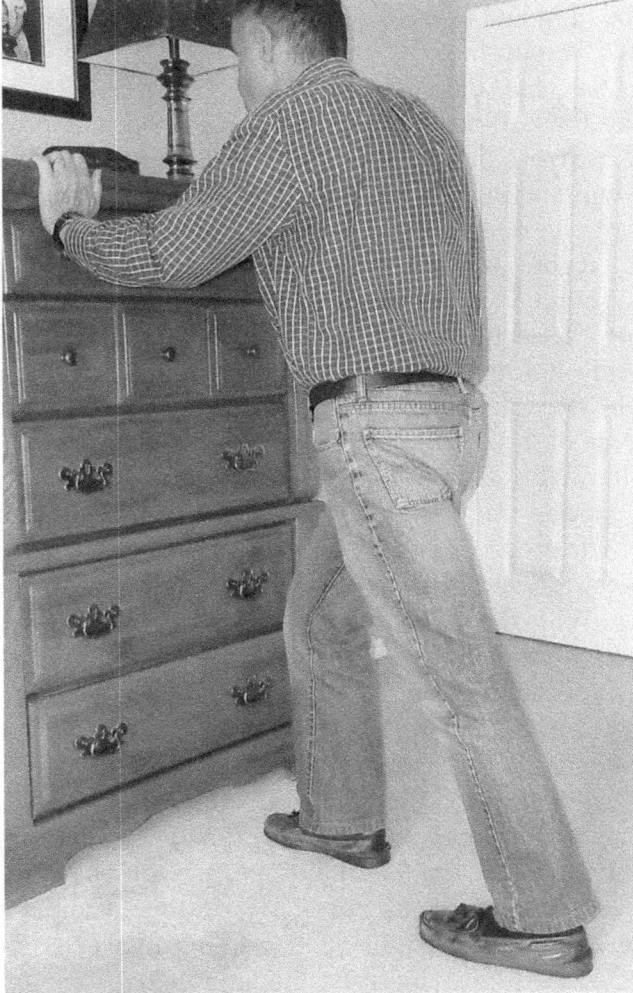

Picture 4, Runner's stretch

Instead of hurting it, give it time or warm up in other ways. Try light strengthening of the muscles as a warm-up (light active resisted motion). For example, light strengthening of the calf muscles can done by going up on the toes in a sitting position. We can also do it by going up on the toes in the standing position with a little controlled weight bearing on the involved side. As a warm-up, we use 5 to 6 repetitions for light strengthening. The muscle contractions for strengthening should be light and easy. Too much will cause calf tightness or more muscle injury.

After the light strengthening warm-up, go back to stretching the calf and Achilles tendon to notice improvement after the next 1 to 2 repetitions. Noticing an improved range of motion without pain is very gratifying. Being able to do it within a few minutes after only a few easy strengthening warm-up repetitions is also very reassuring. Any muscle or muscle group can sometimes become so irritable and resistant to motion that active or passive stretching will not work even after giving it some time. Instead, try contracting the muscle with light strengthening. It became useful for my patients in many areas of the body.

In 2009, I saw a 25-year-old new patient who had limited motion in his forearm after his wrist fracture had healed. The stiffness persisted even after having had 6 weeks of physical therapy elsewhere. He was discouraged and very worried. With the little finger side of his hand resting on a table and with the elbow at his side, he could not turn the palm of his hand down flat on the table. In turning the palm down, his range of motion was only 35 degrees out of a normal of 90 degrees using the muscles in his forearm (active forearm pronation). Even with the help of his opposite hand, he could not go any farther (passive forearm pronation). Tight muscles and joint stiffness limited the forearm and wrist range of motion (supination contracture). From the same position, however, he could turn his palm up normally 85 degrees, actively and passively (forearm supination).

After x-rays and at the end of his first office visit, I asked him to experiment with light strengthening warm-up exercises. He was to turn his palm up with light resistance from his opposite hand (active resisted supination). After 5 to 6 warm-up repetitions, I asked him to go back to turning the palm down with help of the other hand. After 3 repetitions in that direction, he went about 60 degrees, out of the normal 90 degrees. He had easily improved 25 degrees within a few minutes. He needed light strengthening for the moderately stiff forearm muscle group and associated joints that were limiting motion (supinators). Both he and I learned how quickly tight muscles and joints can relax when we put them in the right circumstances.

Because the patient had not been making progress with his motion over the last 3 weeks of physical therapy, he was excited with the new possibilities. Two weeks later, he was even more excited when he came back because his forearm motion was normal. With his elbow at his side, he could easily put his palm down flat on the table both actively and passively 90 degrees. He had followed instructions, had remembered them often and saw the rewards. I had learned some fine-tuning of active and passive motion that some physical therapists may already use.

In April of 2010, I was picking apricots in our backyard, using my old 6-foot aluminum ladder. I had used it for years to put up Christmas lights and pick fruit. Our apricots that year were delicious and larger than average (Picture 5). Birds were leaving most of them alone. A few old gopher holes were under the tree, so I was careful with the footing of the ladder. However, I was standing on the step next to the top and was picking apricots with my right hand. I was holding onto a large branch with my left hand.

The 5-gallon plastic bucket of apricots was nearly full, hanging on a hook at top of the ladder. When the front left leg of the ladder gave way, the bucket fell to the ground. I hung on to the tree branch with my left hand. As all my weight went to the left hand, I twisted towards the right, wrenching the index, middle and ring fingers. The branch broke slowly at its base, and as I fell in slow motion, my left chest hit and broke the plastic bucket. It must have been a funny sight with me on the ground and a tree branch in my left hand.

I did not hurt anywhere until I tried to move my left fingers actively. The two end joints of the left ring finger hurt every time I stretched them out straight or bent the fingertip near the palm. Passive motion with help of the other hand was only slightly better. The pain was mostly in the left ring finger middle joint (proximal interphalangeal joint). My fingers had no swelling or deformity. As I moved them, I was thrilled with their normal alignment.

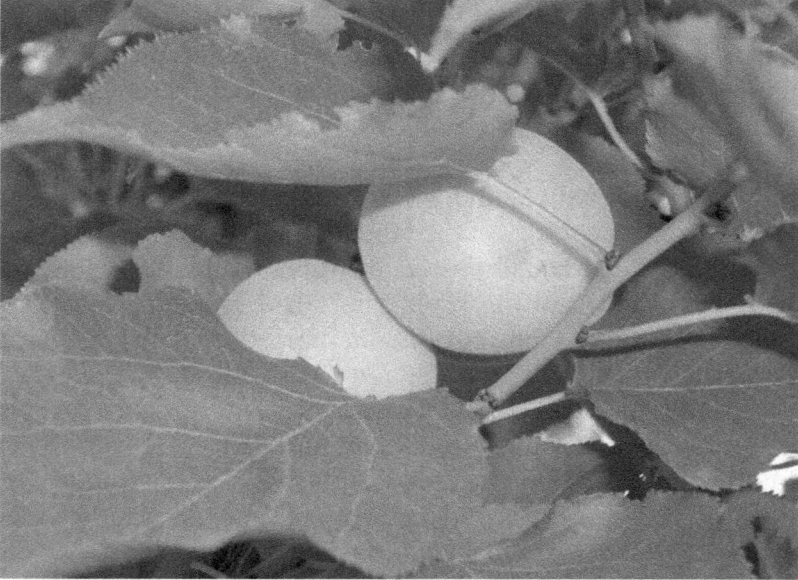

Picture 5, Large, delicious apricots, April 2010

The mid ranges of active motion were without pain. Within a couple of minutes after the fall, I remembered that I needed to take my wedding ring off. So far, there was no swelling, but I knew it would come. The motion of the ring finger was easier with the surrounding fingers for support. With full extension and near full flexion, the pain stayed about the same. I was sure that I had a nondisplaced fracture of the left ring finger near the middle joint. There was no cracking with movement and no initial tenderness. Pain limited my use of the left hand. Because of the findings, I did not need x-rays at that time. I buddy taped the left ring finger to the middle finger and avoided using the hand.

The plastic bucket cracked in multiple places, but the apricots were okay. The next day, I could not get my ring on the left ring finger. The middle joint swelled more than the end joint (distal interphalangeal joint). Tenderness was on the palm side of the left ring finger middle joint. But there was none at the sides of the joints. Within 4 days, the swelling began to go down. Swelling still limited movement, but moving it felt good, especially with help. If warm-ups were slow enough with 4 to 5 repetitions, both extremes of passive flexion and passive extension felt good.

After 3 weeks, tenderness was gone at the left ring finger middle joint. The swelling was down only slightly. The extremes of motion were full although still tight. I stopped using buddy taping, except with use of the left hand or when there was a risk of catching my finger on something. My wedding ring did not fit until 2 months after the injury. At that time, I could only get it off with soap. Another month passed before I could get my ring off without soap. The swelling was gone, but stiffness was still present at the extremes of motion in the morning. At this point, healing was going as expected, so except for curiosity, there was still no reason for x-rays.

After 5 months, if I warmed up the left ring finger for 30 seconds at least 4 times a day, tightness was gone. Normal passive range of motion had led the way for full active motion as expected. By 8 months after the injury, I began forgetting about warming it up. Even after heavy use, there was no stiffness, pain, deformity or other residuals compared to my other fingers.

For arm or finger injuries, we should do the following:
1. Check active or passive range of motion after a possible fracture.
2. Remove rings as soon as possible after an arm or shoulder injury.
3. Monitor swelling and observe for any deformity.
4. Monitor range of motion without pain. Gentle passive motion leads the way for active motion.
5. Do not ignore the injury. We can make it worse.
6. If there are any questions, get x-rays.
7. For definitive answers or if questions remain, see an orthopedic surgeon early.

8. Allow time for fracture healing. It takes 3 to 4 weeks for a finger and 6 to 8 weeks for most other bones in the arm.
9. After bone healing, work stiffness out within 2 weeks before using. Recovery of basic use and strength takes another 4 to 6 weeks.
10. Use gradually as it feels strong enough if stiffness stays resolved. Full arm recovery and maturation with no residuals takes 6 to 8 months.

So, a wrist fracture takes about 6 weeks for the bone to heal (distal radius). As in other bone fractures, the soft-tissue healing and maturation begin after bony healing finishes. We should recover soft-tissue flexibility as well as basic use and muscle strength in another 6 weeks. Therefore, for a wrist fracture, basic recovery time should be about 12 weeks.

Being able to keep within the usual, normal period for healing is reassuring. Healing may easily take longer, but healing is never much shorter than expected time frames. For all injury healing, timing is everything. In our busy world, taking advantage of the normal time for healing an acute injury or fracture is critical. When healing of injuries goes longer at any stage, many things can be the source of the delay. Clive Staples Lewis (1898–1963) wrote about timing in our fragile existence and noted a parallel for the hatching of an egg. He commented, "We are like eggs at present. And you cannot go on indefinitely being just an ordinary, decent egg. We must be hatched or go bad."[72]

After any bone heals, an orthopedic surgeon can estimate how long basic injury recovery and full use should take. A large thigh bone fracture can take 4 to 6 months to heal the bone (proximal femoral shaft). Full recovery of use easily takes another 6 months. For every injury recovery, full use without residuals is less predictable than bone healing, and there are always risks along the way.

---

[72] C. S. Lewis, <u>Mere Christianity</u>, Macmillan Publishing Company 1960, page 155, © copyright CS Lewis Pte Ltd 1942, 1943, 1944, 1952.

Chapter 20

Hope to Heal

A broken bone that does not heal is called a nonunion (pseudarthrosis). The most common cause of bony nonunion is too much movement or stress at the fracture site during healing. That causes excessive amounts of new bone healing in the wrong places that does not do any good (hypertrophic nonunion). Less commonly, little or no new bone forms at the fracture site when there is too little stimulation (atrophic nonunion). Nonunions allow abnormal movement of the bone and are usually painful.

Before exercise or real muscle training can begin, a broken bone must heal with a solid bony bridge (bone union). Then soft-tissue flexibility, strength and maturation can be developed. The same is true for a surgical joint fusion in the neck or low back (spinal arthrodesis). The bone needs time to heal. If we use hardware to help the bone, it is a race between the bone healing and the metal breaking (fatigue fractures of pins, rods, screws or plates). Recurrent injury or misuse limits healing in bones, muscles and ligaments and if so, they usually stay painful.

Does hope play a role in healing an injury, illness or surgery? When we feel hopeless, we tend to make decisions differently and make decisions more for the present. We have no view of a bright future. We are more impulsive and tend to want things now even at a higher cost. If we have patience and hope, we are willing to wait, and we will productively work for the future. How do we obtain hope? First, we desire it. Then our hope increases as we learn to trust what is right.

In 1993, a 27-year-old patient Peter Gardner, came to my office about 6 weeks after breaking his right upper arm midway between the shoulder and the elbow (midshaft humerus fracture). I had not seen him before. He was not having any pain. He also said that he thought there might be something wrong because "there was movement." I asked him to show me what he meant. The patient quickly took off his arm fracture brace and did it so nonchalantly that it sent chills up and down my spine. What happened next was worse.

The Miracle of Pain

Without hesitation or pain, he moved not only his shoulder and elbow but also, disturbingly, the fracture site between the elbow and shoulder. It was a repeated, sickening 30 degree bending motion. With my hand and fingers, I felt his arm at the fracture. There was no soft-tissue swelling or pain to the touch. I could feel only a small amount of new bone formation at the fracture site. I asked the patient to put the fracture brace back on. He did it quickly, easily and still without pain.

The x-ray films showed vivid signs of a bone fracture nonunion at the mid upper arm (short oblique humeral shaft fracture hypertrophic nonunion). There was a small fracture gap and scattered new bone in the wrong places. Hard, white bone was at the fracture edges. The alignment and length of the bone on the x-rays was okay. He had the right brace, and it fit well. However, his use and misuse of the arm in and out of the brace had contributed to the lack of any real bone fracture healing. I told Peter that if he wanted the fracture to heal, he needed to change what he was doing. He had the indications to have surgery, but it was so early that I gave him both options. The first option was surgery with an internal rod inside the shaft of the humerus bone. The second option was no surgery, and he would wear the brace correctly.

Because the nonunion was still early, theoretically it could still turn around and heal. Though I had seen many nonunions of the humerus, I had never seen one heal without surgery. The usual treatment is surgery with hardware that holds the position of the bone fracture until it heals (internal fixation with a metal intramedullary rod or plate and screws). I asked each of my orthopedic surgery partners what they would do. Each of them said that they would do surgery. They, also, had never seen one heal without surgery.

Peter decided that he wanted to try to change what he was doing, leave the brace on and give it a chance to heal. Since the patient was obviously active, I knew I had to give him things to do for the arm. They might take the place of his inappropriate use of the arm. In addition, I also had to tell him what not to do. For his biceps and triceps muscles I gave him a few, very simple exercises to do in his fracture brace. They were light enough not to cause angulation at the fracture and were motionless exercises (isometrics). The exercises were in different degrees of elbow flexion. I also gave him exercises with the help of his other hand (active-assisted motions). I also gave him light strengthening exercises (gravity-resisted motions). After showing him the exercises, I asked him to do the exercises before he left. It took a little time and practice for him to get the involved muscles to contract lightly without causing angulation or motion at the fracture site. He was to do the exercises often. When he was good at them, he could do them every few minutes.

I wondered if he was going to remember the arm exercises and be consistent with them. He had no stiffness or limitation of motion of the fingers, wrist, forearm, elbow or shoulder. I added passive motion exercises for his shoulder to keep him from developing a frozen shoulder (adhesive capsulitis). I told him to stay out of the sun to minimize sweating. He was not to take his arm brace off for anything, even for bathing. He was to keep it clean and dry by not doing anything heavy, even with his legs. He needed to avoid any use of the right arm or hand.

He came back for an appointment 3 weeks later, which was about 9 weeks after the fracture. The amount of new bone forming on his x-rays amazed me. It was consistent with about 6 weeks of bone healing. He was catching up quickly and was only about 3 weeks behind where he should have been. I asked the patient what he had been doing, and he said, "I just did what you asked me to do." He stopped using his right hand and arm but was not afraid to do the appropriate movements and simple exercises. He had obviously changed his attitude and modified his behavior.

The patient had taken to heart, both things to do and the precautions I had given him. The brace did not change, but he began to wear it faithfully and was more careful in the brace. When the patient returned after another 3 weeks, 12 weeks after the fracture, the x-rays at that time showed a large, strong, complete bridge of new bone (mature bone callus). The healing had caught up to where it should have been by 12 weeks after the injury.

The density of his bone healing was stunning. He was not having pain. When I pushed on the fracture site with my fingers, he still had no pain. Even better, I felt no movement at the fracture, and it felt solid. Again, I asked the patient, "What have you been doing?" And he said, "I just did what you told me to do." The change in direction and speed of bone healing that had occurred impressed me. Over the next few months, the bone and soft-tissue healing finished maturing. The use and strength of his arm returned to normal.

I learned at least four things. 1) Things that I think will not heal have a possibility of healing if I can talk the patient into doing appropriate things and not doing the wrong things. 2) The time I spend with patients explaining their options and having them do the exercises before they leave the office is not wasted time if they show an interest and if they use them. 3) Simple options are sometimes as good as or better than surgery. 4) Many large structures in the body can heal well if we put them in the right environment.

I did not see Peter again until about 8 years later when he was working as a student nurse on a hospital orthopedic unit. He said that his arm was fine, and he had no trouble using it normally. He told me that he was so grateful that his fracture had healed that he had decided on a nursing career to help others. I have described his story to many other patients who were struggling to find hope and needed encouragement. How well our bodies can heal is miraculous. Even if we think our bodies will not, many times they can heal.

Earlier in my practice, I also learned a lot from another patient who was a 30-plus-year-old female with a common, simple broken ankle (nondisplaced oblique distal fibula closed fracture). After placing her in a short leg walking fiberglass cast, I told her to elevate it often. I encouraged her to put weight on the foot of her cast when the pain was gone and gave her a cast shoe to walk on. At 2 weeks after the injury she was doing well. The x-rays showed excellent position of the ankle fracture and nothing unusual. It was too early to see new bone healing on the x-ray. I encouraged her to gradually progress to full weight bearing over the next 4 weeks if she had no pain. She was to elevate her leg and move her toes often to control swelling and stiffness.

When the patient returned in 4 weeks, she said that she was doing well. However, when she went down the hallway on her crutches to get x-rays, she held her hip flexed and her knee straight with her cast awkwardly out in front of her. The heel of her cast was about 6 inches off the carpet. She told me that she was afraid to put weight on it. The cast was clean and looked nearly brand new. She had not put any weight on the bottom of her cast during the entire 4 weeks. The x-rays showed perfect position of the fracture, yet there was no new bone healing. At that time, there should have been a lot of visible bone healing on the x-ray.

It took time and patience to get her to start putting weight on her foot before she left the office. Because she was overprotecting her ankle, the foot was more sensitive than it should have been. I told her to not be afraid to put more weight on her foot gradually and progressively. She was also told to keep the time up on her crutches short for the next 3 weeks. When the patient returned in 3 weeks, x-rays showed that the fracture had completely healed. We removed her cast. Her recovery progressed normally from that time onward and she regained full use of her ankle.

Because these two patients had a complete change of direction in a very short amount of time, they are unusual. Most patients who have bones that are not healing take more time to learn and go in the right direction. Sometimes they need surgery. I was in awe how quickly our bodies have the capacity to heal. To get a patient to turn around is difficult when they are going in the wrong direction within the first few weeks after an injury. It is also difficult to get a patient to turn around when they have been going the wrong direction for several months.

Many patients who have missed appropriate healing times ask, "How long will it take now?" Reasonable minimum time frames for most musculoskeletal problems are 3 weeks to see a difference and 3 months to notice a big difference. But actual times vary and depend on several things. It depends on how well a doctor explains things to the patient and how well the patient understands. It also depends on how consistently the patient does what the doctor explains, and it depends on what the patient learns as they continue. For the patient to apply and use what they learn is always difficult. Healing also hinges on how well the patient avoids doing things they should not be doing.

After we have told patients what to do and what not to do, many more healing variables are up to them. Types of activity, levels of activity, duration and weight bearing are choices they make constantly. The patient has control over a multitude of choices they make hour by hour throughout the day. Those decisions are among the most important variables that influence healing. Other influences include family support, physical therapy expertise, insurance benefits, insurance deductibles and concurrent conditions such as obesity, emotional problems, depression and diabetes. High blood sugar levels may slow down healing, but they alone will not stop healing, unless the levels are life-threatening.

Since 1999, I noticed a disturbing trend with simple ankle fractures. Getting them to heal was harder, both with and without surgery. The trend was especially noticeable with simple outside ankle fractures (lateral malleolus fractures of the fibula). Some of them were turning into delayed unions and even a few nonunions. This was occurring though I was providing the same diligent treatment I had always given them. I applied fiberglass casting for nondisplaced fractures, and I performed surgery for displaced fractures (internal plate and screw fixation). While working with these patients, it took me a while to figure it out. Some had overdone their activity. On the other hand, some had been afraid to do things they should have been doing. I found many of these patients getting into trouble at both ends of the activity spectrum.

Spending more time with these patients turned out to be the best answer. They were doing too many of the wrong things and not enough of the right things. What are the wrong things? Being up too long is the most common mistake, either at one time or total time per day. Being up means any upright position where the ankle is below the level of the heart, which causes swelling. Another mistake is using the body part before bony healing, either with activity or physical therapy. The body needs to heal the bone before physical therapy starts and that has been known for many years. Some physicians have forgotten or pushed that knowledge aside. Doing so creates problems with delayed bone healing and nonunions.

However, early physical therapy can be important when a patient is struggling with the use of crutches. Good therapists will help them catch on to the use of crutches with the right amount of weight bearing, based on instructions from the doctor. Some stable ankle fractures need a controlled, limited amount of weight bearing for stimulation of fracture healing. In that situation, no weight bearing is a mistake. On the other hand, too much weight bearing or no immobilization are other big mistakes. For unstable ankle fractures, there should be no weight bearing until cleared by an orthopedic surgeon.

What are the right things to do? Movement of joints that do not need immobilization such as the toes helps lessen stiffness and swelling. To an orthopedic surgeon, good toe motion is always encouraging. Movement of the knee also increases ankle healing with increased blood supply. Elevation at or just above the heart level also helps lessen swelling and stiffness. Some weight bearing helps some fractures.

Warning signs can give vital direction during the later phases of bone healing. Signs that are equally important as pain are swelling, stiffness, discoloration, limping, tingling, numbness, muscle tightness or spasms. After pain is gone, the more subtle, earlier warnings become important to monitor and avoid.

Evaluation of the progress of bone healing with x-rays at appropriate intervals is reassuring for the patient and the physician. It allows the doctor to give the patient direction and helps avoid pitfalls. Knowing where the patient is helps a doctor encourage better patient behavior during different stages of healing.

The Miracle of Pain

Many patients with an ankle sprain have mistakenly said, "I wish I had broken my ankle." They express that wish out of frustration, because their ankle sprain is taking longer than expected to heal. The wish is a mistake because a bigger injury is not the answer for healing. Taking good care of what we have is the answer. Almost all ankle sprains heal well within 2 to 6 weeks. An ankle sprain involving a ligament that has a complete tear still only takes 6 weeks for basic healing. A high ankle sprain, which involves torn ligaments between the ankle and the knee may take 8 weeks.

If an ankle sprain is not healing within 6 to 8 weeks, something is usually wrong with what the patient is trying to do. The control a patient has over the right and wrong things to do is the same for an ankle sprain and for a nondisplaced ankle fracture. The need for surgery in ankle sprains is rare and is only for persisting gross instability that we can prove on x-rays taken with stress testing. Nondisplaced ankle fractures do not need surgery.

In crush injuries of the hand or foot, the soft tissues can be more injured than the bone. After bony healing finishes, the soft tissues must then heal, which is equally important. The soft tissues can take longer to heal than the bone. There can also be crush injuries without broken bones. In all cases, we should not dismiss the injured soft tissues. Healing requires time, elevation, limited activity and range of motion in the right directions. After the soft tissues have healed and swelling has resolved, the bone and soft tissues need opportunities for strengthening, maturation and toughening together.

Healing of soft tissues is just as reliable as bone healing when we take care of the soft tissues well. In about 2003, a 48-year-old patient described pain in his Achilles tendon. On exam, the tendon had a painful, large, firm lump from chronic tendinosis. It was 1¼ inch long, ¾ inch wide and ½ inch thick. The x-rays showed only mild calcific deposits. He said, "At my age, things do not heal as well, right?" I told him what I have told others, that if he was going to have trouble healing things because of age, then I was in real trouble. I told him that he had a chronic soft tissue injury of the tendon fibers with

204

degeneration. He had not ruptured the tendon apart, so I could reassure him that it should heal. It would take time and would depend on how he treated it. He came in because he had recent pain, not because of the swelling or the lump. He had ignored the swelling and the lump for quite a while. Swelling, a lump or pain are always warning signs. The patient could use those warning signs as guide posts as he tried to do what I recommended.

There were things for him to do and not to do. I also told him that because I can get an 80-year-old patient to heal a hip fracture, he can heal his Achilles tendon. A hip fracture involves a large bone, and it takes a long time to heal (femoral neck). It is a much bigger injury than his tendon. After surgery for the hip fracture, it takes a year for the healing to fully mature, including the surrounding soft tissues. The 48-year-old patient with the degenerated Achilles tendon resolved his pain. The tendon healed without surgery. Within a year, he had no swelling or lump compared to his opposite normal side. Age is a small factor compared to other more important determinants for healing.

Some specific areas of bones have a propensity to not heal. This poor healing is independent of what the patient does. It occurs because a that area of a bone has less blood supply than other areas of the same bone. So, we adjust what we do to help them heal. One example is a fracture of the upper part of the long bone in the midfoot on the little toe side (proximal fifth metatarsal shaft). It tends to heal very slowly over 8 weeks. The fracture may not heal if a patient bears weight on it. On the other hand, progressive weight bearing using crutches helps heal a fracture of the lower end of the same bone in 3 weeks (distal fifth metatarsal neck).

One of the small bones in the wrist is also slow to heal. In 2003, I had an opportunity to do a pro bono consultation for a missionary when an orthopedic surgeon in South America recommended surgery for a wrist fracture. On February 6, 2003, I received an email from an orthopedic friend who needed to decide whether or not to give approval for the surgery in South America. He asked me to advise him regarding treatment for Elder Perez, who fell off his bicycle on an outstretched hand. X-rays showed a fractured navicular bone at the wrist. The surgeon said he recommended a long arm thumb spica cast, but he preferred instead to operate using a navicular bone screw with early elbow range of motion to limit stiffness.

I had the benefit of the history and x-ray images via email but no physical examination. Within those limitations, I gave the following opinion. "…A long arm thumb spica cast for 3 weeks, then a short arm thumb spica cast for 3 weeks should work well for a nondisplaced carpal navicular mid-waist fracture…[73] I have noticed more physicians here [in the United States] wanting to operate on nondisplaced fractures as well. I have also seen more patients not taking care of their fractures very well and tend to go on to nonunion. In response, I have learned over the years to aggressively teach patients to avoid prolonged or heavy use even in a cast. This has reversed delayed unions and nonunions about 80-90 percent of the time if I have been consistent with my encouragement and the patient is compliant."[74]

The need for compliance keeps reappearing. When patients do it, it is amazing how well things heal. Being compliant means listening to good sources, including their body and the doctor. Hope gives us a reason to be compliant. The creation of our bodies and their astonishing healing capacity are inspiring many times. Their marvelous capacity is far beyond what most of us, including physicians, realize. All can have hope, no matter what our limitations or disabilities are. Though we should not ignore facts, we should never take hope away from patients or their families.

---

[73] The carpal navicular bone (scaphoid) is one of the eight small bones of the wrist and is located near the base of the thumb. A fracture tends to heal slowly. The bone is shaped like a peanut shell. At its waist, where fractures in this bone frequently occur, the blood supply for healing is marginal and easily compromised. Nonunions occur with or without displacement of the fracture. A long arm thumb spica cast extends from high above the elbow to the palm crease in the hand and to the tip of the thumb. A short arm thumb spica cast starts from just below the elbow.

[74] Personal email sent February 8, 2003.

Chapter 21

Quick Relief for Back Pain

At home after dinner in December 2008, I noticed that one of our guests Elder Charles was leaning backwards while standing. He hyperextended his back by pushing on the low back with his hands. He was a 20-year-old missionary. I asked him if he wanted some simple things to help. He said he would let me know. At church on a Sunday 8 days later, he told me that he wanted some help for his back pain. I asked him to call me the next morning at 8:00 when I had time in my schedule. I did not want to charge him to see me in the office because he did not yet need x-rays.

It had been 10 years since I had helped a friend over the phone with acute low back and leg pain. This time, I wondered if quick relief might also be possible over the phone for chronic low back pain. He would later likely need an office visit and x-rays. For the phone call on Monday I asked Elder Charles to use a hands-free phone to allow him to move fully and freely. The following paragraphs are from my notes.

Dr. S: First, I don't remember what you already told me. I need to write it down. After a few basic questions, then we will go further. When did your back pain start?

Elder Charles: I flew over the handlebars of my bike 9 months ago.

Dr. S: Has there been a time when the back pain was gone?

Elder Charles: No, maybe less pain.

Dr. S: So it is still constant?

Elder Charles: Yes.

Dr. S: What makes it worse?

Elder Charles: Lifting. I have to lift to move boxes, furniture and sometimes a few other things.

Dr. S: Have you spoken with the mission nurse?

Elder Charles: Yes, she gave me some stretches that helped a little and some Motrin.

Dr. S: Are you still taking the Motrin?

Elder Charles: No.

Dr. S: Have you had a doctor's evaluation or x-rays?

Elder Charles: No.

Dr. S: Does it hurt when you stretch?

Elder Charles: Yes, but it feels better afterwards.

Dr. S: Are you sitting right now?

Elder Charles: Yes.

Dr. S: Scoot forward on the chair so you are sitting on the edge of the chair. Let one leg go straight. Does that hurt?

Elder Charles: No.

Dr. S: Lift that same leg a few inches, keeping your knee straight and your ankle relaxed. Does that hurt?

Elder Charles: No.

Dr. S: That is a straight leg raise. Do it 5 to 6 times in a row. If you feel pain when you get to a certain height, keep the next repetition lower. If you do not feel pain, you may gradually increase the height. Can you visualize what I am talking about? (Pictures 6 and 7)

Elder Charles: Yes.

Dr. S: You may do that same exercise often with 5 to 10 repetitions at least every hour if it does not hurt at the time or afterwards. Does that make sense?

Elder Charles: Yes.

Dr. S: The next exercise is a knee-to-chest motion, bringing one knee to your chest by using your hands around the knee. Bring your knee up only partially, and then lower it slightly. Then, gradually raise it further if there is no pain. When you relax and let it down a little, each time is another repetition. Do the same number of repetitions as the first exercise if you do not feel pain at the time or afterwards. If it gets tight, then progress more slowly. You don't want to go too far or too fast. (Pictures 8 and 9)

Elder Charles: Okay.

Dr. S: These first 2 exercises were in the direction of flexion for your hip and back. While still sitting, do a third exercise in a different direction which is extension. Simply arch your back by sticking your chest and abdomen out. Use the principle of going slow and short, the opposite of going too far or too fast.

Elder Charles: Okay.

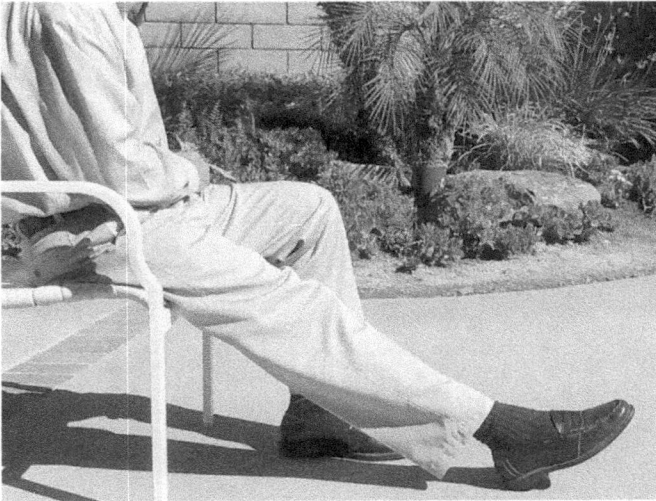

Picture 6, Straight Leg Raise, starting position

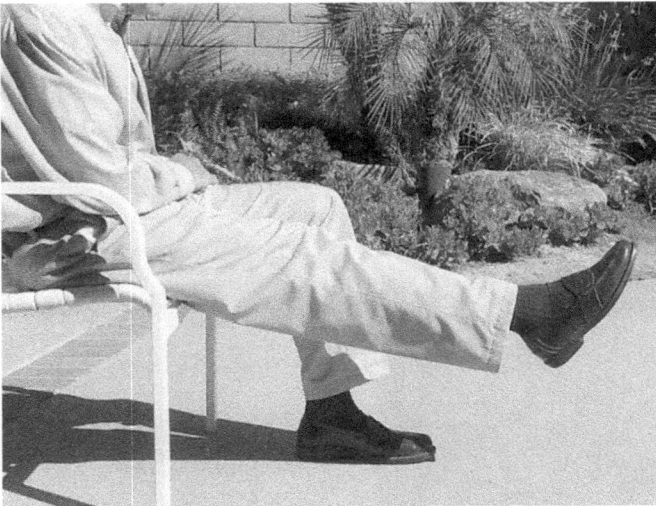

Picture 7, Straight Leg Raise, repetitions

Dr. S: Extension can also be done from the standing position. Go ahead and stand for the fourth stretching exercise. Separate your feet with one foot out and forward by about 12 inches or so. Then, put more than half your weight on the forward foot and arch backwards again. Putting your hands on a wall or table for more stability is a good variation of the same motion. Are you trying it?

Elder Charles: Yes.
Dr. S: Does it feel okay?
Elder Charles: Not much pain.

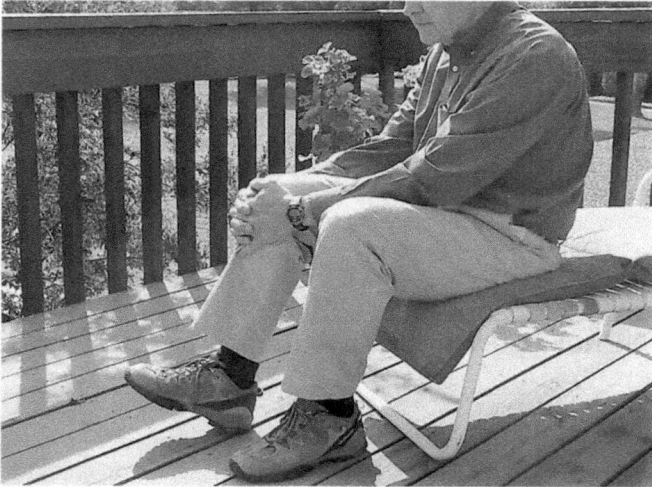

Picture 8, Knee-to-Chest Motion, starting position

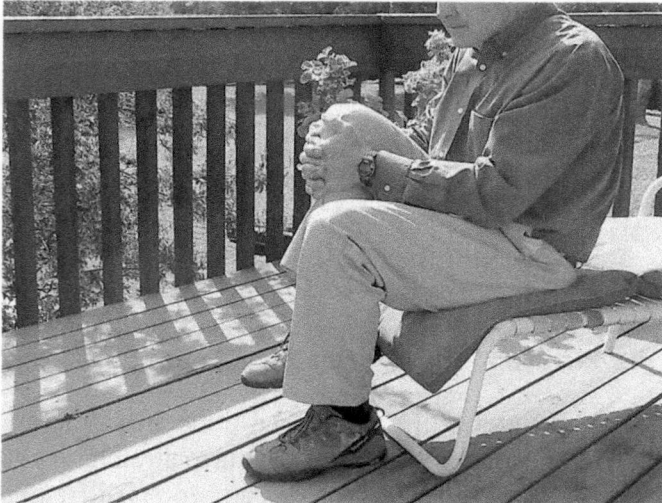

Picture 9, Knee-to-Chest Motion, repetitions

Dr. S: Slow down and keep the movement shorter, so you do not feel pain.

Elder Charles: Okay.

Dr. S: Try a few repetitions right now, and see if it feels good. That means no pain.

Elder Charles: There is no pain with that.

Dr. S: So far, the movements we have done are 4 stretching exercises for the low back in 2 directions, flexion and extension. There are also movements in rotation and lateral bending directions. You eventually want a total of at least 5 or 6 exercises that feel good and do not hurt. Do you have any questions?

Elder Charles: Should I do some of these on the floor?

Dr. S: Yes, you can. Lying down on different surfaces is helpful during the day even if only for 5 to 10 minutes at a time. Just don't go to sleep. A horizontal position is one of 3 positions you can use during the day. Finding ways of doing the exercises in the other two positions, standing and sitting, is just as important as doing them while lying down.

Elder Charles: How many repetitions and how often should I do them?

Dr. S: It should be 5 to 10 repetitions at least every hour. If any of the repetitions hurt, then modify the degree or amount of movement you are doing. Many times, small amounts of motion are enough to relax muscles. If they still hurt, then change the position. Sometimes the same movement in a different position will not hurt and will instead feel good. Good luck, and let me know how it is going. Please ask questions about anything that is not making sense.

About a week later, Elder Charles had some questions.

Elder Charles: I did think of something. I had to do some lifting that I could not avoid, and it flared up. What do I do now?

Dr. S: You must be more forceful in saying what you will and will not do. That is an obvious but very important answer. Less obvious is the necessity of respecting or thinking of your back much more often even when it is feeling better.

You must think of it more often to monitor it, to learn from your experiences and to keep out of trouble.

At our home 6 weeks later, Elder Charles told me that he had spoken to the mission nurse, Sister McCall, and she had approved coming to my office for x-rays. I gave him my secretary's phone number. Though he was arching his back less often as I watched, he was not doing any other stretches spontaneously. I asked Elder Charles to experiment with 3 other easy variations of the 4 stretches I had already given him, and I asked him to report back to me when he came to the appointment.

The first of the 3 new exercise variations was a standing single hip extension with the foot behind on the same side, the toes resting on the floor and straightening the knee. The next 2 exercise variations were a standing straight leg raise and a standing knee-to-chest motion using both hands while leaning back against something. He was to do 5 repetitions at a time and do them carefully so that there was no pain, either at the time or afterwards.

At the appointment, he reported that the 3 new stretching variations were helping. He went for a maximum of 12 hours at one time without pain in the last week. After my exam and x-rays, the diagnosis was chronic low back sprain. At the end of the appointment he had some excellent questions. They are paraphrased in the following paragraphs.

Elder Charles: How often should I do the stretches?

Dr. S: You should do them at least every hour, 5 to 10 repetitions for each stretch. That is why you do not want to do stretching exercises that hurt. Better than 90 percent of the time, they should feel good.

Elder Charles: If the original injury was in extension, which is more important, flexion or extension?

Dr. S: That is one of the best questions a patient has ever asked me. You have tended to stretch in extension frequently, and it tends to help. But how far have you gotten with that? When you stretch in flexion, it is stiff, limited and tends to hurt. Both flexion and extension are important. How you do them is critical and will determine how effective they are, more than which stretches you do. If you avoid flexion, that direction will stay limited and stiff. If you stretch in either direction until it hurts, both will stay tight. If you stretch infrequently, both will stay tight.

Elder Charles: Okay.

Dr. S: Do not be afraid to stretch in flexion often, at least every hour. When stretching, keep how far you stretch short, about 50 percent of what it takes to cause pain. Do about 5 to 10 repetitions at a time if you can do them without pain. Later, after you have warmed up, you can stretch as far as you like when it does not hurt at the time or afterwards.

Elder Charles: Okay.

Compared with where he was initially, Elder Charles had improved a lot. He would undoubtedly experience more ups and downs as he learned what to do and what not to do. He needed to become more consistent with frequent position changes, stretching exercises and avoiding heavy lifting. I did not hear from him after he completed his 2-year mission and returned home. Longer periods of time without pain would help him towards a full recovery with no recurrences.

After being without back pain or limitations since 1993, I had pain in a different part of my low back in March 2009. It started after an endurance test to my 50-plus-year-old body when I was on 24-hour call for orthopedic surgery trauma cases at Riverside Community Hospital. I took emergency room orthopedic trauma calls about 3 times a month. While doing several outpatient surgeries on a Wednesday morning, I received a call from one of the trauma surgeons Dr. Wallace Hill about a 25-year-old male who had been in a motor vehicle accident.

The patient had bilateral open thigh bone fractures, a right kneecap fracture and bilateral closed lower leg fractures (femur, patella, tibia and fibula). These major injuries needed urgent attention (multiple trauma or polytrauma). I asked my secretary to reschedule my afternoon office patients to another day. When the call came, I was on my last scheduled surgical procedure for the morning and finished it without difficulty. I headed over to the emergency room. An operating room was available and within an hour of the call, I started piecing back together this young man with many injuries. Fixation of all the fractures took the rest of the day and evening. I finished the surgery that night at 1 AM after almost 12 hours of standing on my feet in the operating room.

I was tired and a little sore in my feet and entire body. I was able to get to sleep at home by 3 AM. Soreness in my feet resolved the next morning, but it persisted in my low back. I got dressed to see patients in the office. As I warmed up during the day, the soreness resolved. With no persisting pain or soreness for 2 days, I went outside Saturday to prune our apricot tree. After a couple of hours, I had finished pruning about a third of it. Then, I spent several hours sitting at my computer finishing a medical report. After finishing it, I noticed some back stiffness and pain that did not go away.

The next day, Sunday, it took a long time to warm up in the morning and to stand up without pain. At church, I moved and stood like a very old man. After sitting for an hour during the first meeting, my back was stiff when I tried to get up. I could not stand up straight and had pain in the low back if I stretched too far or too fast. That afternoon I tried lying down often, a few minutes at a time. The pain was present less often and was less intense.

By evening, I was having a few hours at a time without pain. It still hurt during the night if I turned a little too quickly or stayed in one position too long. What could I learn from it? This new reoccurrence was humbling. It was reassuring, in a way, that the pain was in a different place in the low back. That meant that my back strain in 1993 had healed well. Because I had reinjured the back, but then was better again, had I found another quick cure for another low back strain?

Then the next day, on a Monday, I was on orthopedic trauma call again for the hospital starting at 7 AM. After spending plenty of time warming up that morning, I felt pretty good and had no pain. After some paperwork that morning at home, I went to the office and still felt fine. That evening, I received a call about a 23-year-old female with multiple injuries of both legs when her car hit a tree. The patient had closed bilateral thigh bone, bilateral kneecap, bilateral lower leg and bilateral open ankle fractures (femur, patella, tibia and fibula, trimalleolar ankles). Her severe injuries were equally as bad as those of the 25-year-old patient with multiple fractures I had repaired 5 days before.

In surgery, it felt like I was operating on a female version of the 25-year-old patient. The work was heavy and prolonged. The funny thing was that I continued to feel fine as I worked into the night and finished the 10-hour surgery, early the next morning. I worried that I might be feeling okay because of the adrenaline or endorphins from the challenging puzzle I had put back together. This time, as I worked, I paid more attention to my back by squirming and stretching frequently during the surgery as well as afterwards. The stiffness and pain did not return.

Then in March 2010, I wanted to clear out some magazines from my home office. My wife wanted them in a big box, so I started loading them. After the box was nearly full and over 60 pounds, I realized it was too heavy, bulky and awkward for me to pick it up from the floor. I was in too much of a hurry to think of unloading the box before moving it. So, I pushed and pulled as I slid the box across the tile floor. When I tried to move it past the rug near the door to the garage, I felt and heard a sickening "crruuunchh" in my low back.

I had immediate sharp pain in my low back and felt a little faint, so I sat down next to the water heater in the garage. In a bent over position, I went back into the house. I rested, changed positions and stretched. The pain was in a different location, left more than right, but was another acute low back strain. That night, I felt better enough to go for a ride with my wife in her car. After we rode for 15 minutes, I could not get out of the car very well. I struggled more on the trip home, and every bump in the road seemed to be magnified in my back. Fortunately, I had no leg pain or numbness. In the next few days, I stood, sat and lay. I was changing positions so often, I felt like a yo-yo.

As I recovered again, I thought about what I was learning with this episode of recurrent pain. I had not been careful or smart enough to avoid it and avoid aggravating it. However, numerous steps were working as I quickly and fully recovered. To help me remember, I wrote them down:

Change positions frequently.

Use several different surfaces to lie on.

Lie down frequently.

Use positions that feel good and experiment with them.

Dress warmly.

Take a single deep cleansing breath occasionally.

Stretch short of what it takes to cause pain.

Keep upright postures short.

Short, light strengthening to warm up often helps a tight muscle that will not relax.

Squirm frequently.

Do not do things that hurt except lying down, and do not wait too long to lie down.

Occasionally stretch other nearby joints and body parts well. Do not worry about strengthening.

Use gentle traction. When sitting up, push down on the chair with the hands to partially lift the body up from the chair.

For another form of traction when lying face down on the stomach, hook the toes and feet over the edge of the mattress. While keeping the knees and hips straight, raise the ankles to stretch the body (ankle dorsiflexion).

Look for things you can do that lessen the pain.

Short periods of heat are okay, but heat may not be necessary.

Make changing positions frequently a good habit.

Hold back on doing things.

In a few days, the back pain was gone, and the morning stiffness was gone a week later. I appreciated my wife's concern. Within reason, I tried to test my limits. I began doing many things again without pain such as sitting at the computer for several hours at a time. I stretched before getting up from sitting or lying down positions with a few repetitions on each side using a single knee-to-chest motion and a straight leg raise. My wife and I went for a 90-minute drive to Joshua Tree National Park and an easy hike down a dry river bed from

Cottonwood Spring Oasis. We stopped many times to rest, stretch and photograph the wildflowers. For a few months, I was careful not to sit too long or walk too far.

Knowing how well our bodies can heal when we allow them the opportunity is not only reassuring, it is exciting! That knowledge gave me courage to continue writing. Because the stresses of life go on, those may not be my last episodes of low back pain. Some worry about, "a calm before the storm." There may be some truth to that. However, how our problems turn out depends on how many times we keep reinjuring it, how well we rebuild it back up after it heals and what we are doing during the "calm" period.

No matter what their age is, many adults tell me that their doctor says that they "have arthritis." That sounds wrong because they have no signs of arthritis on the history, exam or an x-ray. Also, many are told that their problems are because they are "getting older." Age can be important, but age does not cause bursitis or a strain. Age makes us more susceptible. Age does not prevent healing. Disease can slow healing but will usually not stop healing. What we choose to do or not do are the biggest impediments preventing injury healing.

Patients often ask, "How long do I have to stretch?" Another good question is, "Do I have to stretch the rest of my life?" After 2 to 3 months of being okay, we usually do not have to stretch as often. Nevertheless, like paying taxes, we must stretch and change positions until we are dead and gone, resting in peace. We are not designed to stay in one position very long. We get into all kinds of trouble by not paying attention to that simple truth.

Our bodies are marvelous creations and will often heal quickly if we are paying attention to and learning from the pain. Quick relief for back pain is okay, but it is not the best or final answer. We must learn to avoid the mistakes that cause back pain in the first place.

Chapter 22

How Do I Help A Sister-in-law?

At the end of 2007, I received a phone call from a relative Ken Duncan about his wife Lisa, my sister-in-law. He asked me if I was willing to look at her medical notes and MRIs. Her doctors were offering her the possibility of surgery for her chronic back pain. Her husband was wondering if it might help, and Lisa was considering the surgery. He said that she had been having lower back and right leg pain for many years. Traditionally, doctors often refer their relatives to other doctors to avoid any potential conflicts. Many doctors believe that relatives can be difficult to treat.

After hesitating a moment, I asked Ken if he knew what the diagnosis was or what procedure the doctors wanted to do. He said, "It has something to do with a disc in her low back." I also asked Ken what type of doctor Lisa was seeing. He said the medical doctor who was offering the surgery was a physical medicine and rehabilitation specialist (PM&R). He was at an academic spine center in Minnesota and was sending her to an orthopedic surgeon for further evaluation.

I told Ken I would be happy to review the notes and studies that she had done, especially recent studies including x-ray films and MRI scan films. She did not have a claim for Workers' Compensation. In December 2007, I received 17 pages of records from her doctor but no films or images. At this point, acquiring the images would take at least several more weeks. I decided to go ahead and work with the records I had already received.

The most recent notes by the doctor, from a few weeks before, said that, "she had responded well to epidural injections, but the effect wears off" (corticosteroid and anesthetic). The notes also indicated that the patient was taking 2 to 3 tablets of Ultram per day, a synthetic opioid (tramadol). The physical exam was unremarkable. The January 2007 MRI scan films were described by her doctor as, "showing a broad-based right sided disc protrusion at L4-5." The working diagnosis from her physician was descriptive and nonspecific, "acute on chronic low back right buttock pain."

The options given to her at that time were "injection therapy," a pain rehabilitation program, a surgical opinion and an updated MRI scan.

After looking at the previous MRI scan report by a radiologist in January 2007, it appeared likely to me that there was no significant disc abnormality. There were several reasons for me to come to that conclusion. First, the MRI scan disc signal intensity showing water content was not described as either normal or abnormal. Water fluid in a disc is a normal finding that adds padding between the bones of the spine. Second, the MRI scan report suggested mild broad-based disc bulging towards the left at L4-5, not towards the right. Lisa's symptoms were on the right.

The report of a follow-up MRI scan by a different radiologist in November 2007, again, did not describe the disc signal intensity. It described a right sided, small broad-based disc bulging at L4-5 slightly increased compared with the prior MRI scan. There was a contradiction of the side of the disc bulging in the first and second MRI scan reports. Both descriptions suggested a small broad-based disc bulge. Even if there was a consistent right sided disc asymmetry, it appeared likely that the size of the disc bulge was small, and it was surgically insignificant.

A report of plain x-rays of the low back from March 2007 suggested a slight backwards offset of the bones of the spine (posterior subluxation from L2 to L5). It also stated that there was "degenerative arthritis" of the lower lumbar facet joints. However, it gave no indication of the severity of the degeneration or arthritis. No other x-ray findings in the report supported the description of facet joint arthritis.[75,76] The findings of the x-rays and MRI scans did not demonstrate or even suggest a problem that needed surgery.

---

[75] Facet joints are the two small joints behind the spinal canal at each level of the spine. They are like the two small wheels of a tricycle. The large front wheel of the tricycle is like the spinal disc joint in front of the spinal canal at each level of the spine.

[76] Arthritis is joint surface wear with roughening and thinning of the cartilage surface, often associated with cartilage craters, hardening of the bone, joint swelling and joint deformity.

The Miracle of Pain

After reviewing all the above medical information, I called my in-laws back as planned. I told them my impression was that the surgical indications were very weak. At this point, I asked her a few more questions. I asked my sister-in-law how much information she wanted. She told me that she wanted as much information as I could give her. I asked them if I could call them back in a few days because I needed an hour or two to go over the diagnosis and what to do and what not to do. I told her that part of the plan to get her better, would be to get her off her medications.

I also explained to her and her husband that they could stop my evaluation or my explanations at any time if they had no further interest. I did not want to waste my time or theirs if she was not interested in my opinions and explanations. Lisa expressed an interest to continue with the plan. Before ending the phone call, I asked her a few other strategic questions. Her answers helped me understand that her right low back pain was constant and had been constant for several months. She was having frequent right leg pain to the knee and occasionally to the inner aspect of the right ankle. She told me that she had no numbness.

Her doctor had already scheduled another low back epidural injection for her in 3 days. She and her husband were leaving for Hawaii in 8 days to celebrate their thirtieth anniversary. She was taking two 50 mg Ultram tablets every morning, two more tablets an hour later and occasionally another tablet during the day. She also occasionally took ibuprofen 400 mg during the day. She was lying down an average of an hour and a half at a time, less than once per day. She indicated that her doctor was also proposing a discogram at a later time.[77]

My short, over-the-phone physical assessment was with her in the sitting position. She could perform a straight leg raise and a knee-to-chest motion with the right lower extremity without pain, though it was tight. Both the brief history and

---

[77] A discogram is an outpatient x-ray study using an injection of a local anesthetic in the skin and soft tissues and then an injection of contrast dye into the discs of the lower back spine.

the brief physical assessment allowed me to have some perspective for her current status. That, together with her recent records, gave me a sense of the direction that she was heading. I again told Lisa and Ken that I wanted to call them back when they could be on the phone together. I needed to be able to some spend time with them on the diagnosis as well as my recommendations of what to do and what not to do.

During the next phone call to them within a couple of days, I gave her multiple diagnoses. She had a chronic right low back strain with muscle spasms, disuse and multiple medication dependency. I discussed each part of the diagnosis at length with them, and their questions were answered. The first word of her diagnosis was "chronic" because the pain had lasted more than 3 months. That did not imply it could not improve. It meant that the pain could improve once she changed basic things like positions, position changes, exercises and activities. After making changes that allow pain to improve, resolution of chronic pain takes longer than if the pain had started less than 3 months before.

The words "low back strain" indicate that the problem is a muscle fiber injury that can heal if put in the right circumstances. If not put in the right settings, the low back muscles will continue to be reinjured (re-strained). The words "muscle spasms" indicated that the muscles were irritable and more easily reinjured. They would have difficulty healing until they can relax. The "disuse" meant that she was not doing enough of the right things to help her back and right leg. In addition, she was doing too many of the wrong things that were irritating or aggravating it. That disuse pattern can happen in the same day as well as within the same hour.

The "multiple medication dependency" also gets in the way of her recovery because of the masking effects of her medication. She cannot tell when she is doing something bad or when she is doing something good. She was not told until now that Ultram is a synthetic opiate. Its continued use, I told her, will have characteristics not only of dependency but also of addiction. I explained to her that the dependency was more important to focus on than the addiction because her dependency is obvious. By using enough of the tools that I would give her, she would not need to continue to depend on the medication. I also let her know that she would go through withdrawals at some point within a few days, and that may include severe pain, anxiety, hallucinations, muscle spasm, writhing and restlessness.

The first basic thing I told her to do was to avoid stretches that hurt. Also, she was to rest in horizontal positions frequently for a maximum of 10-15 minutes at a time as often as she felt a need to do so. She was to taper off her pain medications, both Ultram and ibuprofen. I told her that she could use the ibuprofen temporarily but only if needed. She was to warm up often and gently with movement. She could use local heat if needed to help muscles relax. Her movements were to be in all 3 positions: sitting, standing and lying. She was to use all 6 directions: flexion, extension, right and left rotation and lateral bending to the right and left. The direction that was the toughest was to be done easiest but most often.

She was to avoid prolonged positions, and she was to change positions at least every 5 minutes. She was to avoid any heavy use, and she was to continue to follow up with a physician whose opinions made sense with the above diagnosis and recommendations. It could be her physical medicine and rehabilitation physician or an orthopedic surgeon. I also encouraged her, if possible, to cancel the trip to Hawaii. She would be much better able to control her environment at home. At a later time when she was not having pain, she would enjoy the trip much more. She was to call back within 2 weeks, so I could help her figure out where she was. The follow-up is what most patients need to help modify what they are doing and to keep the progress going.

I did not hear from Lisa again for a long time. I thought maybe she did not want to try the recommendations after all. I did not know if she had the scheduled epidural corticosteroid injection or if they went to Hawaii. About a year later, I heard my wife talking with her on the phone. After the call, I asked my wife how she was doing. My wife said that she was doing fine. Her back and right leg were doing well.

That was great news, but I had no other details. I did not think to ask any more about it at the time. I knew I would eventually have another chance to talk to her and ask her.

In the fall of 2010, I could not wait any longer. I knew that I needed better follow-up for what had happened with her pain. I called my sister-in-law, and she told me that she was doing well. She said that she put the recommendations I had given her into action. Ever since then, she was very happy with her progress. She said that none of her doctors had ever explained a diagnosis or what was wrong with her in the way I had. Before that, she said that she could not understand what was wrong. She said she understood after I explained it because, "it makes sense." She explained that about three times per year she has small reminders with pain. She also said that the pain goes away quickly with stretches and the other tools I had given her.

She told me that her low back pain had been going on for 14 years. It started in 1993 with the difficult delivery of one of her children. It was a natural birth delivery, and she said that the contractions would not stop. She described feeling pain into both legs at the time. She felt that she could not breathe for 45 minutes and needed more oxygen. With the births of her children before 1993, she described having back labor or low back labor pains. After the 1993 delivery, with the help of a different obstetrician and epidural anesthetic injections, she says that she did okay with the back pain associated with the births of her last two children.

To get over chronic pain after 14 years of suffering is extraordinary. My sister-in-law told me that she went ahead with the planned epidural injection before her trip to Hawaii in January 2008. She felt that the shot helped her back and right leg. However, while they were hiking in Hawaii, her husband sprained his ankle and was on crutches for the rest of the trip. She says that she got into a little trouble with her back because she had to carry their luggage.

Lisa stated that she applied my recommendations when she got back home from Hawaii. The recommendations kept helping more and more. She remembered them from listening and trying to understand during our phone conversation. I made notes before, during and after the phone call. She and her husband did not take notes. For them, that may have helped their understanding on the phone and afterwards more effectively. Everyone learns in slightly different ways. She said that she was able to get off her medications and did go through withdrawals. Now, she rarely has pain in her low back or right leg since 2008.

My sister-in-law's follow-up history suggests that she took 6 to 12 months to stabilize her pain. She had good resolution of pain and only infrequent minor reoccurrences. Turning the chronic pain around so well after so long is impressive. She did it within reasonable periods of time. I hoped that she would do well, but chronic pain is often unpredictable, and I did not know what would happen.

Ninety percent of chronic pain patients did well in my practice within a few months to a year, but that was with frequent follow-up, guidance and encouragement. My sister-in-law did much better than average by continuing to learn and by being consistent during her recovery. It was very reassuring to hear how she was doing. After reviewing my follow-up notes of what she told me, I decided to ask her a few more specific questions.

Question #1: How long did it take to get off Ultram?

Answer: After talking with me in January 2008, she stopped Ultram immediately. She went through withdrawals within 2 to 3 days. Lisa said she decided that she did not want to be dependent on the medication, and after going through withdrawals, she went ahead with the epidural injection. She and her husband then went to Hawaii a few days later.

Question #2: Have you had any pain medications in the past year?

Answer: She stated that she rarely takes ibuprofen. The last time was 5 to 6 months ago, and she took 600 mg at that time. She takes two Tylenol Extra Strength (ES) tablets about once per month. For her, it has about the same effect as ibuprofen. The amount of medication she has taken in the last year has stayed about the same.

Question #3: How long has the back and right leg pain been about the same now?

Answer: She stated that she had significantly reduced pain after January 2008. Since then, she feels that she continued to improve with less pain overall gradually over the next 2 and a half years. She feels more confident, and she is able to manage any pain that occasionally occurs by using the recommended stretches and other tools.

Question #4: What other tools besides stretching and medication do you use?

Answer: She stated that when she is not having pain, she is much more aware of how much she is doing. However, she acknowledged that she still, at times, tends to stay at the computer too long which means 2 to 3 hours. She said that 3 hours at the computer will make her back start hurting. That also means that her back gets tight. Then, she is okay within an hour if she lies down and stretches. Tools that she uses when she is having pain are resting and lying flat more often for 30 to 60 minutes at a time.

Question #5: Have you had any doctor visits since your trip to Hawaii?

Answer: She has not had any visits to an orthopedic surgeon or a pain management doctor since her trip to Hawaii in January 2008.

Question #6: Have you had any injections or other procedures since the trip to Hawaii?

Answer: She has not had any injections or other procedures for her back or right leg since the trip to Hawaii.

After she reviewed this last question, Lisa's written comment was, "Yipee! ☺"

The Distractions of Pain and Tragedy

Soon after I retired from medical practice in January 2010, I had more to learn about pain. Because I had severe pain in my right shoulder, I could not use a keyboard for several weeks, so I dictated instead. The following paragraphs in quotation marks were dictated and explain the injury. At the end of the month, when the pain subsided, I stopped dictating and typed the rest of the chapter on my computer.

"It is January 14, 2010. Seven days ago, on Thursday, January 7, 2010, I was tired after pruning our Asian pear tree when I sawed off a 4-inch diameter central limb at shoulder height. That evening as I drove to a Boy Scouts of America district roundtable, I felt moderate pain and muscle weakness in my right shoulder. The pain occurred when reaching for the gear shift lever on the steering wheel of my car. That night and the next morning, I felt more pain in my right shoulder.

"I thought that the pain was in the shoulder rotator cuff tendon from the sawing I had done. Before showering the next day, Friday, I glanced at what I thought was a small pustule or blemish on the outside of my right elbow. The raised, yellowish spot had a tiny black spot next to it. The elbow had no swelling or redness. After the shower when I took another good look at my right elbow, the blemish was completely gone. In its place were two small, flat, reddish marks. They were triangular and 2 mm apart. They were symmetrical, and each side of the triangle was about 1.5 mm long.

"I thought then that the marks on the right elbow might be a spider or tick bite, but I had no associated swelling, rash, redness or tenderness. I washed the wound well several times, and within a few days, it healed without any residual. In the right shoulder, however, pain gradually increased the first night. The entire deltoid muscle was in muscle spasm. There was tightness in the surrounding shoulder muscles, weakness with use and generalized soreness in the whole right arm.

"I wondered if there were calcium deposits in the rotator cuff that accounted for the pain (calcific tendinosis). My wife noticed asymmetry of my right shoulder blade. Its lower end was sticking out, away from the chest wall (shoulder blade winging). That was a sign of nerve damage, and a spider bite was the most likely source. As my wife and I sat through a Friday afternoon movie The Blind Side, my whole right arm became extremely uncomfortable. Later that night, the shoulder was more painful.

"When I woke up Saturday morning, it was a little better. I could dangle my right hand and shoulder to get some relief. I could also raise my right hand with the help of the left hand (passive shoulder abduction and flexion). When I tried raising my right hand on its own, the muscles surrounding my whole right shoulder hurt. As I tried to get relief with movement, rest and stretching, the muscle spasm became worse, and the muscles would not relax. I took two regular aspirin tablets, and within a half hour, I felt much better.

"In the late afternoon, I felt I was through the worst of it because the pain stayed at a low level after the aspirin had time to wear off. After my shoulder warmed up, the pain was gone, but the muscles were too weak to reach out or up. It hurt when I tried to finish pruning our apricot tree. After the pain resolved again, riding my mountain bike was tempting. I pulled it down from the garage ceiling hooks without pain and decided to go twice around the block, about 1 mile.

"After that, I felt good and continued up Gainsborough Drive on a short, steep eighth of a mile section of the street that I have biked up many times before. At the top, I continued east, up the hill on Overlook Parkway, a long gradual climb with little traffic. Looking north at the top of the parkway, the air was cool and clear with a fabulous 180-degree panorama of the San Gabriel and San Bernardino Mountains. I turned south on Crystal View Terrace going uphill again. When I reached John F. Kennedy Drive, I turned around. The long downhill ride home allowed lots of speed, and I felt great.

"I had accomplished more than what I was hoping by going 10 miles without pain. I needed to do a 10-mile bike ride to be ready for the next scout outing as a Boy Scout leader. We were planning a 52-mile bike ride along the Santa Ana River Trail. In the past year, I have easily done two 26-mile rides and two 15-mile rides with diverse terrain. However, after the 10-mile ride 6 days ago, as my muscles cooled down, pain returned. More aspirin helped, and I was able to rest that night. The next morning, I had a lot of trouble with pain and spasm of the right shoulder. It seemed to be coming from the shoulder and not the neck. My diagnosis is still a spider bite, but I will need shoulder x-rays if the pain continues.

"Over the next few days the pain improved during the day. Painful tightening at night was a common pattern. I finished pruning our apricot tree yesterday and had weakness with raising the right hand, but I had no pain at the time or afterwards. I also played Wii Sports baseball without pain with my son and his fiancée. To be safe, I batted left-handed, but playing three games with sudden movements was too much. I was easily tempted with games. I should have known better. I allowed problems to accumulate with activities that were prolonged or sudden.

"When on the computer for an hour that night, I noticed pain with using the mouse and with resting the right hand in my lap. A slight, painful pop in the right shoulder occurred with changing positions. Dangling my right arm with gravity helped again. Helping the right hand up with the assistance of the left hand also helped. Since nights had been the toughest, I was unconsciously hesitant to go to bed. Instead, I watched a PBS special about Paul McCartney, 'Back in the USSR.' After an hour of that, I noticed that my shoulder was getting worse, and I realized that I might eventually get some relief from resting in bed.

"I recognized that I had done practically everything I told my patients not to do. Over the prior 24 hours, many of my choices should have been better. By 1 AM, I had to get up because I was so uncomfortable. Position changes were not helping. Every time I moved my shoulder, it became worse. If I held it still, it became worse. I took two more aspirin tablets. Now, 7 hours later, I have not had to take any more aspirin. But waking up and warming up in a cold house was tough. When I started, I could not dangle my right arm without increasing the pain significantly. Now, it feels good to dangle my right arm and stretch it all the way up by sliding my right hand forward horizontally with the help of the left hand.

"Since my bad choices are evident, I am hoping for better insight. Over the last 7 days I learned a few things: 1) Pain is very distracting when trying to get things done. 2) Pain is distracting for a reason. 3) With pain, it takes longer than usual to get anything done. 4) Pain makes it very difficult to get anything done, so do not worry about it. 5) When I am having pain that does not respond, my confidence is gone. 6) It is easy to have thoughts of, 'What if this will last forever?' 7) I might need right shoulder rotator cuff surgery. 8) I need to re-learn more patience.

"It is now January 16, 2010, 9 days after the onset of the pain. Because of pain, I am learning to change positions often and avoid sudden or full movements. The pain is controllable but severe at times. There is less pain if I move easily and slowly, especially with dangling my arm. I also get temporary relief from raising my right arm with help. Reaching forward against resistance seems to make it worse (a 'speed test' of the long biceps tendon upper end). Reaching out makes the pain worse (a test of the rotator cuff tendon). X-rays yesterday showed arthritis bone spurs in the large ball and cup joint of the shoulder, but no calcium deposits were in the tendons or shoulder bursa.[78]

"Because there was no temporary full relief as usual from the aspirin I took at 3 AM, I knew today was going to be a challenging day, and it has been. To see if aspirin will calm the arthritis down, I am going to take it regularly every 8 hours. During that time, I will avoid all activities and motions that aggravate it, especially those that I notice when I am off the medication. I have been able to get a few things done with aspirin. But using the medication to cover things up and get things done is not a good idea. That is true for aspirin, acetaminophen and other over-the-counter or prescription pain remedies.

---

[78] X-ray findings were mild to moderate glenohumeral osteoarthritis with slight irregularity of the joint surfaces, mild joint space narrowing and mild bone spur formation at the bottom of the cup, the inferior glenoid.

The Miracle of Pain

"Maybe some things I am still doing are irritating to the shoulder. I tend to stay at the computer a little too long, which is 10 to 15 minutes at a time. I am experiencing pain about 75 percent of the time. The pain is bothersome enough that I cannot concentrate on much. I have stayed away from my bike now for 7 days and pruning trees for 3 days. In the shower, the pain was there only 20 percent of the time. After the shower when the muscles cooled down, the pain is constant. I am trying to reduce forward reaching while showering and while hanging up clothes. I also changed the Kleenex box on my desk to the left side to avoid reaching with the right shoulder.

"I have been too cavalier about using my right hand. Except for protected motions that decrease the pain, I am trying to eliminate all use. Over the last 8 days, feeling aches and pains extending to the right hand and chest is disturbing. The right shoulder pain is located on the outside and in front (lateral and anterior aspects). With movement and gentle stretching of the fingers, hand, wrist, forearm, shoulder girdle, neck and mid back, the pain has lessened.

"It is Monday, January 18, 2010. Yesterday I noticed that I need to modify daily tasks at or above eye level. I am forced to unbutton my shirts rather than pulling them off over my head. Long periods of rest or lying down increase the level of pain as does sitting, reading a book or using the computer. Changing positions of my arm did not prevent the pain from accumulating with reading.

"Today, the right shoulder is extremely sensitive with muscle spasms easily stirred up in the front, side and back of the right shoulder. The arthritis must be a small source of pain since aspirin did not provide any enduring effects with its use. Therefore, it would not solve anything to continue aspirin or change to a different anti-inflammatory medication. For that reason, I am staying off medication and will instead use only mechanical helps. Avoiding prolonged lying down, sitting, standing and walking has been difficult but helpful.

"To be useful around the house, I tried emptying the dishwasher and loading the wood burning stove. However, when I reach, there are short 1 to 2 second intervals of pain.

Although the pain goes away, I notice lasting effects that accumulate with doing things. Today, the pain level varies from a 0 to 10 out of 10 and comes in waves, lasting 15 to 20 minutes at a time with level 8 to 10 pain. Lying on my back is only temporarily okay if I do it less than 5 minutes at a time. The lying down position is allowing the muscles to tighten up in the entire shoulder and is the hardest position to get temporary relief. I discovered that I have not been lying down often enough and for short enough periods to help the pain. I will need to use that position more often during the day to keep from having a backlash at night.

"It is hard to change positions and move enough at night. I worry about waking up my wife, but she knows I need to change positions. She even said that I was not squirming last night. Using my left hand to help my right arm up helps empty excess blood out the veins of my right arm. Stagnation of the blood in the veins of the arm would increase the risk of clots forming in the veins (venous congestion leading to phlebitis or venous thrombosis). However, after injuries or surgeries, clots in leg veins form more readily than clots in the arm veins because of gravity.

"Today is Tuesday morning, January 19, 2010. Resting last night was difficult with the aching, burning and throbbing pain. I cannot hold a heavy book with my right hand without immediate pain. Even using two hands, a paperback book irritates my right shoulder within 2 to 3 seconds because of the irritability of the shoulder muscles. The only way I have been able to read 1 to 2 pages at a time is in a kneeling position, so I can let my right arm dangle. If I try to sit and read, I have trouble getting through a paragraph without more pain.

"With all this, I feel pitiful and worthless, but the 5 to 10 minutes at a time I have now without pain are rays of hope. The little things that I am learning along the way are welcome sunshine. My wife's care, concern and occasional hugs are like a soothing blanket. I do not know how long she can put up with my nonsense. She has gone from care and concern, to anxiety and many suggestions. Then she went back to care, concern and some listening skills, which I value greatly.

The Miracle of Pain

"It is now Wednesday, January 20, 2010, and I am still off all medication. It has been difficult to focus enough to do any writing or earn continuing medical education credits (CME credits). Those activities will just have to wait until I am more consistently without pain. I found a keyboard shortcut that is easier than using a computer mouse to go to saved websites. That has cut down on the shoulder popping and the 15 to 30 seconds of ache that occurred from turning the right shoulder inward to put the right hand back in my lap after using the mouse (internal rotation).

"It is Friday, January 22, 2010, and yesterday was a good day. The longest period without pain was 1 hour. Last night was difficult, but I am doing much better this morning. I was able to sleep well in the early morning and was not forced to get up out of bed because of pain. When getting out of bed today, there was no pain, which is a first!"

Starting today, which is January 29, 2010, I am no longer dictating. Though the pain is better over the last 2 weeks, I still have pain about 25 percent of the time, usually early in the morning. I am doing limited things during the day. When use of the computer mouse is necessary, I turn my whole body, so my shoulder does not pop and ache. I have also learned to get up and take a break more often. Getting up from sitting also helps to avoid reaching. Learning to delegate has been a necessity. Today, the other registered adult leaders of our scout troop were willing to take our scouts on this month's campout for the 26 to 52-mile bike ride. I could not have slept in a tent because I cannot stay in any position. The longest is flat on my back for 10 minutes at a time.

When I turn on the right side, the right upper outer arm hurts after 10 seconds (deltoid insertion). When I turn on the left side, the right shoulder blade sticks out compared with the left and then hurts after 5 seconds, no matter where I put my right arm. In upright positions, I am regaining some limited ability to reach. Turning the shoulder out seems to help the pain (external rotation). Another favorite is dangling the arm. Others are upwards and backwards shoulder shrugs (superior and posterior). Shrugging forwards is not helpful (anterior). It

232

feels good to accumulate several different movements that help consistently.

Today is February 22, 2010, more than 6 weeks after the onset of pain. I have been without shoulder pain now for about 1 week. I can sit down at the computer and concentrate better. This last Friday and Saturday I was able to go on our scout annual snow campout, and the cold did not cause pain in my shoulder. We camped in our local mountains in 1 to 2 feet of snow. Raising my right hand is about 80 percent but is still weak and awkward. With hands behind the head, turning the right shoulder outward by bringing the elbows together feels good (an external rotation variation).

Today, I found a black widow spider bite photograph online that looks exactly like the bite marks I saw on my right elbow.[79] With all the evidence, I think that my shoulder rotator cuff tendon is okay and that all the pain was from the black widow spider bite. In California, black widow spiders are common. It was not a brown recluse spider bite because I had no skin damage or soft-tissue loss (necrosis).

It is now June 2010, 5 months after the spider bite. With a full range of motion, I have had no shoulder or right upper extremity pain for over 3 months. I have had nearly full use of the right shoulder for 2 months. I can raise my right shoulder to 170 degrees out of a normal of 180 degrees (active motion). But the movement is awkward past 135 degrees. Right shoulder range of motion with help is easy to 180 degrees and without stiffness (passive motion). I have been on bike rides and scout outings without difficulty. The mild to moderate winging of my right shoulder blade is less than it was 3 months ago. Because of good improvement, I do not need a nerve test (electromyography/nerve conduction velocity studies or EMG/NCV).

It is now March 2011, about 14 months after the black widow spider bite. I have good right shoulder strength and a full range of motion. The shoulder blade winging was caused

---

[79] Photo by David O'Connor May 12, 2007, Slide 5 of the "Bad Bugs Slideshow," www.webmd.com/allergies/ss/slideshow-bad-bugs, accessed February 22, 2010 and again May 9, 2018.

by the spread of the venom from the spider bite (envenomation). The bite was at the elbow with a toxic nerve injury at the armpit (right long thoracic nerve). That nerve controls the muscle on the inside of the shoulder blade, and its normal function prevents the shoulder blade from winging (serratus anterior muscle). Mild winging of my shoulder blade persists. The nerve was not cut, so it will likely continue to recover.

Today is Sunday, September 11, 2011, and my right shoulder pain has been gone for a year and a half. With the initial pain, I observed that pain distracts us from getting things done, which helps us focus on the pain. In the face of pain, our choices can help healing and recovery, or our choices can inhibit them. In 2001, I noticed that distractions and inability to focus can also be significant when tragedy occurs.

Exactly 10 years ago today, as I was driving to the hospital to do a scheduled total knee replacement, I heard on the radio descriptions of airline plane attacks on two tall buildings in New York City. I remember that infamous Tuesday morning well. The scheduled surgery I was doing that morning was for a short, obese female patient with massive thighs and a moderately severe knee inward bowing deformity (valgus deformity). She had decreased her weight to 220 pounds before the surgery as I had required, but I still expected the surgery to be difficult because of the shape of her thigh and the deformity of the knee joint.

I wondered if the operating room would continue with its usual schedule. When I arrived, the operating room head nurse said that we were going ahead with the scheduled procedures. Dr. Alma Woods, the anesthesiologist, had already seen the patient, but the nurses in the pre-op holding room did not know where he went. I spoke to the patient, and she was ready. Then I went looking for Dr. Woods. I looked in the operating room where the surgery was scheduled, but he was not there. The last place I checked was the doctor's lounge. There, he was glued to the TV and the unfolding events of that day. With encouragement, he agreed to start the case and with the nurse, took the patient to the operating room.

Chapter 23 - The Distractions of Pain and Tragedy

During the surgery, Dr. Woods continued to talk about the news and tragedy that had occurred that morning and was still unfolding. The chatter by Dr. Woods at the head of the table was annoying and distracting. Because of it, I found myself not able to concentrate on what I was doing. I knew that not focusing on the surgery I was performing presented a danger to me and the patient. As the surgeon and operating room, "captain of the ship," I asked him not to talk about anything except the surgical case that we were doing. He objected, but fortunately he relented after I explained the distraction and insisted that he stop.

We kept a constructive collegial relationship, and the case went well despite being as difficult as I had expected. With the ability to focus on the procedure, I finished within the time scheduled for the surgery. Afterwards, one of the nurses who sensed the danger thanked me for taking control of the atmosphere in the operating room. Tragedy, like pain, can be stressful and distracting in varying degrees with different reactions among various personalities. Fortunately, the patient did well, and she was pleased with her new knee. There were no problems during her full recovery. Her long-term results were excellent at 5 years after the surgery.

With the challenges we face, it is crucial for us to be calm, kind and influence others for good. We can do that by setting a good example and by firmly speaking up when needed. We can focus on good things, and we can encourage others around us to do the same. Remember a universal airline safety instruction: put on your oxygen mask first, and then look to help others who are near you. Despite the distractions in the face of tragedy and pain, good things can happen when we focus on helping ourselves first, so we can then help others around us who are in need.

Chapter 24

Why are Patients Called "Patients?"

As a noun, the word "patient" has been around since about the thirteenth century.[80] The word is not an invention of modern medicine. I do not remember being taught in medical school why we refer to patients by that term. Over the years since then, I have thought of many reasons. In the busy course of our practice of medicine and surgery, we usually do not teach patients why we call them "patients."

In about 2001, the administration of our community hospital decided that everyone, including nurses and doctors, should start using the word "client" instead of "patient." Fortunately, that did not go well. The entire medical and nursing staff just ignored the directive. There have always been and probably always will be tug-of-wars between the administration of hospitals and the medical staff on some issues. Fortunately, most are amiable. Within a few months, we never heard anything else about it. Our hospital administrators may have used the word "client" for a few weeks. They must have soon become aware of the unique and appealing aspects of the venerated, established term "patient." Since then, hospital statements reassuringly describe being committed to quality care and the expectations of patients.[81]

The Middle English (1100–1500) word *pacient* is both a noun and an adjective. The word "patient" as an adjective comes from the Latin *patiens*, which means to suffer. An older meaning of the word "suffer" is "to allow." The adjective "patient" means tolerating pain or challenges quietly and wisely over a period of time.[82] Having patience is a good attribute. Upset or combative patients who thrash in agony in an emergency room will often compound their injuries.

---

[80] Dictionary.com, "patient," Dictionary.com Unabridged, Random House, Inc., www.dictionary.com/browse/patient, accessed May 9, 2018.

[81] Riverside Community Hospital, Riverside, California. "Patients & Visitors," www.riversidecommunityhospital.com/patients/index.dot, accessed May 9, 2018.

[82] Merriam-Webster, Inc., "patient," Merriam-Webster's Collegiate Dictionary, 11th Edition, 2016, www.merriam-webster.com/dictionary/patient, accessed May 9, 2018.

Chapter 24 - Why are Patients Called "Patients?"

The Greek Oath of Hippocrates for physicians was written in 400 B.C. Translated into modern English, one of the sentences states, "I will prescribe a treatment according to my ability and judgment, which is for the benefit of my patients, and abstain from all that is deleterious and mischievous." The plural noun "patients" is a translation of the original Greek word *kamnonton*, which is "of the sick." The present participle of *kamno* is, "to be sick or suffering." The same sentence of the Oath with a literal word for word translation is, "I will use diets for the assistance of the sick according to my ability and discernment; but also to keep away injury of health and injustice."[83]

Patients with challenging injuries or illnesses quickly find out why we call them patients. It is because they and their families are called upon by nature's God to have a measure of patience to allow the body time to heal or to merely deal with the challenges.[84] In addition to patience, a patient needs to trust that the body will heal, thereby motivating good choices. By using patience and trust, patients avoid inhibiting the healing and recovery unwittingly because of poor choices.

Patients also need to have patience with their doctor as the doctor tries to explain what is wrong, what it means, what can be done and what cannot be done. Likewise, a physician needs to have patience with a patient, explaining and listening carefully, then patiently answering questions about a diagnosis and the treatment plan. We should repeat answers to repeated questions as often as needed to help the patient understand.

Early in my practice, patients who asked questions over and over again were irritating. I understood, soon however, that they were not questioning me. They only needed to understand by having things repeated a second or a third time. Or, they could not remember the information they wanted to

---

[83] Howard Herrell, "The Hippocratic Oath, A Commentary and Translation," A Literal Translation, 2000, utilis.net/hippo.htm, accessed May 9, 2018.

[84] The term "Nature's God" is from the first paragraph of The Declaration of Independence, a unanimous declaration of the thirteen American colonies on July 4, 1776 by the Second Continental Congress, meeting in Philadelphia, Pennsylvania, which severed the colonies' ties to the British Crown.

remember. Occasionally, elderly patients and others asked me to write things down for them, so they could remember the basics of what I had told them. I was happy when they asked. Those patients were then more likely to remember and try what I had asked them to do.

If patients try to remember as much as they can, that will usually be good enough. Often, if I gave them exercises, I asked them to do the exercises for me before they left the office. At a follow-up appointment within 2 to 3 weeks, they let me know what their experiences were, and we could then compare notes again. Then, they could ask all the questions they needed to. Anything they tried that was not working or that did not make sense is fair game to ask.

At follow-up visits, I often asked patients to show me the exercise they were doing at home that they liked the best. If they had not improved, they were often doing an exercise incorrectly or the wrong exercise. They were overloading the injured part. Often patients did not remember what they were supposed to do once they got home. That was especially true when they waited until the next day to try what I had asked them to do. The sooner I could detect those kinds of mistakes, the faster their resolution of pain was.

Rarely, repeated questions were raised if the patient or their family disagreed with my diagnosis or the treatment plan. That is okay too because they can have their opinions, especially with the pervasiveness of internet medical advice. I simply ask them to try to understand my opinion. If we still disagree, it is okay. We can still part friends, and they can find another doctor if they want.

In our busy society with the influence of HMOs, doctors often do not spend adequate time on a first visit to understand patients. They take even less time on follow-up visits. No wonder some patients become frustrated and impatient. They have no idea what the doctor just told them. For both doctors and patients, we have an epidemic of impatience in California and elsewhere. That adds to the mounting epidemics of anger, drug abuse, obesity and insulin resistant diabetes (type 2). People tend to want things now.

Many do not understand what saving or working for something is like and therefore accumulate problems or debts. For many young individuals, working towards something good like a usable career is becoming a lost art. Instant gratification has become more important than long-term goals. They lose the opportunity to feel the joy that comes with work, responsibility, service to others and earned respect. Unless they change, they have no idea what earned success is. Impatience may also be a prominent part of the reason for an increasing incidence of painful syndromes from disuse.

"Can I exercise?" is a common question. For those patients, resting and waiting for things to heal is hard. They want to "do something." They want to keep up their aerobic capacity and strength. They worry about getting weak. They want to exercise another part of their body that is not injured. And they also want to forget about the problems with the injured part. If I say "Yes" to be agreeable, then correctly qualify and clarify my answer, the only thing most patients hear is the "Yes." It is like a race horse out of the gate and impossible to hold them back. Sometimes, patients will tell me that they "will go crazy" if they cannot exercise. When patients tell me that, I tend to believe them. Worry can feed into anxiety, anger and other emotional baggage. Impatience and anger are a dangerous combination.

The best answer to the question "Can I exercise?" is "No." Patients should focus on resting the injured body part. Ignoring the injured body part is never a good idea and will always slow recovery. They should use occasional easy exercise for surrounding joints to keep stiffness out. These easy passive exercises should be at a lower level than patients would like but are critically important for helping the healing process. They keep stiffness out by lowering muscle tension in the region. Movements of the surrounding areas should always feel good to the injured area, or they need to be modified.

For the question, "Can I exercise something else?" the answer should be, "No, not your usual exercises." Exercise in other areas, or activity in general, easily becomes a distraction. The injured body part needs more time, not less time, with simple, easy, boring things such as elevation and keeping stiffness out of surrounding joints. With an injury, the body preferentially directs the blood supply to the injured part during healing phases. If the patient exercises an uninjured body part, the body short circuits (shunts) the blood supply away from the injured area to the body parts that we are using or exercising.

Is there a way around this? Yes, but the exercises need to be light, easy, infrequent, varied and of short duration. They should be easy warm-ups for the body in general and not distract from paying attention to the injured part. Infrequent means only occasionally or less and to keep exercises for variety, not for regular exercise. After hearing that, someone with an injured ankle might think, "Okay, I will just do some arm curls for my biceps muscle. Because I am exercising the arm, it will not hurt my injured ankle."

If they keep the biceps muscle exercises light, occasional and short, it would be okay. That assumes the injured ankle continues to make progress with healing in reasonable time frames. If the ankle is not improving or the swelling is not resolving, it means that other activity is getting in the way. While doing arm curls, cheating is easy to do unconsciously with heavy free-weights. It is using the back and legs to help, even if we use an elbow support to prevent cheating. That can easily overload the injured ankle in addition to shunting blood to the biceps away from the ankle.

Keep it light. Because a little exercise feels good, increasing weights with exercise is tempting. By using heavy arm curl repetitions, an injured ankle will easily develop stiffness or swelling. Keep it occasional. Boredom may tempt us to exercise other parts of the body. Not learning and using what the injured ankle needs also adds stiffness or swelling. Keep it short. Too many arm repetitions or going too far is tempting to do because after we have warmed up, it feels good. That contributes to ignoring the injured ankle and also adds ankle stiffness or swelling.

With an injury to an arm instead, patients will often ask, "Can't I exercise on a treadmill?" The answer can be,

"Yes, but it is easy to go too far or too fast." When patients are struggling with an injury or ongoing pain, look at the choices they are making. Many of them complain of increasing swelling during the day or a continuing need to warm up in the morning for several hours. Keep activity and exercise for other areas of the body light, occasional and short.

Many patients also complain of increased pain with cold temperatures at night and in the winter. These are common patterns across many different body parts, including the arms, legs, neck and back. Most of my patients live in the Los Angeles basin of Southern California. The climate is temperate and void of extremes along the coast. Patients living in the high deserts and San Bernardino Mountains have snow and some extremes of winter temperatures at elevations of 2000 to 8000 feet, up to 100 miles away from the ocean. However, their low temperatures are not much below freezing. The ocean has a tempering effect with an average winter water temperature of 57 degrees Fahrenheit.

When patients complained of pain and stiffness with chilly winter temperatures, I asked them, "What would you do if you lived in Minnesota?" Most patients shuddered at the thought because they knew that they would be in more trouble with more stiffness and more pain from the bitter cold. Midwest winter lows can be less than 0 degrees Fahrenheit and even colder with the wind chill. Many of my patients were not sure how they would survive and said, "Oh, I could not do that." If visiting northern Midwestern states, those patients would either move their joints and muscles more or freeze to death. Our bodies normally acclimatize within a few days to a change in climate.

However, some patients have ongoing challenges with a cold climate each year. They will do better if they do a few basic things. First, move the injured body part more often. Second, shiver, wiggle and squirm. Third, put on more layers of clothing. Fourth, find a warmer place in the house. Fifth, frequently put the injured body part in a warm protected place. Sixth, frequently elevate an injured part at heart level or one pillow higher than heart level. Elevate continuously if needed to control swelling. Seventh, avoid elevating the part too high for more than 30 to 60 seconds at a time to keep from increasing the pain and making it harder for arterial blood to get to it. Eighth, stay well hydrated with water to improve blood circulation. Warm drinks are helpful but optional.

Visiting or moving to Minnesota in the winter would force patients to do most of those things. Doing good things, however, before our body compels us to do them is usually better. I encouraged my patients to do all eight of the above things without moving to a different state. They should be grateful for the Southern California temperate weather. By learning to deal well with climate challenges, patients will notice immediate beneficial effects, and they will usually improve each winter. If they do not, their pain or stiffness may remain a problem for them each winter.

Over the years that I have practiced orthopedic surgery, I have helped many patients who have struggled to heal. They may tend to describe their complaints almost too well and sometimes in intricate detail. They seem to have difficulty shifting from profuse complaints to asking questions. They often throw out complaints as fast as they can because they know that most doctors will cut them off. They fear that if they miss describing one little detail, I will not be able to decipher what is wrong with them. It seems that they are also trying to avoid asking questions. That may be because they fear that we will not have good answers. A competent doctor will listen to the complaints for a few minutes and then ask directed questions, based on the complaints. The questions are also based on what he thinks might be wrong. The answers help the doctor come to a preliminary diagnosis.

The doctor collects and tries to understand the story of the symptoms, which is "taking a history." We should not delegate it solely to a "historian," physician assistant or nurse practitioner. The history is the most important part of the exam. The process helps the doctor determine how likely the preliminary diagnosis is or if there are other possibilities. The physical examination and lab studies confirm a diagnosis or suggest other possible diagnoses. The doctor should, at the very least, be able to give a most likely diagnosis the same day as the first exam. If many uncertainties remain, the doctor may give a list of diagnoses (differential diagnoses). But a list is much less helpful to the patient than a most likely diagnosis.

The change by a patient from complaints to questions about the diagnosis and what to do about it, is terribly important. Good questions could be about what they are feeling, why they feel it and how long it will last. The patient can ask questions about the diagnosis and any problems they experienced from past treatment. Questions about what to do and what not to do are critical because the doctor will not know very much about what patients are doing at home, work or for recreation. Anything that does not make sense is vital to ask. Other questions should be about reasonable treatment options, their rates of success and risks.

A respectful doctor will spend time answering questions. Good questions do not always have an answer. A good doctor will admit it when they do not know. Medical science knows a lot, but there are many things we do not know. If a doctor does not have the answer, they should say the dreaded words, "I do not know." The doctor should try to help find the answer if there is an answer. If a good answer does not exist, it is okay, and the doctor should acknowledge that they do not have a good answer.

To me, it seemed odd that many patients who were struggling would not ask questions. It appeared that they could not form the questions in their mind because they were so accustomed to complaining. It seemed that complaining had become a bad habit. Such a habit may be part of a syndrome that has become known as "disability sickness." Their frustration and lack of hope, curiosity or initiative may feed into the "sickness."

The questions asked by a doctor while taking the history can prepare a patient to ask good questions after the diagnosis is made and treatment is prescribed. In the middle of treatment, my questions continue. If I ask patients how they are doing after a few days or weeks, many had no difficulty describing their complaints in great detail. To understand them better, I question patients about their persisting complaints. I also ask them if they remember and understand the diagnosis. I ask them if they remember what to do and what not to do. If they do not, I give a condensed version of the diagnosis again, what they should do and what they should not be doing.

By asking patients good questions, I am giving them an example that they can follow. Then I ask, "Do you have any questions?" Many chronic pain patients will say "No" even though they do not see a path forward. This pattern became so common and predictable that I needed to teach and encourage those patients how to ask questions. They needed to regain a natural curiosity for what they feel, what the diagnosis is, what they can do and what they should not do. They should not fear what they are feeling and should not ignore it.

Are there bad questions? Many say that the only bad questions are the questions that are not asked. That may be true in many respects. However, many individuals or attorneys ask questions to confuse issues or expose weakness. They want a response, but they are not really looking for an answer to the question. Some also ask questions incessantly with a devious intent to bring out inappropriate behavior. Almost all patients are not devious. But the difference between poor questions and good questions is vital. If a patient wants to know something, a bad question is one that they ask over and over without listening to, understanding or remembering the answer. Other bad questions are those asked of an inappropriate health care provider or of a friend who tends to promote fads or give sensational, misleading information.

Patients who question everything show a lack of trust. Finding a doctor you can trust is important. The degree of trust may depend upon how well the physician listens. Trust also depends upon trying and testing what the physician tells you. Asking questions to help learn how to modify sources of pain is extremely helpful. Asking questions to understand, reflects an attitude of learning. I treasure that attitude most in a patient who has struggled. They ask questions to understand what they feel. They also ask questions about what is working for them and what is not.

Poor questions by a patient can dishearten them even with a perfect answer. There is no good answer to the question, "Why did this have to happen to me?" Rather, the patient should ask, "What can I learn from this?" Or they could ask, "What can I change?" Or they can ask, "Is there someone else I might help if I have courage?" Another poor question is, "Will I ever get better?" This is especially true if the question was asked after the diagnosis, prognosis, treatment and treatment options were fully explained. Often the answer is, "Usually yes, but it depends upon what you do."

A better question is a specific question such as, "What is a back sprain?" or "Can it heal?" or "Why does my leg tingle after I walk for a quarter of a mile?" The more specific the question is, the better it is. Another good question would be, "Why am I still feeling pain after 3 months if I only have a back sprain?" The doctor should have an answer to that question, but they will need the patient's help. The patient needs to describe what they are doing or what they just finished doing when they feel recurrent pain.

Another example of a better question is, "What about heat or ice?" A good question should be about anything that is unclear or does not make sense to the patient, especially after the patient has tried to do what the physician or physical therapist has suggested. The better the questions are, the better the potential for learning is. Learning and wisdom are learning to ask good questions. Medical knowledge is power, and it takes patience to learn, both for the patient and the physician.

To help a patient ask good questions, first I need the patient to stop ignoring the pain and to stop excessive worrying about the pain. Next is using the good habit of listening to the pain. How often is it there? Is it constant? Where does it start? How far does it go? What can I learn from the pain? What am I doing when the pain increases? What am I doing when the pain decreases? Am I having periods of time without pain? Lastly, I must enable changing behavior, both habits of activity and inactivity. As I am talking with patients, noticing what they do in my office gives excellent clues to what they are doing or not doing at home. Are they spontaneously moving or stretching? Do they tend to keep still? Do they stretch until it hurts? Because I cannot see their behavior at home, work or play, a patient's observations and good questions will always be a crucial advantage for both of us.

Many patients commented that there should be an owner's manual for our body. Well, I did not tell many of my patients this, but we do have one! The writings in The Holy Bible describe many individuals who are good examples and others who are bad examples. The accounts give us insight and guidance for our body, mind and spirit. Job's wife saw the losses, troubles and misery Job was enduring and encouraged him to, "curse God, and die."[85] Thankfully, most spouses are better than that.

Also, Job's friends judged him incorrectly, chastised him and then abandoned him. In 36 pages, The Book of Job in the Old Testament gives us many truths about dealing with pain. Job's trust in the Lord God was unshakable. If we learn to have patience and other characteristics like Job, our trials and challenges will be less oppressive. He declared, "For I know *that* my redeemer liveth..."[86] If we trust in our Creator as Job did, we will, as he did, look to a brighter future, whether in this life or the next.

Because they recover well or endure patiently, many around us are good examples. If we listen to them, we can learn from them. We may also help to sustain them because we have listened. Patients will be rewarded with greater patience and hope if they can resist the misinformation sold in the world. When we feel physical, emotional or spiritual pain, we can improve if we have patience, seek proper help and listen to good sources.

---

[85] The Holy Bible, Authorized King James Version, The Church of Jesus Christ of Latter-day Saints, 2013, Old Testament, Job 2:9, www.lds.org/scriptures/ot/job/2?lang=eng, accessed May 9, 2018.
[86] The Holy Bible, Old Testament, Job 19:25, www.lds.org/scriptures/ot/job/19?lang=eng, accessed May 9, 2018.

Chapter 25

Early Warning Signs

Though pain can be the earliest warning sign of injury or disease, other warning signs may appear earlier. If there is no pain, many of us ignore subtle, early warning signs such as stiffness, swelling, tingling, numbness, tiredness, restlessness, limping, weakness or a lump (a mass or tumor). These are only some of many examples, but each may be important and may be precursors to pain or other problems. Nevertheless, pain is the first sign of trouble that we, as patients, tend to pay attention to and go to the doctor for. We may find common reasons for pain, but there may be unexpected or unknown reasons for pain. Knowing what pain is from gives us power and perspective.

Itching and discomfort are often early warnings that patients are not sure whether to call them pain. Some say that itching is an annoyance and is an exception to being a warning sign. Itching may be less of a warning sign than others, however, it accompanies many abnormal problems. Itching or pain at the site of a recent bruise is due to tissue damage or increased swelling that can occur over a few minutes or hours. If we ignore the causes of warning signs, pain can turn into burning pain. Sharp stabbing pain can also develop from associated muscle spasm. Each of those warning signs reflects some damage or physiologic abnormality.

Many of us have felt discomfort from a prolonged soak in water that causes damage to skin. The damage is visible with wrinkled, whitish skin, known as skin maceration. The skin may itch, and if contact with moisture continues, it can hurt. Tissue damage also occurs with itching or pain that happens inside a cast. Urgent doctor visits for problems with casts are common for an orthopedic surgeon's office. If simple things do not solve discomfort or itching immediately, taking a cast off and looking at the skin is the best answer. Not only can there be maceration of the skin under the cast, we can also find coins, pencils, toys or other interesting objects.

In my office years ago, I found the usual cause and cure for itching inside a cast. It is from prolonged moisture on the skin. The itching goes away by using air at the edge of the cast from a fan, air hose, hairdryer without heat or other source of air. The itching stays away by decreasing activity, staying out of the sun and keeping the skin under the cast dry. The moisture can be from sweating in the cast or from leaving a cast wet after bathing or swimming. Drying out a cast is a lot of work, but it is worth the effort.

Even without a cast, itching in the legs can occur from stagnation of the veins in the soft tissues (venous congestion). With greater symptoms or warning signs, abnormalities of the veins and surrounding soft tissues are greater. Leg aching or a pressure sensation is from increased muscle or soft-tissue swelling. Burning is from stagnant waste products in muscles (lactic acid and other metabolites). Pain from muscle spasm can occur in a small part of the muscle. Severe pain with a muscle cramp can involve a larger part of a muscle. Soft-tissue damage occurs with many different manifestations.

Many people, including physicians, say that itching of a wound or a surgical scar is a sign of healing. That explanation has been passed down by surgical residents to each other and to patients who ask about itching. The answer usually works for most patients. They leave the wound alone, and the itching goes away. For a few years, I used that answer. Then, I found it to be not entirely correct. There is a more accurate, though hard to understand, physiologic answer. Itching is a warning sign of skin or soft-tissue damage. Itching of a wound can be from venous stagnation, swelling or prolonged moisture with persisting sweating.

All these problems can resolve with basic wound care by keeping the wound elevated more often, leaving the wound alone and keeping it clean and dry. We can also help itching in a scar by holding the scar with the whole hand. We can do it over a bandage or clothing. We can do it on bare skin after the wound has healed. Holding the scar decreases irritation and will usually afford some immediate relief of itching or associated pain. Moving the hand, bandage or skin area may also help. Holding it for extended periods will not help, but coming back to it often will help and can solve itching. If we scratch, the itching usually comes back with a vengeance. With time, the problems with continued scratching become more apparent. For that reason, eventually, most people learn to not continue scratching.

Some patients tend to touch a skin wound that has healed with their fingertips even without it itching. This is an unconscious tendency that can become a habit. If I noticed a patient touching a wound several times, I would point it out to them. They frequently rationalized it by saying, "Doc, I am just checking it." The itching of a scar can also be bothersome enough for a patient to touch it, check it, rub it, scratch it or dig at it. Any of those habits irritate the scar at the skin or the scarring in the underlying soft tissues.

Whether consciously or unconsciously, a scar may draw the patient's attention to it. Some will touch it or poke at it with their fingertips, merely to see how the scar is doing. Unfortunately, that repeated bad habit over time can lead to the formation of a thicker than normal scar, which is called a keloid. The tendency or habit of touching a scar with the fingertips usually develops a few days after we remove stitches or staples, which is when a keloid tends to form. Patients are normally hesitant to touch a wound with staples or stitches still in. Therefore, staples and stitches are an effective, temporary barrier for the abnormal, irritating habit of touching or poking.

We can teach patients, instead, to replace the bad habit of touching with the good habit of holding the scar. During healing or after the scar has healed, they can use the whole hand. Then later, they can use gentle, general rubbing. Then, keloids will not develop even in a patient that tends to form keloid scars. A history of forming keloids does not mean that there is a genetic disorder. Keloids frequently form from the consequences of unconscious choices or habits. When it feels good, general rubbing of the entire area of skin with the whole hand can be added. That is a rub using gentle, random, non-repetitive motions.

Rubbing helps reestablish normal motion of the skin over the underlying soft tissues during healing. In a normal way, holding and rubbing of an area increase blood supply to finish healing and maturation. If rubbing does not feel good, then do it easier or wait to try it later. General rubbing motions should be light and firm but not deep. Deep massages are popular with some individuals and health practitioners because they occasionally feel good, especially when they stop. Just like scratching, they are counterproductive. Deep massages are more irritating than they are helpful. That is why tightness or other symptoms will tend to keep coming back.

Remember that nearly everything in the body stretches, including ligaments and scar tissue. The denser the scar tissue is, the longer it takes to stretch out. The key is patience. Give a skin wound time to heal and stretch normally, so it moves like the surrounding skin. Remember, scar tissue is healing tissue. If we are doing something that irritates our scar, it will thicken, and a keloid will tend to form. If we are irritating a keloid that has already started, a larger keloid will tend to form. On the other hand, the keloid can become smaller and more like the surrounding skin by simply holding it. Later, we can gently rub the area with the whole hand. It should feel good at the time and afterwards. If not, we must change how we are doing it.

I have learned from many variations in the formation of keloids. In patients with multiple scars that need to heal at the same time, if keloids form, often only a few of the scars will keloid. The scars that tend to keloid are visible to the patient or reachable with their fingertips. After surgery, one of my male total knee replacement patients had the usual long scar on the front of his knee, above and below the kneecap. Only the upper half of the scar was keloided with a thick, dark scar. Below the kneecap, the lower half of the scar was normal, perfectly healed and barely visible. He tended to touch the upper scar. But he ignored the lower part of the scar that was just a little harder to see and reach, allowing it to heal normally. Leaving a scar alone is always a great idea.

Using a principle of general rubbing and no poking of the soft tissues has also helped pain for different conditions in many locations, such as the back, knee and elbow. Earlier in the 1980s, I discovered the principle from an experience with another male patient. He had a firm lump in the soft tissues under one of the three knee arthroscopy scars 2 weeks after the procedure. The skin had healed normally. He had no sign of infection or keloid of the skin. The scar was only ⅜ of an inch long and barely visible. The lump underneath the skin was about the size of a marble. It was not painful, but the patient insisted repeatedly that I take the lump out. I felt that the lump was scar tissue and encouraged the patient to ignore it.

After several weeks, because the patient was still insistent, I took the tumor out in outpatient surgery with a slightly larger incision. The pathology report showed that the mass was benign scar tissue as I had suspected (fibroma). By the time the pathology results were available, the patient's surgical skin wound was again well healed. Nevertheless, he was already concerned that the tumor under the skin was coming back. As we were talking and as he described his concerns, I noticed that he was touching the spot with his index fingertip. When he did that a second and a third time, I asked him to stop touching it. Later in the same visit, I noticed him touching it again.

It seemed to me that the patient had a habit he was not even aware of. At his next visit, the habit of touching his wound and the lump with his fingertips was still there. After reminding him several times not to touch it, I realized that I needed to give him something to do to replace the habit. I also recognized that eventually he needed to be able to touch the area. So, I encouraged him to hold the area with his whole hand and then gently rub a bigger area, again with his whole hand. It seemed to work for him because the second lump did not grow further, and he seemed to deal with it better. He was happy with the ultimate result for his knee.

Over a period of several years, it surprised me to find other patients doing the same abnormal things. They were struggling with sore spots in various locations. With other patients and different areas of the musculoskeletal system, I learned how to fine-tune my instructions. Thus, the principle of general rubbing and no poking was born. Fine-tuning the principle included keeping the rubbing firm, light, random, short and coming back to it often. Avoiding repetitious movements and prolonged use or positions was also important. Muscle relaxation is a nice side effect of general rubbing and no poking that can be very helpful for pain, pressure, pulling, itching and other warning signs.

I later rediscovered the same principle for my own muscles and soft tissues. In the early 1990s, I had a small spot or trigger point on my left upper back that itched and then hurt on and off for a few months. At first, I ignored it. I could barely reach it with my fingertips. Poking at it temporarily helped. But it tended to come back quickly. If I rubbed my back muscles against the door frame, the same thing happened. It helped, but the symptoms quickly tended to come back. Soon, I found that when I rubbed up against the broad, slightly textured wall surface in my office, the relief seemed to last a little longer. Gradually, I learned not to do the rubbing against the textured wall repetitiously because the relief was longer if I did it in a gentle, random fashion.

After a few weeks of trying to get the painful spot to go away, I realized that the muscle tension or spasticity at the trigger site was probably coming from my neck (referred pain). I did not remember having any neck pain. When I felt the pain, or before feeling it if possible, I tried to lie down for a few minutes. I could not always prevent it, so I continued to learn more about general rubbing. Wiggling or squirming on different, large surfaces was effective, such as the back of a chair or the floor while lying flat on my back. I also found that poking with an S-shaped rod or stick did not work any better than using my fingertips.

The reasons why poking helps only temporarily are interesting to look at. Though poking may give temporary relief, it tends to force the muscle to relax. Because the poking is also irritating, muscles will tend to tighten back up readily. If I continue to poke a friend in the shoulder, eventually they will stop me, poke me or may even strike back. Muscles are no different. We need to value them, respect them and encourage them. We should not force muscles to relax either with poking or with over stretching, both of which are irritating. The pain and itching in that spot of my left upper back never returned after I fine-tuned the rubbing I was doing and took care of my neck. I believe the trigger point resolved because I addressed it with a variety of good tools. Though challenging to learn, I found ways to avoid irritating it, and I found productive ways of dealing with it.

A few years later, experimenting with pain in another area proved to me again the general rubbing and no poking concept. With kneeling, I suddenly had right knee pain at the front and lower end of the kneecap (inferior patellar pole). I had no swelling or redness, but I could not kneel. An inflammation of the soft tissues was causing pain between the skin and the bone (pre-patellar bursitis without effusion). Because it hurt, I quickly learned to not touch it and to avoid kneeling on it. After a week or two, it was still there if I knelt on it. I wondered if general rubbing would help.

While rubbing it, I did not feel anything. However, after I rubbed it for 60 seconds, I could kneel on it without pain for 1 to 2 minutes. The bursa had warmed up, and afterwards for a brief time, the pain did not return. After a few weeks of frequently using the same general rubbing technique, I discovered that I no longer needed to warm it up before kneeling. The bursitis and pain were gone. I had not used any medication. The soft tissues of the bursa had regained their ability to move and to be used without being irritated. When done correctly, general rubbing and no poking is a warm-up technique that we can use often.

Pain can be an early or a late warning sign. Pain is also a warning sign that is frequently sandwiched between other early and late warning signs. If pain persists, we may find late warning signs such as muscle atrophy, varicose veins, skin and soft-tissue pressure sores (bedsores, ulcers and decubiti), bone and joint deformity (bunions and hammertoes), loss of joint motion (contractures) or enlarging tumors. After having pain for 3 months, pain becomes a late warning sign. It may be aching, burning, stabbing or constant pain at higher levels. Even minor pain such as discomfort, pressure, soreness and itching can contribute to late warning signs. Getting over an early warning sign is much easier than getting over a late warning sign.

When recovering from an injury or disease, if a patient begins to have time without pain, other early warning signs often remain. To recover fully, patients must learn to resolve all early warning signs, such as swelling, numbness or tingling. Painless early warning signs are easy to ignore. They may vary minute to minute and are more difficult to monitor and understand than pain. If we ignore them, we have a higher risk of persisting warning signs or recurrent pain. Ups and downs, however, give a patient many opportunities for learning what helps and what aggravates a warning sign. To learn most effectively, the patient should pay attention to one or two early warning signs at a time. If the patient is going in the right direction, the area size, intensity or number of the warning signs will lessen. Resolving all early warning signs minimizes the risk of pain coming back.

When a family member sees the effects of pain or other warning signs, they often wonder if they can help by reminding the patient. Though encouragement by a friend or a family member is good, only the patient can feel the pain or early warning signs soon enough to keep going in the right direction. If a patient always relies on a family member or a friend for reminders to stop doing things, the patient will wear them out. If a patient does not learn to move more often or do other helpful things, progress will stop. The best help by the friend or family member is to be encouraging, loving and positive.

Someone loving us enough to try to help us is always good, but it will never be enough. The patient is the only one who must fully learn to deal with it. When a patient is paying attention to early warning signs before their pain comes back, improvement and resolution of all symptoms are more certain. On the other hand, if the patient puts up with and ignores early warning signs, the warning signs and recurrent pain will more likely continue. Therefore, it is important for the patient to be willing to change what they are doing to learn from and avoid early warning signs. If a patient does not get over pain fully, it directly impacts the rest of the family as well as friends. Fear for the future is often part of it. Fear is why some family members try to control the patient or the pain. Chronic pain affects friends, activities, memories, employment and much more.

With time, pain becomes easier to put up with and ignore. Then, we suffer the consequences, and we will more often stay limited because of pain. We should not give up trying to learn from the pain we experience. Learning is what life and being a patient is all about. After paying better attention to early warning signs, the patient should feel more in control. Patients who choose not to pay attention are enabling their recurrent or continuing warning signs, often without realizing it. For them, painful aggravations are inevitable.

Family members and friends are often very supportive early on. For that support to fade is normal and okay, but love should not diminish. Part of that is letting the patient live with the consequences of their choices. As the patient can take more responsibility, help should diminish. If help does not aptly diminish, friends and family members can be unwittingly enabling poor choices. The patient can develop unnecessary dependencies. Enabling is cruel to all involved. To become self-reliant, the patient needs to take responsibility for learning along the way and for pacing limited activity. As long as insight is gained and lessons are learned, mistakes are okay.

Often, when I ask a patient how they are doing with their pain, they tell me, "I am not getting any better, and the pain depends on what I am doing." They usually do not understand the strength of their statement. Then I ask them, "Do you realize what you are saying?" What they are saying shows they have more control over pain than they recognize. Helping them see at least the little control they have is a start. If a patient gives the impression to others by their description of symptoms that they have no control of the pain, they are expressing a degree of hopelessness. They may say, "I do not know why, but I have an excruciating pain." Instead, they should be saying, "I am trying to understand why I have this excruciating pain." In reality, control over pain only comes if we pay attention to it and become wiser along the way.

The Miracle of Pain

If a patient wants to accept pain or another warning sign as it is, wants to ignore it or wants to put up with it, then I have to wish them "Good luck." They, in essence, are complaining about something, but they are not willing to do anything about it. I can do little for them, except listen. About 10 percent of patients with chronic pain, will have to live with it, no matter how good a doctor's diagnosis, instructions and treatment are. C. S. Lewis wrote, "But pain insists upon being attended to. God whispers to us in our pleasures, speaks in our conscience, but shouts in our pains: it is his megaphone to rouse a deaf world."[87]

There are many reasons for pain that we should pay attention to and learn from. Nevertheless, there are patients whose chronic pain or other suffering we do not understand, and there is no known solution. Again, we can listen. The good news is that 90 percent of patients with chronic musculoskeletal pain and other warning signs will do well with the right help, support, direction and encouragement. Many chronic pain patients need a lot of guidance. A few need only a little redirection, and they do well. When they can be pointed in the right direction, continue in the right direction and never turn back, that is unusual. Physicians pray to have those kinds of patients.

On the other hand, many patients pray to God for physicians who will honestly and clearly tell them what the diagnosis is and what they should and should not do. For early warning signs that do not hurt, resolution may take less time. However, resolution of them can often only come with the same amount of diligence it takes to resolve pain.

---

[87] C. S. Lewis, The Problem of Pain, HarperCollins 2001, page 91, © copyright CS Lewis Pte Ltd 1940.

Chapter 26

The Miracle of Swelling

Swelling in the shoulder and knee is usually about the same on the first day after a similar outpatient arthroscopic surgery. However, on the second day, there is routinely little swelling in the shoulder compared to moderate swelling in the knee. Though the procedures in the knee or shoulder may be similar with 3 to 4 tiny incisions, there is more swelling in the knee, and it lasts consistently longer. Occasionally knee swelling can be severe. For the knee and shoulder, the only constant variable that accounts for the differences in swelling is elevation. An elevated body part is above the level of the heart.

For a shoulder after surgery, automatic elevation above the heart level occurs in sitting, standing and most other positions. The patient naturally avoids lying on the same side as the surgery. That is the only position where the shoulder would be below the heart level (dependent lateral decubitus position). When the patient is lying on the opposite shoulder, the surgical site is above the level of the heart. Lying flat on the back is a position with the shoulder at the same level as the heart (supine position). Therefore, patients are elevating the shoulder for most of the positions they would tend to use.

When sitting after surgery, knee patients often prop the leg up on a stool and a pillow in front of a chair. If the knee is below the level of the heart, they are not elevating the knee. If not elevated, a knee after surgery will tend to swell (dependent swelling). Being upright too early or too long with crutches is tempting for knee patients. If a knee arthroscopy patient elevates their knee after surgery the same amount that shoulder patients do naturally, swelling of the knee resolves just as quickly as shoulder swelling.

Elevating the knee at or above the heart level is easy on a bed, on the floor or in a recliner. The right kinds of knee movement, if allowed and encouraged by the surgeon, will also help minimize swelling. Like pain, swelling is an important early warning sign. But swelling is often subtle, easy to ignore and frequently does not hurt. Painful swelling means that the swelling is increasing rapidly, staying too long or is causing other secondary damage such as nerve compression, vein clots or muscle irritability.

In normal, controlled amounts, swelling and bleeding at an injury, fracture or operative site are early parts of the healing process. However, if swelling or bleeding is an abnormal amount and stays longer than normal, it will delay or stop healing. Swelling in abnormal or persisting amounts are often a reflection of too much activity or continued reinjury. Swelling is a warning sign that should resolve, but it usually resolves after pain from an injury or surgery is gone.

If we are doing what we should after an injury or surgery and the pain resolves, any remaining or recurrent swelling will guide us if we are watching and listening. Your doctor should be able to tell you what the average time is for pain and swelling to resolve after a specific injury or surgery. Swelling that is resolving is evidence that a patient is learning to do what is appropriate. Resolving swelling as soon as possible helps the healing stay at a normal rate, including bone fracture healing. Our bodies are much more capable than we give them credit for. Because we cannot completely avoid life's experiences of pain and swelling, we should plan to learn from them.

In March 1992, I attended a week-long trauma and sports medicine conference with my wife in Snowmass, Colorado at the former Silvertree Hotel. The medical lectures were early in the morning and later in the evening, which allowed day time hours for skiing. The hotel had ski-in, ski-out access to the ski slopes, which is a skier's dream. My wife was on skis, and I was on my snowboard. On the third day, we were out on the slopes together as usual (Pictures 10 and 11). After lunch, I returned to the slopes while she read a book and took a nap. Snowmass is a huge ski resort, and there was a foot and a half of new, untouched powder at the top and back of the resort.

Since 1989 when I first learned to snowboard at Snowbird, Utah, I have always enjoyed powder. With the new powder at Snowmass, the broad double black diamond runs were easy. My snowboard was an all-terrain board, perfect for powder. After riding on powder for an hour, I rode down to an easier run, a wide, groomed, single black diamond. Half way down that run, I hit a small patch of ice and twisted awkwardly. I felt a crack in my left ankle and without falling, slowed to a stop. Still strapped into the bindings on my board, I stood there for a minute. I tested my left ankle by putting more weight on it to see if it hurt or if I was okay.

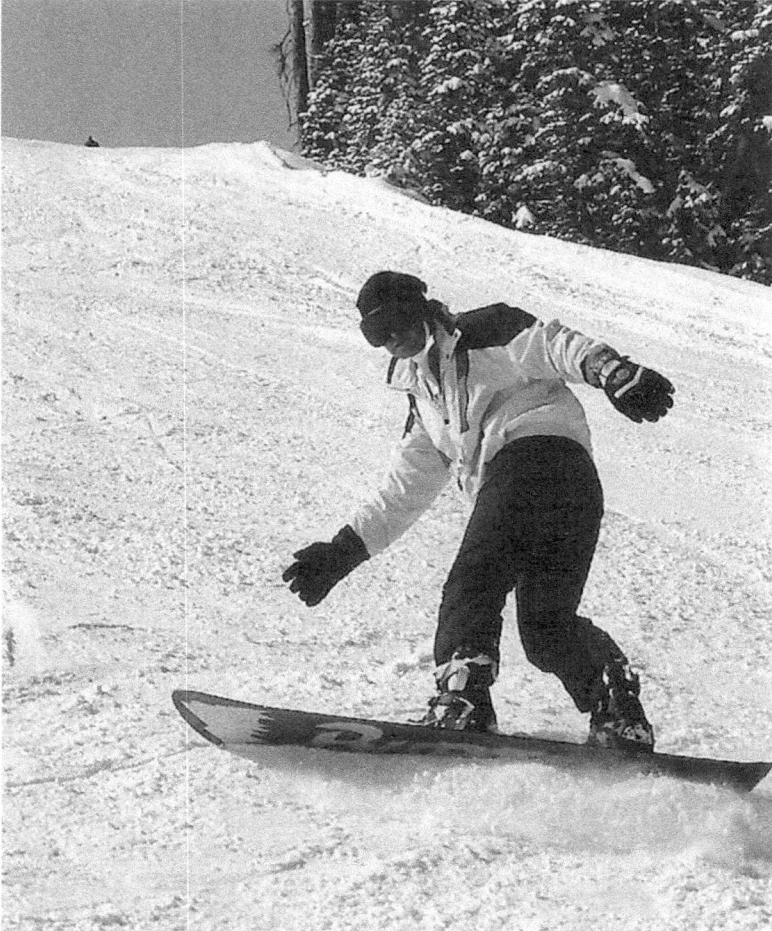

Picture 10, David, 1992, Snowmass, Colorado

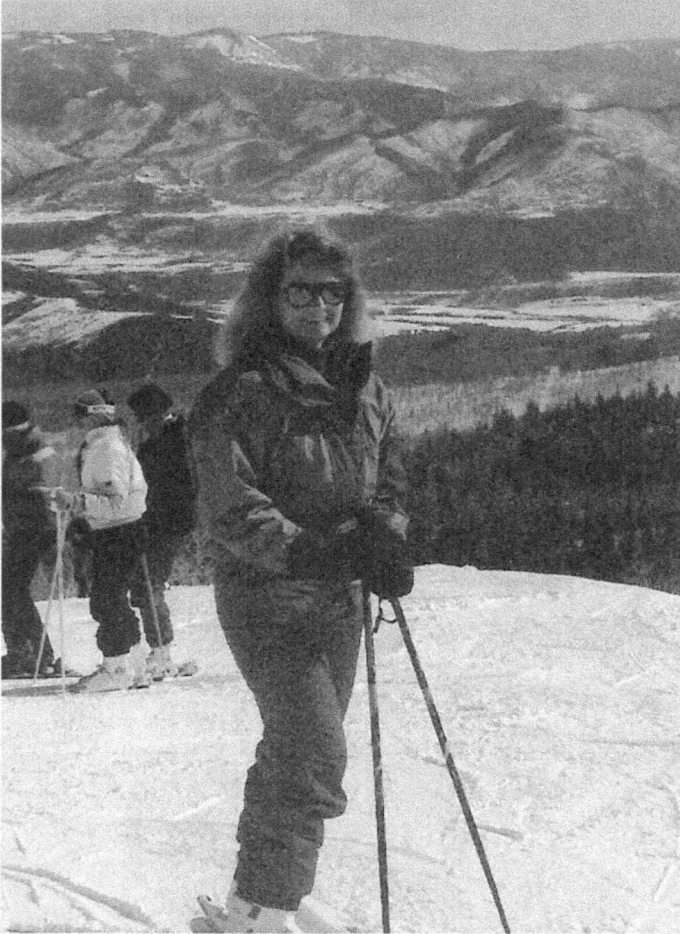

Picture 11, Tamera, 1992, Snowmass, Colorado

The pain was minimal, so I thought I might be okay and started down the hill again. Riding regular footed, I could turn to the left balancing on my heels. However, I could not turn to the right. Every time I tried it, the inside of my left ankle hurt. Still far up on the mountain slopes, I knew I could not make it down safely. If I tried, it would jeopardize the position and stability of a probable fracture in my left ankle. I flagged down another skier and asked him to call the ski patrol. That was the only time I have needed first aid from the ski patrol, and hopefully, it will be the last.

The ride down the slopes in a toboggan and then on the back of a snowmobile was comfortable but humbling. The ski resort emergency clinic x-rays showed a nondisplaced left ankle fracture on the inner side (medial malleolus). The fracture line started at the upper inside corner of the joint and went upwards at an angle of about 60 degrees, involving a larger than usual amount of the bone (medial tibia). I was relieved that the fracture was nondisplaced. By the time I called my wife, she had wondered what was taking me so long to get off the mountain.

Because my injury was a joint fracture, I expected bleeding and swelling in the joint. When the doctor wrote a prescription for Vicodin, I asked for milder narcotic pain pills instead, Tylenol #3 (codeine and acetaminophen). I was not having much pain. However, that night, despite the splint and elevation, the pain was excruciating. The pain pills helped some. Later, because elevation was not helping, the pain forced me to find better positions for the ankle. The higher I elevated my ankle, the worse the pain got. If I did not elevate it, it also hurt. If I hung it down, that also hurt. After struggling with it, one or two pillows of elevation seemed to be the best with the least amount of pain.

Still later that night, because the elastic bandage around the splint seemed tight, I asked my wife to loosen it. After she loosened it, I could move my toes better and was able to get some relief. I was fortunate that I had not covered up the pain more with Vicodin. A tight splint through the night would have created bigger problems in the muscles and surrounding soft tissues. I was able to reduce my use of Tylenol #3 the following day. After the first 24 hours, I did not need it at all. The pain and swelling stayed under control though I attended the rest of the medical conference on crutches. I became adept at using them. At the airports, I asked for a wheelchair to minimize swelling.

When back in my Riverside, California office, repeat x-rays showed that the fracture was still nondisplaced. I could move my ankle up and down half way without pain. I used a hard-plastic stirrup ankle brace (Aircast). The brace helped me avoid any twisting motions. I used partial weight bearing on crutches for the first 2 weeks. Then, I gradually progressed to full weight with the brace and crutches until the bone had healed, 5 weeks after the injury. Later, the joint space stayed normal on weight-bearing x-rays with no evidence of arthritis (no bone spur formation or joint space narrowing).

I continued to build flexibility, and then gradually I worked on the strength in my left ankle. Within 3 weeks, I was able to return to work, and I returned to the operating room in 6 weeks to do cases where I could sit. After 3 months, I could do surgeries that I needed to stand for. I did not do spine surgery cases with prolonged standing until 5 months after the injury. There was no continuing pain or swelling. I resumed full activity and regained full strength in my left ankle.

The experience allowed me to learn what being dependent on crutches is like. I learned how to safely negotiate stairs at home. For years afterwards, some of my patients reminded me of the time that I was on crutches. It gave me a bond with other patients on crutches that I had never felt before. When I was on crutches, I still remember how long the hallways at the hospital seemed. I learned how to wean myself off the crutches and limited activity enough that the pain and swelling stayed resolved during physical rehabilitation.

I made a full return to skiing and snowboarding. Then, in February 1994, less than 2 years after my left ankle fracture, I went heliboarding in Utah with Snowbird Powder Guides (Pictures 12 and 13). We wore transmitters, so they could find us if an avalanche occurred. The helicopter landed across the crest of a high, snow-covered mountain ridge on a small packed landing. Earlier, the helicopter had packed down the landing pad, about 8 feet long and 8 feet wide. Before we climbed out of the helicopter, the guides reminded us to keep our equipment on the east side of the ridge. If any of it slid down the west side, we would have had a long walk to retrieve it. They matched me with other skiers and boarders who had a similar ability level.

After each run, during the helicopter ride back up to the top of the ridge, we rehydrated with water and reenergized with trail mix and beef jerky. After a full day with seven long exhilarating runs in deep powder, I was tired but elated with the experience. My left ankle was fine, and my wife was thrilled when I returned to our condo without another injury. It was for me a fun, once-in-a-life-time, expensive opportunity. It was also a delightful reward for a full recovery.

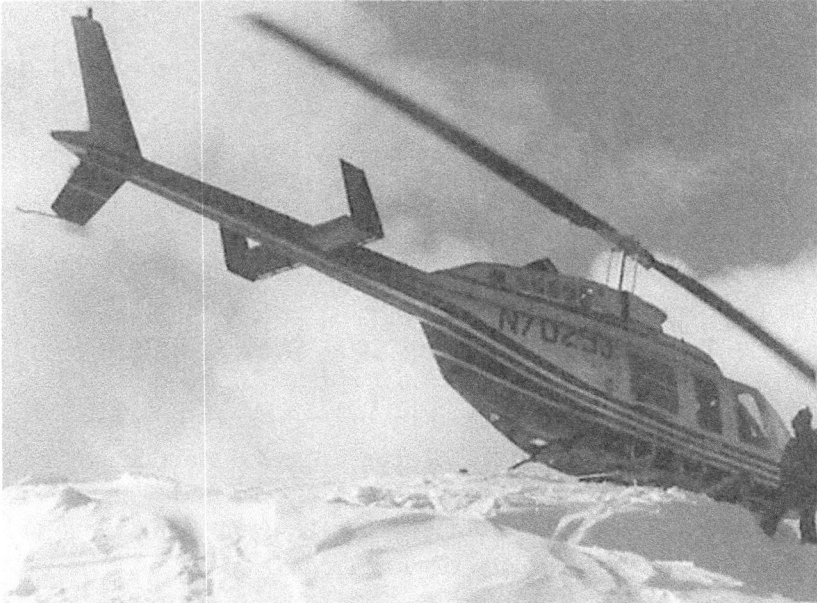

Picture 12, Heliboarding, 1994, Snowbird, Utah

Without a full recovery, persisting swelling creates many problems after an injury, fracture or surgery, especially in the legs. Both early and late manifestations of those problems are important to guard against. Early effects include pain, tingling (nerve irritation), numbness (neuritis), clots in the veins (phlebitis), poor healing of wounds (dehiscence), skin pressure spots, infection and poor fracture healing (delayed union). Late effects may include worse pain or pain variations like burning, varicose veins, chronic swelling (lymphedema), deep vein clots (deep vein thrombosis), discoloration of skin (stasis dermatitis with brawny pigmentation), chronic skin ulcerations (decubiti), lack of fracture bone healing (nonunion) and sometimes lethal clots extending to the lungs (pulmonary embolism). These examples are not a complete list.

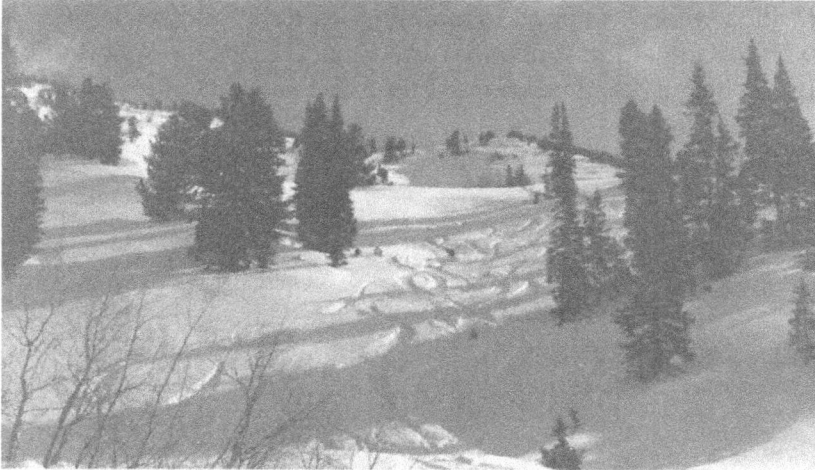

Picture 13, Heliboarding, 1994, Snowbird, Utah

Mechanical tools used by most orthopedic surgeons to prevent clots in the legs are an accepted basic practice and may include movement, activity, stockings and pneumatic intermittent compression devices. Surgery may limit the lethal effects of dangerous clots already formed (vena cava filters). Blood thinning medication may or may not be needed as determined by a physician in different settings. The risk of bleeding with blood thinning medications is real. We must use them with care and caution after discussing the benefits and risks with the patient.

Since the early 1990s, I have fostered many simple, finely tuned mechanical tools that help guard against the early and late problems caused by swelling. They do that by minimizing swelling. They help to prevent vein clots and other effects of swelling. We need to obtain the cooperation of the patient for all six of these tools. They are 1) reassurance, 2) education, 3) no prolonged positions, 4) get up early but keep it short, 5) use interval training to progress and 6) look for early warning signs to modify what the patient is doing. These tools are not empty buzz words or phrases. I have given each tool to

264

my patients and have had excellent results after taking time to explain them. Patients used them readily because they made sense to them.

Many physicians routinely overlook the first simple tool. Reassurance means that we should talk to patients early and give them something useful to do. They should move joints that we do not immobilize. Many multiple trauma patients are afraid to move anything until we tell them to move. The early reassurance to move parts that they can move is important. We should give it in the emergency room after the initial stabilization of a patient with multiple injuries.

Also, after surgery, the doctor should reassure the patient in the recovery room that movement is okay. We can do it as the patient is waking up, but we should reinforce it with specific postoperative orders. Though the patient may not remember it, a pattern is set for the nurses and the patient to follow. For example, after knee surgery, asking the patient to move their toes and ankles is a good idea. Also, after a doctor applies a long arm cast, they should encourage movement of the surrounding joints in the cast room, especially the fingers.

We should also use reassurance to help patients who already have blockage from clots in the veins or other consequences of swelling of the arms or legs. Taking the time to show the patient how to move is extremely important. It is important for the doctor to take time to discover with the patient ways to move while minimizing pain. Motion without pain is safer than thinning the blood with medication (anticoagulants). Movement and reassurance are natural. For most patients, if used early, they are better than medical and surgical prophylactic methods.

However, some patients with swelling need reassurance that anticoagulant medication or surgery is okay. They may have had previous vein clots or risk of artery clots (history of phlebitis, vein thrombosis, pulmonary embolism or arterial emboli). These patients have increased inherent risks. With some blood vessel clots, blood thinners decrease acute and chronic swelling, as well as other complications very, very effectively (heparin, warfarin or others). In the right settings, the benefits of the medications outweigh the risks of bleeding, nerve compression or other risks.

The second simple mechanical tool to minimize swelling is the education of the patient, so they know what helps and what does not help swelling. They need to know that walking farther and farther is not good, with or without leg swelling. Instead, we need to educate them about methods of active prevention that are as easy as frequent movement, stretching and elevation. Patients can do all these on any surface and in nearly any position. Frequent elevation for 10 minutes at a time is more effective than most of us realize. Frequent short walks may be okay. Ice does not help swelling from an injury after 48 hours, and ice will worsen the swelling associated with vein clots.

The third of the six tools, is to have patients avoid prolonged positions whether lying, sitting or standing. Though a recliner may be comfortable, drawbacks are real because of prolonged positions. Patients cannot easily turn on their sides in a recliner, so they tend to stay on their back. In a recliner, the pelvis is usually the lowest part of the body. Blood in the large veins can pool in the pelvic area and form dangerous, large clots. Prolonged positions are the enemy! Frequent, short use of a recliner is okay.

The fourth mechanical tool is to get the patient up as soon as possible after an injury, fracture or surgery, but they should not stay up. To avoid adding swelling and muscle tension, keeping it short at first is wise. Exceptions depend on the nature and site of the problem. By the physician making mobility orders clear, health care workers such as physical therapists and nurses, as well as family, can be on the same page. Giving them reasons and following up to make sure the orders are done, and not confused with the usual orders from another physician, is vitally important. For a patient with surgery on a hip fracture or a knee replacement, getting up the first time may be as little as a few seconds to a minute.

For the fifth tool, which is interval training for being upright, we must teach specifics. Both patients and their physicians tend to increase the upright duration too quickly.

Because it is human nature, I tend to do the same thing when I am recovering from an injury. It gets me into the same trouble as anyone else. Gradually increasing the frequency of being up, is safer than increasing the duration of being upright. If the frequency of being up has increased enough and cannot be realistically increased more, the next step is to decrease the frequency and lengthen the duration of the time up.

For example, when the frequency is 10 times per day, we can decrease it to 3 times per day. Then, the upright duration can increase from 10 seconds to 15 seconds. Never double the interval duration. Intervals can be in seconds or minutes. We know the interval training is working if the direction is right, if progress continues at a reasonable pace and if there are no early warning signs. If we are progressing upright duration quickly, watch out. We are an accident waiting to happen.

The sixth tool is looking for and avoiding early warning signs. They are much easier to ignore than pain. When found, we can use the warning signs to guide the modification of the upright activity. To modify, a good rule of thumb is to cut in half the duration of what we have been doing. Decreasing frequency alone is never enough to help. Do not give up and do nothing when the doctor allows upright activity.

I have successfully used the above simple mechanical prophylactic tools in many patients. They have eliminated or minimized swelling and its consequences. Though limited swelling is a normal early phase of healing, healing continues more effectively if we help swelling go away as quickly as possible. Swelling, like pain, is always a warning sign, and it is a fascinating miracle.

❧ *Chapter 27* ❧

What Gets in the Way of Recovery?

When we learn a principle that helps our pain, it does not change. But because we are human, we may forget. We face distractions, and we have weaknesses. If we forget what we have learned, our recovery will be slower. If we remember, we might not keep making the same mistakes. At first, we will not fully comprehend the diverse levels and intricacies of a principle. Our perception of it will change over time.

After we learn something that helps our pain such as lying down or taking a single, deep, cleansing breath, we should not minimize it even if it seems too simple or trivial. We should be excited with its possibilities. That will help us remember it, use it more often and use it more effectively. In addition to learning from our own experiences, we expand our horizons by learning from the experiences of others whom we trust.

The abilities of each patient vary for learning and remembering. I make a valiant effort to show patients each exercise I want them to do. I have them do each one before they leave the office. Few knee patients, coming back for a second visit could perform all 3 basic knee exercises that I had shown them. Patients usually did 1 or 2 of the 3 knee exercises correctly. Knee problems will be worse with exercises done in the wrong way. Exercise repetitions done correctly that hurt even slightly will also perpetuate knee pain. With repeat instructions or modifications to avoid pain, eventually 90 percent of patients do 3 knee exercises or modifications correctly without pain.

When patients do exercises before they leave the office, do them as soon as they get home and do small amounts often, they will usually remember all 3 basic knee exercises. A sheet of exercise instructions with pictures did not increase the number of exercises done correctly without pain. There was a need for individual modification after a trial period. Exercises on an instruction sheet may be okay for a patient with a normal knee but are not individualized enough for patients with painful knee problems. If any one of the exercises hurt, a patient will tend to avoid it and probably not remember it. We need to stop or modify exercises that hurt.

Exercises for the knee should feel good for both the knee and other parts of the body, including the back. Knee patients often have latent back problems. If we do an exercise that helps one area but hurts another, we will be spinning our wheels and get nowhere. Correction or modification of what the patient is doing at home is a normal part of the guidance they need with each follow-up office visit. Basic exercises are more important than higher levels of exercise. They form a foundation that we can use at all levels of recovery. They also build parts of the knee that take time to accumulate strength and endurance such as ligaments and joint surface cartilage.

The 3 basic knee exercises are a straight leg raise, knee-to-chest motion and quadriceps setting. I have already described the first two for back problems (pages 208–211). We can do the third exercise, quadriceps setting, from the same starting position as the straight leg raise. While sitting with the leg out straight in front and the heel resting on a flat surface, we tighten the muscle in front of the thigh (the quadriceps muscle). The muscle pulls the kneecap towards the hip and the knee joint moves down slightly (slight extension). When this exercise feels good, we can straighten the knee fully, which stretches the muscles in the back of the thigh (the hamstring muscles).

Since the quadriceps setting is the most basic of the 3 knee exercises, it is also the most important. It makes the quadriceps muscle contract and work. The straight leg raise also makes the quadriceps work, and orthopedic surgeons use it often. The knee-to-chest motion balances out the other 2 exercises by stretching out the quadriceps, keeping it from staying too tight. Without the knee-to-chest motion, the knee becomes limited due to chronic quadriceps tension and stiffness from unbalanced exercise.

The foundation of 3 basic knee exercises should extend from the beginning of knee rehabilitation to the end of it. We can add many exercises with or without physical therapy. We should do them less than what it takes to cause pain. Some patients will be able to tolerate all 3 basic knee exercises well from the beginning. However, most patients with knee problems will need modifications to keep the exercises from adding to pain. Changing positions is one of the easiest modifications. We can use sitting, standing or lying down positions for all 3 exercises. Slight changes in the degree of rotation of the hip is another easy modification.

If quadriceps setting causes pain or if the knee tends to go backwards, do the exercise with the whole leg on a flat surface with a small pillow under the knee. That will stop an overstretching of the ligaments in the back of the knee (hyperextension). If the patient cannot contract the muscle, trying to straighten both knees at the same time is helpful. Other variations for quadriceps setting are lying down on the side or even on the stomach. The degree of difficulty is different in each position and varies with the patient's specific knee problem. When doing an exercise, cracking or popping is not good. They are less of a warning sign than pain, but when noticed, we should modify or stop the exercise. It is damaging or at least irritating to the structures involved. If 1 or 2 of the 3 knee exercises still hurt or crack after all modifications, use only 1 or 2 of the 3 knee exercises at first.

Continuing to neglect quadriceps setting will set a patient up for ongoing problems with the knee. It does not matter whether the patient is recovering from a meniscus injury, knee ligament instability or total knee replacement. Without the quadriceps setting, the patient will not be able to use the normal knee locking mechanism and may not be able to fully straighten the knee. Locking the knee straight with good muscle control is a resting mechanism when we are active on our feet, standing or walking. Quadriceps setting also helps to maintain a full range of motion, control swelling and builds endurance. Without being able to lock the knee, a patient will develop a bent knee with tight ligaments in the back of the knee (flexion contracture). If you walk around for a few minutes keeping your knees slightly bent, you can experience what it feels like without the resting mechanism of locking the knee. It quickly does not feel good.

The 3 basic knee exercises should be progressed with the goal for each to become equal to the opposite normal knee. If a patient has no ability to do quadriceps setting, we should not increase the other 2 basic knee exercises. If all 3 basic knee exercises cannot be done well, other high-level exercises should not be added. If a patient is running and having pain but cannot do quadriceps setting, they have no foundation. They will struggle to improve and may add another injury. Another common knee exercise mistake is to bend and straighten the knee repetitiously with an ankle weight. That exercise may be okay for a normal knee, but it will wear out the joint surfaces of an injured knee.

After the physician makes a diagnosis, specific guidance in activity and exercise is imperative. If the patient is not improving after reevaluation, then guidance and monitoring by a physical therapist becomes necessary. Physical therapy can be a useful tool for many things and helps if a patient does not catch on to exercises or the use of crutches. It especially helps if a patient needs more attention for higher goals such as competitive sports. Direction and advice from a physician and the physical therapist should be consistent. They should communicate and resolve any discrepancies between them. If confusion remains, the advice of the physician should take precedence. Of course, another opinion is always an option. Regular communication between a physician and a physical therapist is always helpful.

Other issues can also get in the way of the patient remembering. A patient's pride about what they already know is one issue, especially if it includes forms of misinformation. A well-meaning family member, friend, magazine or another physician might add to the patient's confusion. If the treating physician does not address differences of opinion, confusion remains. Most patients and families need to hear the correct information repeated, so they will understand, retain and apply it well after a second or third visit.

Questions by patients often relate to the diagnosis. Some diagnoses are easier to understand than others. What the diagnosis is, what it means and why some activities will inhibit healing are great for discussion. We need to review the specifics of what patients are trying to do to help their recovery. The patient's questions are important. Patients should not be ashamed to ask questions that will allow them to hear things again that the treating doctor has already told them. We are all fallible. We need some repetition to learn, remember and apply what we learn.

It is well known by orthopedic surgeons that depression also gets in the way of recovery from injuries, surgery and chronic pain. Most orthopedic surgeons know better than to operate on a patient with severe depression. Those patients do not do well after surgery. In the face of depression, we should undertake surgery cautiously, only with clear indications and if there are no better options. Depression needs to be under reasonable control and stable according to the patient's family doctor or psychiatrist to expect a good surgical result. When depression is under control, recovery from injury or surgery and resolution of pain are easier.

Depression does not get in the way of recovery because of chemical imbalances in the brain. It directly gets in the way because of the choices a depressed patient tends to make. Their choices tend to lean toward immobility and inaction. The choices we make are huge influences in the recovery from pain, injury and surgery. When a depressed patient finally does move, they tend to move too far or too fast. They move impulsively, despite taking risks. Then, when recurrent pain occurs, there is reinjury. Because of failure and the recurrent pain, they go back to the same vicious cycle of inaction and immobility. That feeds into more pain, stiffness and the depressed patient's self-justification for not moving.

The way out of the vicious cycle is the opposite of moving too far or too fast. Patients should learn to move more often and in slow, small ways so they do not cause pain. They must learn to not be frustrated and start with small motions that feel okay. It may be our choices of inaction and immobility that contribute to the chemical imbalances of depression as opposed to the other way around. We often have more choices than we realize.

Chapter 27 - What Gets in the Way of Recovery?

As an orthopedic surgeon, not sweeping emotional difficulties under the carpet is important in dealing with depressed patients. We need to openly discuss objective observations. Depression is better dealt with and not ignored. Exposure to the light of day and learning what the problems are with open-ended questions such as "Why?" and "How?" are helpful to both the patient and the physician. Depending on the level of depression and the response, a family member, friend or professional needs to deal with persisting depression. Encouragement and support should emphasize options and teach consequences. Seriously depressed patients need professional psychological or psychiatric help. If they need psychotropic medication, a psychiatrist should be consulted.

There is always a chance to affect the choices and behavior of patients with depression with love. Family members and friends should not enable or condone bad behavior. In some situations, rewards could be beneficial to help change behavior. Bribes are, however, never appropriate. The difference between rewards and bribes is that rewards encourage but do not force better behavior. Bribes are an exploitation of power or a gift for evil. When a reward is offered and earned for good deeds, both the receiver and giver are uplifted. Forced behavior is only appropriate when the safety of the patient or those around them is in jeopardy.

A depressed patient otherwise retains a God given right to choose inaction or action. Our choices, however, always have consequences. That is fortunate because consequences are some of the ways we learn. Trying to force a depressed patient is like trying to force a horse refusing to drink water. Forcing a teenager to do something that they choose not to do is similar. It often does not end well. Explaining options and consequences while teaching with love is a better way.

Depression gets in the way of injury recovery and resolution of pain by diminishing hope. It also diminishes trust that our body will heal even if we do good things for it. Without hope or trust, a patient with depression may not move for extended periods of time. Depression, therefore, gets in the way of recovery because it affects critical choices of activity, mobility and immobility that we make minute to minute and hour to hour.

Besides forgetting and depression, many more things delay injury recovery and pain resolution. Numerous studies document that recovery is delayed in government entitlement programs such as Medicaid and Workers' Compensation. We see multiple reasons for this, including generous benefits, secondary gain, limited providers, rationing of resources and corruption. Many of the same problems interfere with other government health care systems, including Medicare, military medicine and Veterans Affairs (VA) health care. "Free" health care has no competition, and it always comes at a higher overall monetary cost. The cost may also be longer wait times, limited options, more missed diagnoses, ineffective treatments or other idiosyncrasies.

In 2015, my experience as a patient with Medicare was especially frustrating. I attempted to get Medicare to pay for the cholesterol/triglycerides (TG) and prostate specific antigen (PSA) screening lab tests I had done. Both lab tests are covered benefits according to the, "official U.S. government Medicare handbook," at the time.[88] I appealed to Medicare contractors twice and then had an Administrative Law Judge hearing. As Medicare requires, I also sent copies of everything to the lab company.

In 2016, after over a year of appeals, the lab company gave in to the bully Medicare system. The lab company reversed the charges for the lab tests, probably to keep me from appealing to Medicare again. Medicare paid nothing for those two "covered" tests. How does this encounter affect health care? Even though those tests are covered benefits, I am not sure I want to have those tests and go through that again. What kind of preventative government health care is that?

Is it surprising that Medicare has an appeals backlog? They do not want to solve it. We cannot motivate them to solve it. They claim that they need more resources, in other

---

[88] U.S. Department of Health and Human Services (HHS), Centers for Medicare and Medicaid Services (CMS), Medicare & You 2015, pages 44 and 55, CMS product No. 10050-02, September 2014.

words taxpayer's money, to staff the appeals that they, in effect, do not want to pay. Based on my experience with Medicare appeals and the experiences of others, Medicare is okay with a backlog and with not paying. The health care systems of U.S. and state governments will never be as efficient or as effective as private care. Why do we keep asking them to be? The U.S. Department of Health and Human Services (HHS) says that they cannot solve the Medicare appeals backlog even though U.S. District Judge James Boasberg in Washington, D.C. ordered them to do so.[89]

Protected by the federal government since 1973, HMO health care is an insurance product. Using HMO coverage can feel like the care is free, especially if the employer is paying most of the premium. A conflict of interest for prepaid HMO physicians is unavoidable. All the incentives are to offer less care. The less care they provide, the more money the doctor owners and company shareholders make. They profit by withholding care, which compromises optimal health care and recovery. HMOs are also a concern because of crowded facilities and their real propensity to keep office visits short and to delay surgery or other care.

HMO administrators nudge their doctors to do less. However, the same administrators often put pressure on nurses, nurse practitioners and physician assistants to do more than they are comfortable with. For years, HMOs, some hospitals and institutions have tended to hire "physician extenders," such as a podiatrist (DPM), nurse anesthetist (CRNA) and physician assistant (PA). They have less training and are less expensive than a medical doctor. An orthopedic surgeon, family doctor, internist, pediatrician and anesthesiologist, all of whom are medical doctors, have the best medical and surgical training and the most experience in their health-related fields.

HMOs, government and private health care insurance carriers are the proverbial bulls in the china shop. For those of

---

[89] Modern Healthcare, "HHS says it can't clear Medicare appeals backlog by 2021 deadline," by Maria Castellucci, March 8, 2017, www.modernhealthcare.com/article/20170308/NEWS/170309902/hhs-says-it-cant-clear-medicare-appeals-backlog-by-2021-deadline, accessed May 9, 2018.

you who are beholden to HMOs because of financial or other interests, I give you a challenge. If you think HMOs are so good, I challenge you and your lawmakers to put them on entirely equal footing with traditional health care insurance products. We will see what can happen with fair competition. HMOs might survive, but they would not be the driving force they are now, pushing us towards mediocrity and health care cost increases. Try moving with your HMO coverage to a part of the United States where they have no coverage. I do not think you will be very happy. "Free" health care is never free. It comes with false promises and a huge price tag for everyone because of inefficiency and corruption.

In the late 1980s, my orthopedic group had a fee-for-service contract with Kaiser, an HMO health plan, at a local community hospital. We learned a lot about HMO health care systems. We knew this would only be until they could staff a new Kaiser hospital they planned to build in Riverside, California. After it was built, we continued working at the new hospital for several years until they could recruit enough orthopedic surgeons. We enjoyed working with the Kaiser patients. While there, we noticed a few attributes of HMOs that are not widely known.

In the operating rooms of the new hospital in 1989, we learned about "Kaiser revenge" from the nurses. If a surgeon worked too fast or pushed the nurses too much, the unionized nursing staff used it as payback. To teach the surgeon a lesson, the nurses purposely slowed down the operating room turnover time for the next cases. It limited the number of cases we could do in a day for each operating room.

I was excited to see new, expensive orthopedic equipment in the new Kaiser hospital. However, finding all the pieces of equipment was difficult for the nurses and us because of inadequate storage. Over time, we noticed that the new equipment was also poorly maintained. At first, this was frustrating and puzzling. With more time, it became clear to me that the incentives were to do less and to put on a good face for public relations. Many HMO characteristics lowered the efficient use of their operating rooms.

An enormous help for all doctors to mitigate negative insurance and government influences, is taking time to do a good job the first time. Also, doing our work efficiently and having good peers to compare cases with are big helps. Reviewing x-rays or MRI scans with peers is another help. Assisting each other in surgery is also a significant safety net, where insurance coverage still allows equal peer assistants. Older and younger doctor partners often have different but helpful insights.

Impatience can easily reverse those positive influences and can be a stumbling block for doctors or patients. Impatience can tempt a doctor to operate too early. It maximizes risks and minimizes benefits. Impatience may also entice a patient to accept surgery too early. It can tempt a patient to do too much, too early in recovery phases leading to a slower recovery. A safe recovery from injuries commonly occurs in a hockey-stick-shaped pattern. That means that there should be no or little progress in activity levels initially for a period of weeks or months. Then, after staying within limits during an appropriate time, the recovery and activity levels can often speed up quickly at the end without repercussions. But remember that any level of recovery always carries a risk of reinjury.

Besides failing to remember, depression, "free" health care and impatience, many other impediments also slow down recovery. Common examples are abusive relationships with family or friends, unsupportive family circumstances, various emotional disorders and financial concerns. We should do the best we can with our circumstances. We cannot avoid some problems. To keep from repeating painful mistakes, we can learn as we go. Do not minimize a truth that seems small, whether it helps or hurts. The truth will not change. What we have learned is worth trying to remember, and if it helps, we need to remember to use it often.

Chapter 28

Can Knee Joint Cartilage Surfaces Heal?

A common sentiment in orthopedic surgery practices and training programs has been that knee joint cartilage surfaces do not heal (articular cartilage). Despite the voluminous amount of research in that area from 1980 to 2010, even with treatment that sentiment persists. In a 2010 article, the authors in a respected orthopedic journal explain, "Although most authors assume that traumatic articular cartilage lesions progress to arthritis, the true natural history of these lesions has not been formally studied and remains unknown." The natural history of a cartilage injury is what happens over time without treatment. The authors list factors for cartilage lesions developing into arthritis. The list includes size, location, presence of arthritis, status of the underlying bone, age, limb alignment, joint stability and body mass index (BMI). They also felt that significant injuries will progress to degenerative arthritis of the joint. They conclude, "Articular cartilage has limited, if any, capacity to heal and/or regenerate."[90]

The authors' list of factors is interesting because patients do not have much control over the items they list. An exception could be body mass index. For treatment options, they list surgical options. The authors do not explore nonoperative treatment or things controlled by the patient. Activity, inactivity, exercise and stretches are among the most important variables for early and late joint surface healing. In my office practice of orthopedic surgery, making a concerted effort to fine-tune these variables helped many patients. Patients often ask about other options they can control such as water intake and diet. However, those are miniscule factors for joint surface healing, unless grossly deficient. Orthopedic surgeons have become proficient with operative treatment.

---

[90] Marc R. Safran, M.D., Kenneth Seiber, M.D., "The Evidence for Surgical Repair of Articular Cartilage in the Knee," Journal of the American Academy of Orthopaedic Surgeons, May 2010, Volume 18, Issue 5, pages 259–266, journals.lww.com/jaaos/Fulltext/2010/05000/The_Evidence_for_Surgical_Repair_o f_Articular.2.aspx, accessed May 9, 2018.

Many have adopted a cursory approach for nonoperative care, which is poorly paid. This is a result of economic forces from several decades of abusive power by insurance companies, including federal and state governments.

Early joint surface damage of the kneecap, which includes softening, fissures and fragments, is a painful condition known as chondromalacia patella. It is common in young teenagers. Patients who take care of it well can be back to normal within 3 months without any long-term sequelae. Joint surface damage, however, progressing to more fissures, flaps, fragments and missing pieces in weight-bearing surfaces of the knee joint is worrisome in patients of all ages. Many in orthopedics think that some cartilage damage might heal, but if it heals, the surface is fibrous and less durable than normal. That in the minds of many rationalizes surgery for implanting joint surface cartilage grafts. They harvest cartilage grafts, with or without underlying bone, from other joint surfaces of the patient (autograft) or from cadavers (allograft). Cartilage surface grafts also result in joint surfaces that are less durable than normal. I saw no advantages but many disadvantages compared to better nonoperative care and other simpler arthroscopic procedures I was already using.

A knee joint has two types of cartilage. There is joint surface cartilage (articular cartilage). The other is meniscal cartilage on the inner and outer sides of the knee (fibrocartilage of the medial and lateral menisci). Since the 1970s, we have treated meniscus cartilage tears very well by knee arthroscopy. Since then, there have been many technical improvements in arthroscopy that allow its use in a wider array of problems. Yet for many orthopedic surgeons, operative and nonoperative solutions have been elusive for knee joint surface cartilage damage (chondromalacia and localized degenerative arthritis).

Arthroscopy has worked well for my patients with all types of significant, localized damage of knee joint surfaces. That includes joint surface fragmentation, from fissuring up to full-blown loss of cartilage with exposed and hardened bone in localized areas of the joint surfaces. Widespread joint surface loss of cartilage contributes to a narrow joint space on x-ray and a much greater risk of no improvement. I found 90 percent good to excellent end results if there was no joint space narrowing on a standing x-ray. A normal knee joint space on an x-ray is almost ¼ of an inch wide between the ends of the bone. It looks smooth and even (Picture 14).

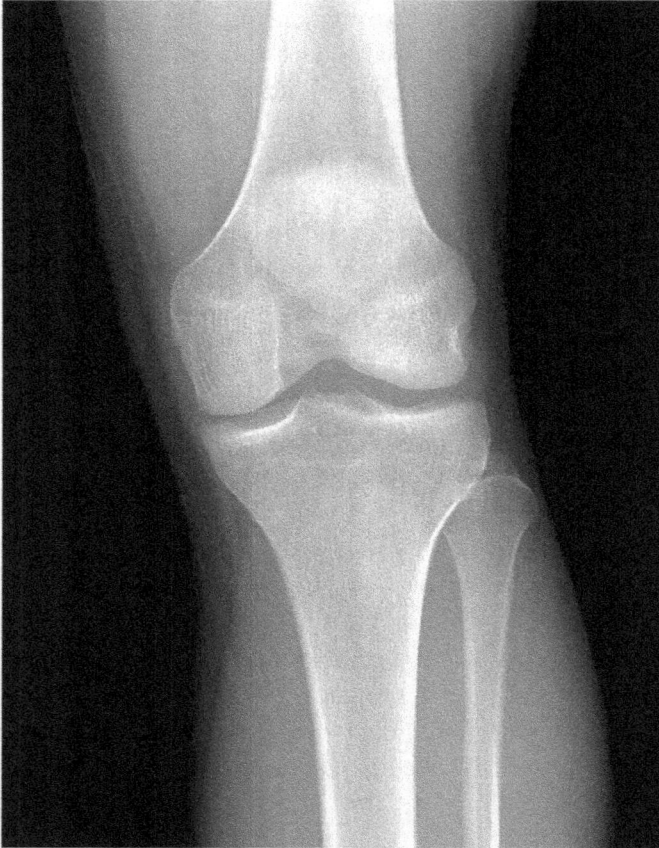

Picture 14, Normal joint space, left knee, front x-ray view (anterior posterior)

A knee with severe arthritis has complete joint space narrowing seen on standing x-rays with bone rubbing on bone. The bone is white, dense and thick, representing years of hardening. Most patients with no joint space will not improve because their knee is worn out and inflamed (osteoarthritis and synovitis). If they have persisting significant pain at an age of at least 55 and their weight is under control, they have the right indications for a total knee replacement.

Basic knee exercises before surgery will help them do better after surgery. The basic 3 are the straight leg raise, the knee-to-chest motion and the quadriceps setting, all discussed previously (pages 208–211 and pages 269–271). A patient should learn to do the quadriceps setting before and after their total knee replacement. After surgery, they will more easily progress to a straight leg raise and have good stability. With good flexibility and strength, forces at the joint are less and pain control is more consistent. When symptoms before surgery correspond to significant findings, total knee replacement has a high success rate of over 95 percent.

Patients who need a total knee replacement based on x-ray findings alone can occasionally have no pain. No pain is more likely if the patient is doing the 3 basic knee exercises or variations of them. If the pain is tolerable, giving it more time before surgery is always an option. Nevertheless, if more deformity develops in a patient with significant pain who waits too many years, the deformity can be harder to deal with. Also, a patient over the age of 90 who has accumulated greater limitations and disability in many parts of the body may not notice as much benefit from surgery.

The right exercises or arthroscopy may resolve pain and delay the need for total knee replacement. That is important because we are seeing younger patients with more joint surface damage from the risks they take with their knees. Choosing less risky activities, having proper training and equipment and avoiding obesity help avoid joint surface damage. A younger patient with a knee replacement will more likely wear it out and have a mechanical problem. A second total knee replacement for the same knee is a total knee revision. It is usually not as good as the first surgery. Though risks increase with each surgery, revisions can be very successful.

Early in my practice, experiences with three knee patients helped me establish methods for relieving pain and healing knee joint surfaces. I learned much from each of them.

The Miracle of Pain

The first patient was an 87-year-old female I treated in about 1985. She came to my office with severe left knee pain. She could barely move her knee. Though she was giving knee movement a good effort, it crunched audibly with small, short, painful, ratchet-like movements. She had no joint space on x-ray and the bone surfaces of the joint were dense and hard, suggesting it had been that way for years.

Even though this patient needed a total knee replacement, she would not accept it. Though I had not given arthroscopy to her as an option, she asked for it. Her family doctor had told her that she was not medically able to undergo a total knee replacement, but she could undergo outpatient arthroscopy. Fortunately, I listened to the patient and her doctor.

With arthroscopy, I found a large torn cartilage flap (posteromedial meniscus tear). The flap was very mobile. It was evident that the flap could have accounted for her symptoms. After I trimmed it out, very little meniscus remained at its attachment (meniscus rim). But then, no meniscus flap would get in her way. She had obvious severe arthritis. Her joint surfaces had widespread, worn, exposed, hardened bone.

Three days after surgery, at her first postoperative visit, the patient was jubilant. I had never seen an 80-plus-year-old patient so excited about the results of surgery. She said that her pain was gone as soon as she woke up from surgery. She was able to walk right away, which she had not been able to do for several weeks. Her swelling resolved. Her range of motion was smooth and without pain. She could also do the 3 basic knee exercises that she had not been able to do before surgery.

At later visits, she kept improving. Because she continued without pain, she did not need a knee replacement. The patient still had knee arthritis, but without the torn meniscus, she had no significant mechanical irritation or pain. I learned that having no knee pain with severe osteoarthritis was possible even after it had flared up. I also learned that meniscus tears as a mechanical knee irritant can be worse than the arthritis.

Another patient who influenced my thinking was a 14-year-old female. She came to my office with a history of pain in both knees for 4 months. She had seen another orthopedic surgeon in our community, whom I respected. He was in another orthopedic group that had signed a contract for many prepaid HMO patients 2 months before. He saw her a few weeks before she came to my office and gave her a diagnosis of chondromalacia patella, which is kneecap joint surface damage. He told her, "to live with it," according to her parents and that there was nothing he could do for her pain. Her parents felt that he did not want to spend the time it would take to help her. They came to my office for another opinion. The x-rays were normal and showed that the kneecaps were stable and centered in the groove in front of each knee (Pictures 15 and 16 are representative and not from this patient).

Patients with the diagnosis of chondromalacia patella have pain and sometimes grinding. They may have cartilage surface fissures, flaps on the kneecap joint surface or loose fragments in the joint cavity. If present, flaps can be the most irritating to the joint and the most limiting. Other associated variables are size of the flap, size of the abnormal area, duration and the patient's age. I explained the diagnosis to the 14-year-old girl and her parents. I told her what to do and what to not do. I told her it would take about 3 months. The exercises I gave the patient were the 3 basic knee exercises. This patient did not need surgery. She did the exercises and got over her pain within 2 months. She resumed her activities within 3 months and had no further difficulties. Most young patients with that diagnosis do not need surgery. That may be why my peer did not want to spend time with her.

The third patient was a 22-year-old male who had a slightly painful clunk every time he bent his knee. I could both hear and feel the clunk at the front of the knee with flexion or extension. With the clunk, the kneecap moved towards the outside of the knee, partially out of joint (lateral subluxation). The x-rays were normal. I felt it might be kneecap cartilage surface damage (chondromalacia patella). I also felt that it could be catching of joint soft tissue (synovial impingement).

The Miracle of Pain

He had an obvious mechanical problem. With arthroscopy, I found a large piece of joint surface cartilage that he had knocked off from the front outer side of the knee joint surface (anterolateral femoral condyle). The undersurface of the cartilage piece had no attached bone, so there was no bony fracture. That was why the x-rays were normal.

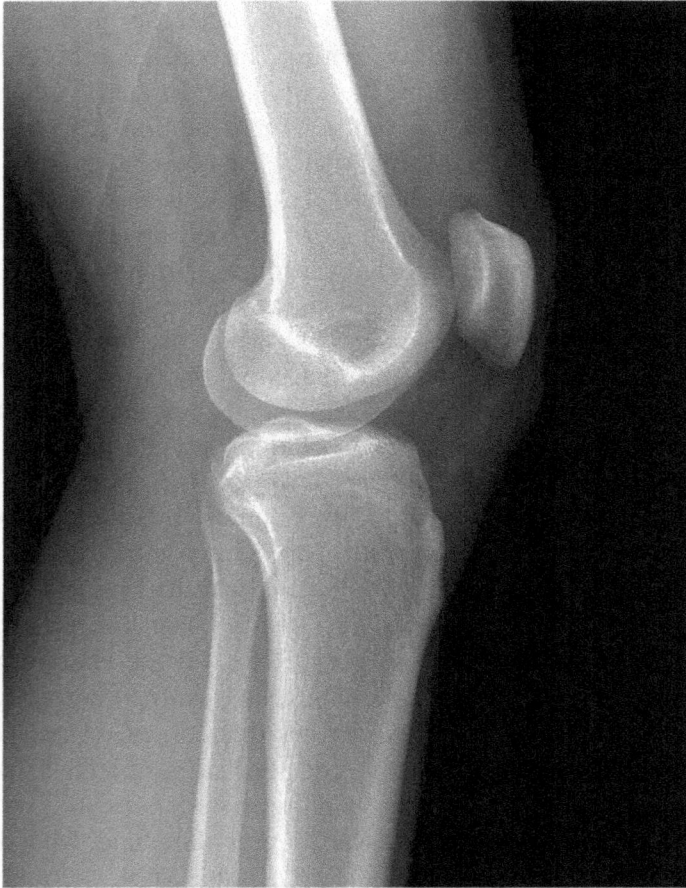

Picture 15, Normal joint space, left knee, side x-ray view (lateral)

His x-rays had also shown a normal alignment of the kneecap in its front groove. Therefore, I knew that the kneecap was in the right position with a straight knee and limited bending. His joint surface crater was 1 inch in diameter and nearly ¼ of an inch deep with a bony base that had minimal bleeding. The injury was recent with tiny, innumerable, bony points on a large, curved bony surface (subchondral bone). There was no indentation of the bone. The edges of the crater had sharp cartilage corners. The kneecap side of the joint surface was completely normal (patellar articular cartilage). Every time I moved his knee to an angle more than 30 degrees flexion, the kneecap ominously fell into the crater.

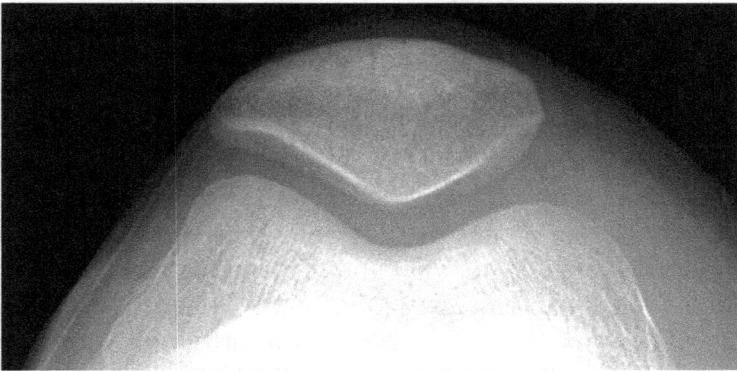

Picture 16, Normal joint space, left knee, Merchant x-ray view (axial)

Reattaching the large, curved, cartilage fragment to the bone surface would not likely heal without complications or the need for more surgery. By breaking it up, I removed it one piece at a time through the ⅜ inch incisions (arthroscopic portals). Taking out the cartilage fragment was disturbing. Then, as I moved the knee and kept a little pressure on the outer area of the kneecap, it stayed in its normal position out of the crater (normal tracking with anterolateral pressure). I used padding after surgery to keep light pressure on the outer area of the kneecap. I put the patient in a knee immobilizer brace, which keeps the knee fairly straight. I hoped that the padding and brace would keep the kneecap away from the joint surface crater while it filled in and healed.

After 6 weeks, I let the patient start to bend the knee. I showed him how to keep a little pressure with his hand on his kneecap to keep it from falling into the crater. Fortunately, the patient was consistent with his use of the pressure. Later, I let him use a patella stabilizer, a knee brace which allows some motion. At first, the body fills in the joint surface crater with a blood clot. It changes to fibrous connective tissue, and then it matures to a new fibrocartilage surface. Much later, it might mature to a more normal articular cartilage surface.

The patient had no persisting pain, kneecap clunking or episodes of the kneecap going out of joint. Within 5 months, he was back to full activity without any problems or limitations. At that time, I asked him to use the knee brace for another 3 months when he was active, to be on the safe side. At the follow-up visit a year after surgery, I wanted to see how well the joint surfaces had healed, so I asked him to accept another arthroscopy (second look arthroscopy). He declined and said that he was doing perfectly well with no limitations.

In the years after the three above patients, arthroscopy has been a valuable tool in young adult patients and older patients with some remaining joint space. It usually helps their pain and limitations. Before and after arthroscopic surgery, we should use the 3 basic knee exercises. Though they are easy for a normal knee, we must modify them to avoid pain in a knee with pain. With arthroscopy, I have seen adult patients of diverse ages who had joint surface cartilage fragments or flaps from many types of wear and tear changes. Some of these patients had a meniscus tear associated with the joint surface damage. When they have normal x-rays and MRI scans, their diagnosis before surgery is usually nonspecific (internal derangement). If I find significant joint surface cartilage fragments or flaps with arthroscopy, I add a diagnosis of chondromalacia. After trimming out fragments or flaps with arthroscopic instruments, patients usually did well. Because of the damaged knee joint surfaces that I saw, I often did not think they would do as well as they did.

Even in the worst of cases, improvement can often be made. In 2005, a 29-year-old female, who had prior knee surgery elsewhere, was having recurrent pain and cracking. She was the daughter of a judge and had very limited motion and function of the knee. Standing x-rays showed slight joint space narrowing. In surgery, I trimmed out extensive partially attached joint surface fragments as carefully as I could (arthroscopic debridement). The 124 arthroscopic photos I took during surgery broke a record in our surgery center. Half of them showed the residual joint surface after I did the best I could with it. She noticed an immediate improvement in her knee. Although the joint surfaces may be better, patients need to know that the surfaces are not normal after arthroscopy. Fortunately, she behaved herself. She did the recommended exercises and held back on activity. That was hard for her because, before surgery, she was very active despite pain.

It is important for patients to know the time it takes for joint surface healing. They should not expect it in 3 weeks, and they should not think that healing will take forever. It takes at least 3 months to heal joint cartilage surfaces after arthroscopy improves them. Patients need something to look forward to at the end of 3 months if they have been good to their knee. If there is disuse, healing will take longer and sometimes never happen. The healing of many joint surfaces in 3 months is realistic and based on my experience.

The quality of healing and the degree of pain relief depend on a lot of variables. How bad the joint surfaces were before and how bad they still are after treatment is part of it. What the patient learns, remembers and does is just as important. If done consistently and without pain, the basic 3 knee exercises are common denominators for patients who do well. The exercises are good for young and old knees. They help before and after surgery with few exceptions and are important for nonoperative knee treatment. A patient may not be able to do 1 or 2 of the 3 basic knee exercises. There may be muscle pain inhibition or simply incoordination.

A patient with a locked knee has a mechanical block, usually from a displaced meniscus tear. The knee is usually partially flexed at 5 to 30 degrees. They will need surgery. If they do at least part of the 3 knee exercises before surgery, they will do better after surgery. If they cannot do quadriceps setting at least partially before surgery, they will struggle to find it after surgery and some limited motion often remains. Without the normal locking function of quadriceps setting, patients tend to have a bent knee and poor quadriceps muscle strength. This combination is disabling, both for a young patient after knee meniscus surgery and for an older patient with a total knee replacement. It occurs because of stiffness, swelling and the lack of quadriceps muscle function.

We should emphasize, teach and monitor each of the 3 basic knee exercises or their modifications until the patient masters them. Patients and physical therapists tend to advance to higher levels of exercises too quickly. Then, the joint surfaces do not get the benefits of easy joint motion that help cartilage surfaces heal. Giving patients copies of the arthroscopic photos is not helpful because most have no idea what they are looking at. They often have wrong ideas thrown at them from family and friends.

On the other hand, a surgeon showing and explaining arthroscopic photos to the patient helps them. If they see how bad the joint surfaces are on photos before and after surgery, patient compliance with the exercises is better. With better compliance, the chances for resolving pain and healing joint surfaces are higher. The 3 knee exercises form a good foundation, and they also offer a good habit pattern for stretching in the future. With them, improvements in the joint surfaces can be sustained.

For patients who struggle with recovery after knee surgery, we can usually sort out the reasons with their help. If they stay upright too long, they cause increased or persisting swelling. Sometimes they forget 1 or more of the 3 basic knee exercises, causing muscle weakness and stiffness. Often, they do the exercises incorrectly. A common mistake is doing a higher-level knee extension exercise against gravity from a flexed-knee position. It is counterproductive, especially with any knee joint swelling, because swelling keeps the joint surfaces soft and susceptible to injury or overuse.

Repetitious bending and straightening of the knee often causes a knee to crack, pop or hurt. It tends to wear out joint surfaces. That motion causes more problems than it helps. It may be okay for a normal knee, but even a normal knee can crack with that type of movement. Cracking or popping are warning signs that we should not ignore. Feeling better soon after surgery easily tempts patients to do too much walking, running or exercise. Sometimes they do too much in spite of pain because they, "thought it would help."

During knee arthroscopy for joint surface lesions, surgeons should remove flaps, fragments and loose edges of craters with a mechanical shaver (arthroscopic chondral debridement). The surgeon should trim loose pieces down to a stable edge or base methodically. When done well, the craters are still there, but no loose edges or partially attached flap fragments remain. It requires common sense and judgment. Removing excess reactive soft tissue inside the joint is important (synovectomy for synovial impingement). Meticulous washing away of loose, floating cartilage fragments during and at the end of the procedure is also important (irrigation for a few pieces or many as in chondromatosis).

As important as surgery sometimes is, the 3 basic knee exercises before and after surgery are at least as important. They help diminish pain, swelling and stiffness. They give patients something to work on early and give them a foundation, so they can be ready for more later. They should not stop the exercises until at least a month after they are able to do the basic knee exercises as well as the normal side. That usually takes at least 3 months. If they think they can do them well earlier, I can often find subtle small differences between the two sides. After showing them the differences, patients can work on them to help the involved knee finish becoming more like the normal knee.

In other words, we should not gloss over the 3 knee exercises even when the patient is able to walk or run. The patient should build up to 10 repetitions at a time. Then they can gradually increase the frequency to every hour while awake. If they do the exercises 15 times per day, it would be 150 repetitions for each of the 3 exercises, or 450 total repetitions per day. At 1 second per repetition, that is a total investment of less than 8 minutes a day. It is usually very effective, but more repetitions are not helpful. Doing 2000 repetitions at a time causes other problems that would detract from what the joint surfaces need. They need an easy, small amount often. If an exercise contributes to pain, popping or cracking, we need to modify it or stop it.

Effective exercise modifications can avoid pain or add strength with the straight leg raise. They use a slightly bent knee, quick repetitions as fast as you can or a slightly outward turned knee and foot (external rotation). Turning the leg inward is not a good variation for biomechanical reasons. It tends to contribute to kneecap instability towards the outside of the knee. Adding 1 pound of ankle weight for a straight leg raise is okay when all the basic exercises are easy. Adding a pound each week, up to 5 pounds, is usually enough to reach full recovery. The amount of weight is not important, but the repetitions are important for healing joint surfaces. The goal is to help quadriceps muscle function become equal to the normal side without the exercises damaging or holding back the healing of the joint surfaces.

Without the foundation of 3 basic knee exercises, progression of other exercises is often more difficult. Using only 2 basic knee exercises is like trying to use a 3-legged stool that is missing a leg. The shortest time for joint surface healing is 3 months, but joint surfaces can continue improving to a lesser extent over another 6 to 9 months. During that time, decreasing to 3 to 8 exercise repetitions at a time 3 times a day for each of the 3 basic knee exercises is still helpful.

The most important exercise position to know and use is sitting because we find ourselves in that position so often. Exercises in the standing and lying down positions can also be effective. Patients, who are conscientious with basic knee exercises, usually experience a shorter recovery time than average. They also often have a greater amount of pain relief when joint surfaces are trying to heal.

Do Supplements or Placebos Help?

Confusion and misinformation is rampant regarding the value of herbal, nutritional, dietary or food supplements. In the United States, the effectiveness of these supplements is not regulated by the federal Food and Drug Administration (FDA). Since a 1994 law signed by President Clinton, the FDA states, "Unlike drug products that must be proven safe and effective for their intended use before marketing, there are no provisions in the law for FDA to 'approve' dietary supplements for safety or effectiveness before they reach the consumer."[91]

If a person is unwise enough to consume a supplement, eat alfalfa or swallow mega doses of vitamins, the FDA, in essence, wishes them "Good luck." After you notice a problem, the FDA encourages you or your health care provider to report it to them by phone or online. They keep records, but your concern does not mean that the FDA will do anything about it. They require a supplement to have a disclaimer in bold typeface on the label if a company markets it to affect the structure or function of the body. The required disclaimer for a supplement is, "This statement has not been evaluated by the FDA. This product is not intended to diagnose, treat, cure, or prevent any disease."[92]

Problems are widespread. Liver injury is increasing with the increase in herbal, dietary or nutritional supplement use in many countries with questionable purity and safety. In an 8-year prospective study reported in 2014, multi-ingredient supplements, marketed for many reasons, were the most common offenders, 58 of 130 liver injury cases. Anabolic steroids, marketed for muscle building, were the next most

---

[91] U.S. Food and Drug Administration, "Questions and Answers on Dietary Supplements... Who has the responsibility for ensuring that a dietary supplement is safe?" Dietary Supplement Health and Education Act of 1994 (DSHEA), www.fda.gov/Food/DietarySupplements/UsingDietarySupplements/ucm480069.htm #responsible, accessed May 9, 2018.
[92] U.S. Food and Drug Administration, "A Dietary Supplement Labeling Guide, Contains Nonbinding Recommendations," April 2005, Questions 45, 46 and 48, www.fda.gov/Food/GuidanceRegulation/GuidanceDocumentsRegulatoryInformatio n/DietarySupplements/ucm070613.htm#6-45, accessed May 9, 2018.

common, 45 of 130. Green tea extract (GTE) with various labeled claims also caused liver damage, 24 of 130. Other liver injuries were from OxyELITE Pro, used for weight loss or muscle building, 6 of 130. This last one is off market since late 2013. Of the 97 implicated supplements that were tested, evidence of GTE was found in 49. Of those 49, GTE was unlabeled in 29. Over a 10-year period from 2005 to 2014, the incidence of known supplement induced liver injury increased from 7 to 20 percent of toxic liver injuries.[93]

Those rates are likely to be low because some who take supplements even when asked, do not report that they take them. Further complicating the assessment of supplement adverse effects is that up to 32 percent of Chinese, Japanese and Indian traditional medicines have significant levels of contaminants, such as arsenic, mercury and lead. They also have adulterants, such as methyltestosterone and ephedrine, or unlabeled ingredients.[94] [95]

If a medical doctor recommends a medication and is diligent, they may tell us that excellent medical studies in respected medical journals support its use. We still need to listen carefully to the risks and benefits. We should express any concerns, especially if taking multiple medications or using supplements. There are many interactions. For treating a vitamin deficiency, which has very low vitamin blood levels, the recommended vitamin replacement should be a reasonable amount. Vitamin insufficiencies, which have borderline low blood levels, are much more common. Often, changes in the diet are enough to solve them.

---

[93] Victor J. Navarro, M.D., Ikhlas Khan, Ph.D., Einar Björnsson, M.D., Leonard B. Seeff, M.D., Jose Serrano, M.D., et al., "Liver Injury from Herbal and Dietary Supplements," January 2017, Hepatology, Volume 65, Number 1, pages 363–373, onlinelibrary.wiley.com/doi/10.1002/hep.28813/epdf, accessed May 9, 2018.

[94] Jonathan M. Fenkel, M.D., Victor J. Navarro, M.D., "Herbal and Dietary Supplement-Induced Liver Injury," Gastroenterology & Hepatology, October 2011, Volume 7, Issue 10, pages 695–696, www.ncbi.nlm.nih.gov/pmc/articles/PMC3265014/pdf/GH-07-695.pdf, accessed May 9, 2018.

[95] National Institutes of Health, "Ayurvedic Medicine: In Depth," January 2015, National Center for Complementary and Integrative Health, Publication D287, nccih.nih.gov/health/ayurveda/introduction.htm, accessed May 9, 2018.

For example, a vitamin D insufficiency can contribute to muscle pain, muscle tightness, weakness or spasticity. We can solve it with reasonable amounts of milk, other dairy products, salmon, dietary fat in addition to sunlight and less sunscreen. The skin produces vitamin D with ultraviolet radiation from the sun, though the amount it makes may not be enough in cloudy weather. Vitamin D is fat-soluble like vitamins A, E and K. We absorb them better with some fat or oil in our diet.

Similar to vitamins and minerals, our bodies require animal and vegetable oils in our diet. Our bodies do not make two essential fatty acids (EFA), alpha-linolenic acid (ALA) and linoleic acid (LA). Good sources are flax and sunflower seeds, beans, walnuts, other nuts, canola oil, safflower oil, other vegetable oils and green leafy vegetables. Longer chain fatty acid molecule derivatives that are helpful but less essential are in salmon and other oily fish, meat, poultry and eggs. Sources do not need to be expensive.

The term "essential oils" for aromatherapy and health issues is a misnomer because they are not essential for our diet or health. "Alternative" therapy advocates use the term "essential" because they use the "essence" of plant oils. Nothing about them is essential. An example is the oil in an orange peel. Their products are only an essence of plant oils. The marketing is therefore clearly deceptive.

If you and your doctor decide that you should take a medication or a supplement before honest studies, you become a guinea pig. That means your doctor, or whomever you allow to advise you, is making you an experiment. If someone is experimenting on you, after they have given you all the known pros and cons (full disclosure), they should get your permission (informed consent). There can be many unintended, unknown or poorly evaluated consequences. Many supplements have been so poorly studied that the provider or the patient often ask, "It couldn't hurt anything, right?" That rationalization is unwise. There are many adverse effects of supplements.

What do the terms "natural" and "organic" mean? The science of all substances in the universe is chemistry and all substances are chemicals. All chemicals are either inorganic or organic. Inorganic matter includes oxygen, carbon dioxide, carbonates, nitrates and granite. Organic compounds are hydrocarbons, such as propane, protein, vegetable oil, sugar or nylon. The FDA, "has considered the term 'natural' to mean nothing artificial or synthetic, including all color additives," but requested comments until May 2016. They will consider the need to make some related regulations.[96] The FDA, "does not regulate the use of the term 'organic' on food labels."[97]

There may be some merit to the term "organic" as defined by the U.S. Department of Agriculture since 1990, though the rules for growers and ranchers are complex. Better foods may be more expensive. But if foods are more expensive, it does not automatically make them better. The more processed a food product is, the more cautious we should be. If substances or foods are marketed as "natural," they may be suspect because no consistent definition is enforced.

In about 2002, a new patient came to my office. After my exam, I discussed the diagnosis and treatment with her. She asked if she should continue the medication her rheumatologist had given her. He recommended glucosamine and chondroitin sulfate. He said that the brand he had was, "the only kind that was effective." He had bottles of the supplement in his office, but they were not samples. He sold the supplement to her. Though she said it puzzled her when he acted like a salesman, she decided to try what he suggested. She tried the supplement for a month but did not notice a difference. She asked me, "Why would he do such a thing?" I told her to stop it. This new, shameless sales pitch stunned me. I had known this established, local medical doctor for years. That was a big change in his practice standards. After that, I did not refer any patients to him.

---

[96] U.S. Food and Drug Administration, "'Natural' on Food Labeling" www.fda.gov/food/guidanceregulation/guidancedocumentsregulatoryinformation/la belingnutrition/ucm456090.htm, accessed May 9, 2018.
[97] U.S. Food and Drug Administration, "Organic on Food Labels" www.fda.gov/food/labelingnutrition/ucm473870.htm, accessed May 9, 2018.

Doctors should recommend medications that have a high rate of success and few risks. They should not dispense or sell questionable drugs, supplements, "nutraceuticals" or other nefarious substances. Patients should always feel free to go to their own pharmacy. If doctors dispense medications, they should be well-studied and appropriate. They can be free samples, or they should be at a price comparable to local pharmacies. County medical societies and state medical boards have looked the other way, allowing dishonest behavior. It has stained all medical professionals. It puts me in the awkward position of answering a patient's valid questions about another doctor that are disturbing. Sometimes there is no good explanation. I must tell the patient that I do not know why the doctor did that, but it is not right.

Another new patient, in about 2007, came to my office with multiple aches and pains in her spine and extremities. When I asked her about medications, she denied taking any. Years before, I had learned to ask a follow-up question, "Do you take any supplements?" She hesitated, and then she acknowledged taking 11 different supplements, vitamins and herbs. After a normal exam and x-rays, I discussed with her my orthopedic diagnosis. I asked her why she was taking so many chemicals? Her answer to my question shocked me. After describing her persisting complaints to her doctor, who was not a medical doctor, she said that, "He told me to take more of the pills that I was already taking."

I asked her to do simple, appropriate things for her aches and pains such as rest and gave her specific instructions for movement. In addition, I asked her to get off all the supplements as soon as possible in the next 2 weeks. She came back in 3 weeks and told me that she was already doing better. At another visit 4 weeks later, she told me that I had "saved" her life. That might have been overdramatic. But while on the supplements, she remembers being in a frightening, downward vicious cycle.

When conspiracy exists between doctors, companies or governments there is dishonesty, corruption and abuse. Since the 1990s, examples of dishonesty are in all medical areas.

That includes the pharmaceutical, insurance, medical equipment and hospital industries and all levels of government, local, state and federal. Governments cite problems like drug abuse, obesity and high costs as an excuse to take over health care. They quickly blame others. They take no responsibility for the problems they have contributed to or created.

Many government entities in the United States have acted unwisely, contributing to dishonesty. We were told that with Obamacare, we would save money. We were also told that if we like our health care plan, we could keep it. If we do not expect truth and honesty in science, politics or advertising, health care will not improve. We should not give a platform or a microphone to dishonest persons, unless they have a change of heart. That means we must be honest and use discernment as we choose wisely.

When we more consistently look for honesty, we can detect what is true and what is not. Good judgment and wisdom follow, and we will understand each other better. Truth will expose lies or propaganda. Elitism is a deception of superiority. Founded in hate, it breeds bullying, statism, socialism, totalitarianism and brutality. Examples are in the Union of Soviet Socialist Republics (USSR) in the 1970s. Other examples are in Germany in the 1940s with the Nazi Party that called themselves the National Socialist German Workers' Party. Pride blinds elitists in any county, including the United States in this century. They are expert in deceiving others. With their intolerance and lawlessness, they may even deceive themselves.

In the socialist, communist Soviet Union, diet and training techniques for elite athletes were done very well during the cold war from the 1950s to the 1980s. In limited circles, athletes, elites and very important persons (VIPs) had access to the best health care available. The same health care and training was not available for most Russians, a common problem in many socialist countries. The totalitarian Soviet government at that time was using real science to gain athletic advantage. Honest scientific research helped Russian athletes to new highs in athletic performance over several decades.

However, in the United States, fads were distracting us. A common fad as late as the 1980s was withholding water from athletes during competition for fear of stomach cramps. Unfortunately, dehydration was the result, which led to leg cramps and greater problems with heat exhaustion and heat stroke. We have also endured ongoing obsessive fads with stimulants, hormones, diet pills, energy drinks and proteins. Some fads go away, but others hang on for years. When they crash and burn with problems, they usually go quietly. Fads come and go at a huge cost with lost time, injury and sometimes death. If something sounds too good to be true, consider the source and how much it costs. Is there any honest science behind it? Fads such as fen-phen, the diet pill combination, had their day in the spotlight because some people and some physicians allowed others to seduce them.[98]

Snake oil, in the American west of the 1800s, was expensive. It was claimed to "cure" everything. When the quackery was discovered, the promoters left town quickly and quietly. Many cultures and nations around the world are plagued with dishonest pseudoscience. We were all told for years that fish oil supplements would help a lot of things. I think we already know that fish is good to have in our diet. So, why do we have to take that knowledge to the extreme with fish oil supplements? One specific type of fish or fish oil is not important. A normal balanced diet will do more for the body than food supplements ever will.

Honest medical researchers evaluating medications, procedures or a device often use a placebo (sham). It is an inert control in an experiment. It helps them understand the effects of doing nothing, compared with the proposed treatment. A medication placebo is also known as a "sugar pill," but it can be any inert substance for research. Only a researcher knows who used the placebo and who used the experimental medication in a double-blind study. The patient and the treating physician do not know.

---

[98] The New York Times, "How Fen-Phen, A Diet 'Miracle,' Rose and Fell," Gina Kolata, September 23, 1997, www.nytimes.com/1997/09/23/science/how-fen-phen-a-diet-miracle-rose-and-fell.html?pagewanted=all, accessed May 9, 2018.

Among physicians and researchers, it is common knowledge that placebos will sometimes help. Occasionally they make a lasting difference. The average placebo success rate is about 20 to 30 percent in most experiments. Why does a placebo occasionally help? Many patients and physicians presume that the limited improvement with a placebo in a medical experiment is "mind over matter." Others might attribute faith or hope to significant improvements that occasionally accompany the use of a placebo.

Those are small things compared to a more prominent, straightforward influence that many of us overlook. When we buy something, we have a vested interest in its success. We have trusted someone enough to pay them money. We have given them some temporary confidence. We are going to hope and trust that it will help. Because of that, we will also, at least subconsciously, do more appropriate things with our activity level. We want to, "at least give it a chance." We may say to ourselves, "I am tired of hurting, so I'm going to give this a real, good try." Another justification is, "I do not want to do anything that would undo the good that this may do for me." We also do not want to look foolish after buying it.

We could, therefore, call the largest part of the placebo effect a buy-in bias. Our willingness and effort to do better puts all the variables in a position to help. It is what we should do in the first place. This easily accounts for most of the 20 to 30 percent improvement with a placebo. This bias incorporates a good attitude, consistency, appropriate behavior and avoiding risk. It includes an effort to, "give it a try." We can also use the attitude to give it a try without using a placebo.

For biomechanical reasons, other conditions may have a higher rate of spontaneous improvement than a placebo effect. This happens often with a total knee replacement surgery for the worst knee in a patient who has severe arthritis in both knees. After the first knee surgery, patients will usually notice improvement in both knees. Patients can put more weight with less pain on the operated side than they could before surgery. Because they can use the operated knee, it takes a significant amount of stress off the opposite knee.

Because the patient walks better, it improves their range of motion and helps the joint surfaces of the unoperated knee. This spontaneous lessening of pain for the unoperated knee is 80 percent. Many times, the improvement will last for years. Pain relief depends on the success of the surgery for the operated knee. "Mind over matter" is not the reason.

The above noted improvement is the first of two reasons not to have total knee replacements on both knees at the same time. The second reason is a significantly increased risk of dangerous clots. They can be in the legs or pelvis (deep vein thrombosis). Occasionally, lethal clots can extend to the lungs (pulmonary embolism). Even when both knees are worn out completely, with no joint space and bone rubbing on bone, we should not do both. Before we do a knee replacement on the opposite knee, there should be a waiting time of at least 3 months. If we see no sustained improvement in the unoperated knee after 3 months, then we can do the total knee replacement without increased risks. I respect the honesty of an orthopedic surgeon who recommends one knee replacement at a time.

Many use the words "alternative medicine" in an effort to legitimize their treatments. Others call these therapies "complementary health care." The words "complementary," "alternative" and "medicine" do not adequately describe the treatments, pills and supplements some are using. The words are misleading and give false hope. Instead, more accurate terms could be "substandard medicine," "marginal treatment," "non-medical care" and "suboptimal health guessing." Those terms would be much harder to advertise. Honest science has no tolerance for clandestine schemes in buying and selling. The potential for abuse becomes worse if religion or government is involved in the scheme. Truth, light and honesty will always eventually defeat deceit and darkness. We need to be willing to look for truth and speak more highly of honest practicing doctors that we find.

Honest science is the only way for meaningful discovery to occur. If medical science is not honest, it will take a long time to catch up to where it should be. Henry Ford, George Westinghouse and Philo T. Farnsworth are good examples of curious, honest scientific investigators. Though he was the inventor of television, Mr. Farnsworth (1906–1971) told his children that he did not want television in their intellectual diets. He did not want his children to be entertained or idle. Rather, he wanted them to be curious and active. He hoped they would learn by trying and learn from honest exploration of the world as he had done.[99]

We can be honest and expect honesty in others. Even under the best of circumstances, the government cannot and will not always protect us from dishonesty. Though enforcing laws will help a great deal, we must look for good sources to find honest information. We should not expect an advertised food supplement to cure what ails us. Why do we enrich dishonest purveyors of food supplements? Why do we trust labels and pills? How trustworthy is a source? Why are we allowing supplements to be untested and unsafe? To make a claim of benefit, companies or anyone selling a supplement should have the same burden of proof that any medicine or drug has. Only affecting structure or function is not a good reason to make exceptions.

Those selling herbal, dietary, nutritional or food supplements should have to prove to the FDA that each part is effective for whatever they claim and that it is safe. Otherwise, the FDA is spending our tax dollars to prove that a problem exists after companies have already sold the supplement in the marketplace. Unfortunately, liver and other severe toxicities will probably continue to increase until we change. To reverse this direction, we should be willing to pay for more time with our doctor, even if it is out of our own pocket, to take advantage of their expertise.

---

[99] Brigham Young High School, "Philo Taylor Farnsworth, Mathematician, Inventor, Father of Electronic Television," paragraph 13, www.byhigh.org/History/Farnsworth/PhiloT1924.html, accessed May 9, 2018.

Chapter 30

Good Tools and Their Misuse

Good tools to diminish pain are resting, position changes, movement, exercise, elevation, a brace, an elastic support, a heating pad, ice, medication, physical therapy, injections and a firm mattress. These are only a few examples, but each is something simple that we should consider using before surgery. Ice can help stop bleeding. A brace can help an injured muscle relax or support an injured joint. A heating pad can help a tight muscle relax. Medication can help stop the vicious cycle of pain and muscle spasm. Physical therapy can help resolve muscle spasm, stiffness, weakness and joint irritation. We can also use some of these tools after surgery. There are many good tools, but we should use them wisely. All can be misused, which turns them into bad tools. Good tools will have a high percentage of benefit with minimal risk. They have an excellent cost-benefit ratio.

It is common knowledge that a firm mattress tends to help us sleep better. What does a firm mattress do, and why is it a good tool? Many manufacturers and retailers pursue marketing fads such as pillow tops, conforming foam or "numbers." They make simple, inexpensive things that work into something that sounds better and is more expensive. Honest science to justify these marketing concepts is lacking. Trying to sleep and rest frustrates some patients so much that they tell me they tried lying down on the floor. It surprised them when they felt a lot better afterwards. What is it about a floor or a firm mattress that helps?

The answer is simple. We are not designed to lie in one position all night. Alcoholics find that out the hard way after passing out with binge drinking. When they wake up, they may find that their arm is numb or certain muscles do not work. With a prolonged position, circulation to a nerve was cut off, and the nerve was deadened (axonotmesis). The nerve had too much pressure on it for too long. If we are sedated or anesthetized in any way, we can create the same problem. Simply staying in one position too long can also do it and can create many other problems. With specific protections in surgery, patients can be okay for a limited time on an operating room table. We place supports and protective padding in locations away from nerves or other sensitive structures.

However, resting on a floor only helps because it is uncomfortable enough to make us turn more often. On any hard surface, we cannot stay in one position very long and will tend to toss and turn more often. We may not sleep soundly on a hard floor. We may feel like we are tossing and turning all night. Even if we stayed awake the whole night on a hard surface, our back or neck pain can often feel better in the morning. It does not work to continue sleeping on the floor because we will develop soreness in pressure point areas.

A firm mattress, firm enough to remind us to turn more often, will tend to have the same effect as a floor. It should be uncomfortable to stay in one position too long. With it, we develop a habit of tossing and turning more often. On a firm mattress, we may not sleep through the whole night. But our mind, muscles and body can feel rested and less pain. On any firm surface, another benefit is taking less energy to turn. It takes more energy to turn on a very soft surface. A cavity on the surface of a conforming mattress may contour perfectly to our body. But rolling up out of it, when we turn, is more work. Because we feel more resistance to turning, it is easier to stay in the same place. We should replace an old, sagging mattress for the same reason. If not replacing it, at least put a ⅜ inch thick plywood board under it.

Sleep studies show that a normal sleep pattern for most of us is to toss and turn all night long. Most of the time, we do not wake up when we turn. People who wake up with a kinked neck often say, "I must have slept hard and fast." Or, they may say, "I did not move much last night." Another common saying is, "I must have slept wrong," which has some truth to it. They probably did not turn enough. They may have used a position too long that they were not used to, such as lying on their stomach.

For those who experiment with sleeping on the floor, they should find comfortable pillows in assorted sizes. They may use several pillows for the head and legs to help create more positions to choose from. Because the floor is cooler, they should stay warm with plenty of blankets. Do not sleep on the floor every night. Remember, the purpose should be to try to change habits and learn to change positions more often in a normal bed. We can use similar efforts to get accustomed to a firmer mattress. There is a happy medium between the floor and a surface that is too soft. Very comfortable mattresses easily become a problem because we tend to turn less often.

Fads by mattress manufacturers are like practices in other industries that try to create new and more complicated things. The purpose is to increase prices and the profit margin. They de-emphasize or stop making good, standard, less expensive items that work. If computers can decrease in price, so can cars, prescription drugs and mattresses. We need ample competition, truth in advertising and no needless government interference. If state and federal governments will enforce laws equally, good things would happen quickly. A lack of competition and the presence of dishonesty and corruption will always compromise a free market.

For the head and neck, a pillow also needs to be firm enough to allow easy turning. But the pillow should not be so firm that it causes pain from pressure on the external ear. A contoured cervical pillow can sometimes feel extremely good initially. Because it inhibits turning, however, it quickly becomes counterproductive. For a problem with neck pain, we can collect pillows with different thicknesses from around the house. Then experiment with them for various positions. Ordinarily, a patient will need a slightly thicker pillow for sleeping on the side. No pillow under the head may work for sleeping on the stomach. For sleeping on the back, an average pillow thickness usually works well.

Patients should continue to experiment with varied positions, so they do not work themselves into a corner with fewer and fewer available sleeping positions. Some patients work themselves down to only one sleeping position. Worse, some are only able to sleep in a recliner. Both situations place them at high risk for stiffness, recurrent injury and an inability to improve their pain. We always need frequent position adjustments. Any sleeping position that feels good can be used frequently. Do not stay there, but come back to it often. If a sleeping position does not feel good, it should be modified, stopped or kept shorter so we feel no pain. If we cannot sleep on our stomach on a flat mattress, we can try sleeping on the stomach in several ways. One way is putting the front of our chest on a large pillow with our head on the downslope of the pillow's upper end. This position gives a slight amount of gravity traction for our head and neck. It can help resolve pain from spinal strains or degenerative disc disease if used for short intervals with other varied sleeping positions.

A few years ago, my wife and I went shopping for a new mattress and box springs. We compromised on a mildly firm set in a middle price range. It stayed firm for a few days before sizable indentations appeared in our normal sleeping positions. It took 10 years for the same depressions to develop in the old set that we had replaced. The new set was poorly made. We returned it and replaced it with a firmer mattress and box springs in a slightly higher price range. The choices for firm mattresses were limited. In contrast, numerous, expensive mattresses with "bells and whistles" had price tags of over $3000. In all industries, we sorely miss good basic tools that work when they are no longer available or changed to new, more expensive versions.

For most recoveries from pain, we need a variety of good tools. If we use only one good tool for pain, such as a firm mattress, a pillow or a heating pad, we neglect others. The patient is not paying attention to other things they should be doing and learning. If so, we easily become dependent on the one tool we are using. When a dependency develops, there is always a negative effect. It can be bursitis, muscle stiffness, muscle irritability, muscle weakness, muscle atrophy, limited or transient relief, diminishing benefit or chronic pain.

An example of dependency with a chronic low back sprain is using a low back brace for 24 hours a day (lumbosacral orthosis). The brace may feel good temporarily, but it will make the low back muscles stiffer and weaker. The patient becomes dependent upon the use of the brace to support their level of activity. That means that despite the use of the brace, relief of pain will be only partial or temporary. Pain will also tend to gradually return. A dependency means that the patient has misused the tool, and progress in the patient's recovery stops.

There are, however, other instances when a patient should wear a brace of the entire back 23 out of 24 hours per day. Under the watchful eye of an orthopedic surgeon, we use a custom back brace for scoliosis. The brace is a holding device for a young teenager to keep sideways curves of the entire spine from progressing. Before spinal maturity in a teenager, a curve more than 20 degrees on an upright x-ray is abnormal. A common form of it is idiopathic adolescent combined thoracic and lumbar scoliosis (Picture 17).

Using the brace for several years is very effective for scoliosis curves less than 40 degrees. It usually prevents a curve from increasing and prevents the need for surgery. When it is time to wean the patient off the brace, around the age of 17 to 18, the weaning should be done slowly in upright positions. The musculature of the spine redevelops with time. Braces or other treatment for scoliosis less than 20 degrees is unnecessary. If those patients have pain, something else is causing it, usually a back sprain (Picture 18). Curves less than 35 to 40 degrees do not hurt or get worse as an adult.

Medication for pain after an injury is another good tool if used as needed for a few days or maybe for a few weeks. We should only use medication to control pain that is not controllable with easy movement, rest and elevation. Rest means to stop the use of the injured body part, but it does not mean to stop movement if the movement helps pain. What is the difference between use and movement? If a patient is trying to get something done, it is use. We also refer to use as activities of daily living. A patient should try to move joints or muscles to test an injury, right after it happens, to see if they broke something. If nothing is broken, they may also move later to try to keep stiffness out. Movement that is helpful is not the same as use. Motion is helpful if the pain improves or if there is no pain at the time or afterwards.

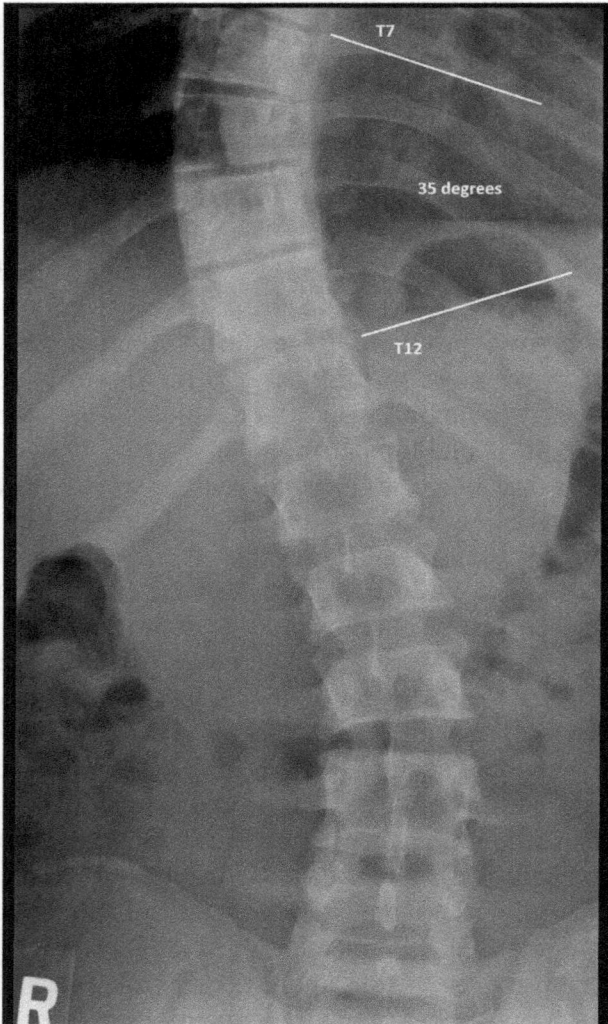

**Picture 17, Spinal scoliosis, front x-ray view,
right thoracic 35-degree curve**

We should stop pain medication as soon as possible, so we can better learn to use movement, rest and elevation as soon as they are effective. Prolonged use of pain medication leads to dependency. Dependency on pain pills is too common and is becoming more prevalent in our society. I have seen many patients with chronic pain from simple injuries that they and their physicians have mismanaged when using multiple medications, especially on Workers' Compensation. By continuing to blindly mask the pain, the patients never learn to deal with it appropriately.

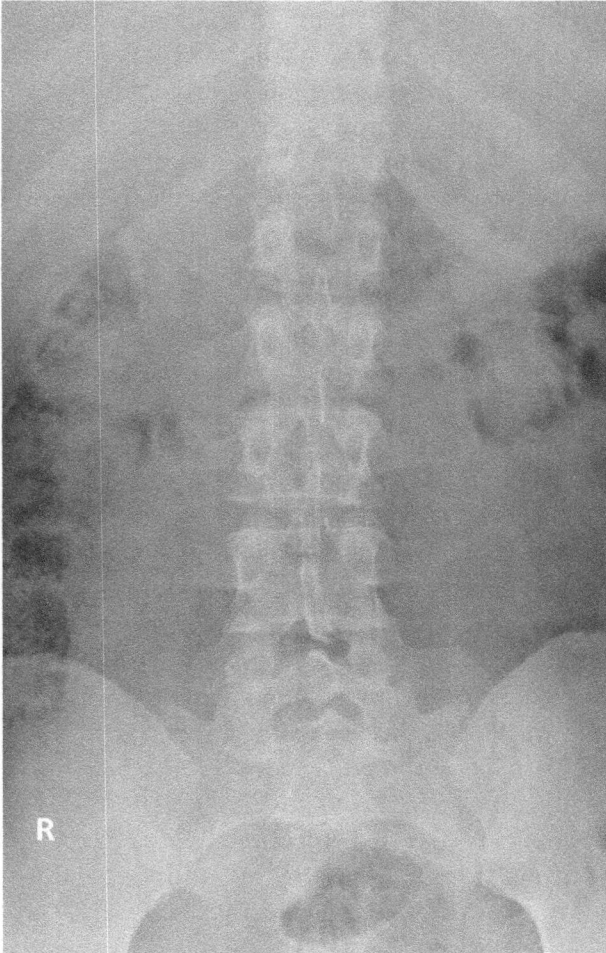

Picture 18, Normal spine, front x-ray view

Learning to deal with pain well becomes a necessity for complex injuries. A foot crush injury may or may not have broken bones, but it can develop chronic severe pain, swelling and stiffness. The sooner patients get off pain medicines after this injury, the better. Though it does not solve everything, they must learn from their mistakes. That allows the patient to make progress with relief of pain and stiffness. A doctor's efforts to get a patient off medication within a reasonable amount of time begins with early instructions. Patients should focus on things that contribute to pain relief and learn the things they should not be doing. That makes it easy for well-motivated patients to get off pain medication after injuries ahead of normal time frames. Even severe injuries may not have ongoing or recurrent pain. The longer a patient clings to a pain medication, the more likely they will become dependent on the medication.

Patients can also become dependent on other good tools such as physical therapy and injections. Physical therapy plays a vital role for many conditions. It can help dramatically in the right settings with attention to detail. The services of many physical therapists have helped the recovery for many of my patients. I value their observations and input if they pay attention to my diagnosis and the patient's descriptions of pain at each therapy visit. The pain should not be staying the same or getting worse with physical therapy. If so, we need to modify or stop it. Registered physical therapists avoid hanging on to patients, which helps to avoid dependency. They are well-trained and do not go beyond their expertise. We can say the same for well-trained, honest medical doctors.

One to three corticosteroid injections are other good tools in many areas of the body. However, we should use them one at a time, separated by at least a few weeks. If the beneficial effects of the first injection last less than 48 hours, a second injection carries increased risk with little added benefit. We should only do the second injection if the first was helpful and if its effects wore off after several days or weeks. We love to see benefits last longer than the effects of the medication. That shows that the first injection had a calming effect on the muscle, joint or bursa (an anti-inflammatory effect).

If we do a second injection and the response is no better than the first, then we should not do a third injection. We might consider a third injection if the benefits are longer with each injection. Just temporary relief of pain is not the goal. The goal is to resolve or lessen pain. Studying the effects of each injection gives essential information to the physician and the patient. The physician should ask and document if the patient felt relief of pain, where, how much and how long. With use of x-rays in an operating room, we should locate corticosteroid injections of the spine accurately (epidural space or facet joint injections). The internal injection site should be the suspected source of pain (a pain generator).

Though injections can give relief of pain and insight for diagnosis, they have risks. With one injection, the risk of an adverse effect is less than 1 percent. With three injections at the same location, the risks triple and the benefits diminish. Risks of more than three injections for recurrent, persisting or increased pain approach 50 percent. The risks include chronic pain, swelling, stiffness, muscle irritability or nerve irritation (neuritis). Scar tissue in muscles or around nerves from repeated use of needles is common. Temporary or permanent nerve damage from a needle can also occur, though it is rare (neurapraxia, axonotmesis or neurotmesis).

The misuse of good tools by patients or physicians accounts for some patients who do not do well. It can be corticosteroid injections, surgery or other established medical treatment. Some ask why they cannot continue receiving ongoing injections that give short-term relief. Think of what is happening to the poor, repeatedly injected muscle or joint. How would you like it if someone kept poking you with a needle? You would get irritated too. Injections, medications, surgery or physical therapy remain valuable tools when used wisely. They have good risk-benefit and cost-benefit ratios. Attention to detail by a physician and the patient during the exam and treatment give a 70 to 100 percent good end result for most orthopedic injuries and conditions.

What about marginal tools? Many different health care providers use tools in this category, such as spinal or pelvic adjustments. They include some medical doctors (M.D.), osteopathic doctors (D.O.), chiropractic doctors (D.C.) and some registered physical therapists (RPT). Marginal tools may help some people, but recurrent pain is common. They provide elements of truth that are often distorted. Misinformation often accompanies marginal tools and confuses the real issues. Patients never really know what is wrong or what to do to resolve the problem causing pain. Because there may be limited or temporary relief, patients can become dependent on the practitioner promoting these tools. Patients are distracted from what is really going on in the anatomy and physiology. Marginal tools delay an understandable and real diagnosis, delay better treatment and may occasionally cause harm.

Occasionally a patient would ask me, "Is chiropractic okay?" or "Is acupuncture or yoga okay?" At times, a friend had told them to try it, making it sound easy, simple and popular. At other times, the patient had already tried it before seeing me. For patients who ask, I tell them that there is a better way. It may take a few more minutes, but the time is well spent. It takes a little more work for me and the patient because they need to pay attention to their pain and learn along the way. The better way is more effective in the short term. In my experience, long-term recovery is more consistent and full.

Chiropractic and osteopathic adjustments often use the principle of stretching in the form of hands-on therapy (manual manipulation). It is a stretch done for the patient by assisting or forcing the stretch. The patient has little or no control over the stretch being done for them. That stops the learning process. Patients say that the practitioner tells them that their joints are "out of alignment." They said they, "put the joint back in." They tell the patient, "just come back when it goes out again."

If we stretch a muscle quickly, soon afterwards it tends to tighten back up. Therefore, the problem tends to come back easily. Manipulation may make the muscle relax, but the muscle is often irritated and occasionally injured. Although a friend may try to reproduce the joint or muscle manipulation for the patient, the results are no better. We can abort the whole recurrent vicious cycle by the patient learning how to stretch independently and more effectively. Getting good at it requires learning, practice and diligence. It is a better way. Some practitioners overutilize and overvalue overstretching, strengthening and popping. The same practitioners also tend to underutilize and undervalue frequent rest and simple stretching that does not hurt or pop.

Cracking or popping is common in joints, muscles and ligaments. It is a phenomenon that occurs normally and sometimes frequently. Most popping is benign. Many assume that cracking is a sign of arthritis. It can be but not usually. The problem is simpler than that. Like pain, popping is a warning sign, but it is not as big of a warning sign as pain. Popping in a muscle or joint is a sign of muscle or joint tightness. Muscles can be so tight that the muscle bundles pop over each other or bony prominences. They can make an audible noise similar to the string on a bow.

An exercise or movement that causes a pop, especially if done repeatedly, irritates the muscle, joint or ligament. The tension and popping will easily come back after a short period. Using a few, short, warm-up repetitions will often keep popping from occurring and from coming back. Then, the muscle has a chance to relax, and in time it redevelops normal tone. Without popping, the involved joint, muscle or ligament tends to have less irritation and less local swelling.

Cracking or popping can feel good temporarily. We may feel short-term decreased tension in the muscle or joint after the stretch. A person who feels a need to pop their finger knuckles has a pressure sensation or an aching that builds up in their finger joints. Knuckle popping is a self-limiting habit. A teenager who does it eventually figures out that popping their fingers only helps temporarily. After a while, it hurts to pop them. Likewise, a person who feels a need to pop their neck or back, often feels a pressure or pain that builds up and feeds into a habit pattern of purposely cracking those areas. They should stretch slower, easier, more often and warm up before stretching. The patient can then receive help from the stretch and avoid the pop, irritation and pressure buildup that follows.

Pain or pressure sensations can be subtle. They can resolve if the patient changes their habits to more appropriate stretching. Hyperflexibility movements, sudden movements and cracking are all irritating to the soft tissues and joints. Doing it right only takes a few more minutes each time, but better movements and habits are always worth it. That way the patient has control of the stretch, and they can continue learning what to do and what not to do. Full resolution of the popping and recurrent pain is much more likely.

When joints, muscles or ligaments crack, the problem is worse if a patient has pain or joint instability associated with it. The pain is often from small injuries of the muscle (strain or spasm) or from joint inflammation (synovitis). Joint instability is common with ligament tears in sports injuries. They may make a noise or a pop with the injury, but many do not.

Cracking of a tendon or a bone is also bad (crepitus). In a tendon, cracking is a sign of tendon lining inflammation, such as ankle tenosynovitis and shoulder subdeltoid bursitis. Cracking can also be a sign of swelling of the tendon itself, as in trigger finger and shoulder rotator cuff tendinitis. Cracking may also be degeneration of a tendon with or without calcium deposits, such as a rotator cuff tear and Achilles tendinosis. In a bone, cracking is one of the many signs of a broken bone.

Yoga is a highly marketed discipline with some truth to it. Stretching is good, but there is a better way to stretch. Overstretching, hyperflexibility and abnormal postures do not cure anything. They may give temporary relief, but they may also cause pain and reinjury. They may give a person a sense of well-being but do not help healing. Class settings induce peer pressure, adrenaline or endorphins. Patients often feel a sense of accomplishment and pride from hyperflexibility and abnormal positions. However, they serve no purpose in resolving pain or injury.

While listening to a Los Angeles, California KCET TV program on yoga for arthritis in August 2010, I shuddered. A yoga instructor, as well as several class members, repeated many times the slogan, "Yoga is my life!" There is more to life and exercise than yoga. Several class members said that they like to do some of the movements on and off during the day. Anything that motivates us to move and stretch more often and more appropriately is good. When a class adds misinformation, however, the exercise or the activity becomes a distraction. When patients develop a dependency, it stops or limits their progress. After a patient pays for a class, it is hard to be objective because of the buy-in bias.

Many tools have limited or no useful purpose. Two examples are rubbing compounds and magnets. The benefit of rubbing compounds is the rubbing, not the compound. Save your money because rubbing with soap, mineral oil or with nothing works just as well. Wrist magnets bear no relation to the magnetic fields of an MRI scan that are useful for testing and diagnosis. Wrist magnets also bear no relation to the low-level and specific magnetic fields of bone stimulators that have been scientifically well-established since the 1980s and are useful for healing chronic nonunions of bone. Wrist magnets are a scam.

With all the good tools available, we might think that the use of anything less than the best tools is nearly impossible. Seeing misuse of good tools in our high-tech society is disheartening. I saw many new patients who had persisting pain though they were dependent on multiple medications. I saw many, who had persisting pain after surgery elsewhere that should have alleviated their pain. Many of them had no idea how to use simple, good tools to help their recovery. Many others had persisting pain or became worse with repeated manual spinal manipulations, exercise overstretching, repeated acupuncture or injections.

Each tool or treatment we choose has varied levels of risks and benefits. It is tempting to misuse a good tool when we feel relief. Misuse of a good tool turns it into a bad tool. I hope for the day when patients use good sources, more common sense and good tools more consistently. If we are willing to learn, we can benefit from many, widely available, good tools and avoid dependency.

Chapter 31

Levels of Injury and Pain

A wide spectrum of musculoskeletal injury severity creates a variety of injury manifestations. Muscle strains and ligament sprains can vary from minimal grade I injuries to complete ruptures or grade III injuries. Ruptures cause a gap in the fibers or separation of the two broken ends under normal tension. Though we do not grade them in the same way, tendon injuries have the same wide spectrum of injury.

Various levels of injury apply to many structures, including bone, nerves and skin. For bone, the lowest injury levels are a stress fracture and a nondisplaced fracture. The fracture lines may or may not be visible on an x-ray, but the bone is still broken. It confuses some, and they ask, "Is it fractured or broken?" A fractured bone is the same as a broken bone. A stress fracture is overuse of one part of a bone over a period of weeks. It results in the bone structurally breaking down. Usually we do not see it on an x-ray, but pain occurs when the patient uses the bone. Nondisplaced fractures occur with an injury and are usually seen on an x-ray. Both stress fractures and nondisplaced fractures heal more readily than higher levels of bone injury if treated appropriately. They are stable because of an intact fibrous layer surrounding the bone (periosteum).

Greater forces produce higher levels of injury to bone causing deformity with angulation or displacement. There may be an obvious, unstable broken bone, which is more likely to need surgery. The highest energy levels of bone fractures cause a higher number of shattered pieces of bone and smaller fragments (comminution). An opening through the skin to a bone fracture is a compound fracture, or an open fracture. In other open fractures, a sharp bone fragment may come out through the skin. Open fractures take longer to heal than closed fractures. They have a risk of infection and are among the highest energy levels of bone injury.

Different energy levels of bone injury are like breaking a cookie with different amounts of force. The least amount of energy is breaking a cookie in half with your hands. At the other extreme, throwing a cookie hard against a wall will shatter it into many pieces. There may be so many pieces that putting it back together might be impossible even if you can find all the pieces. Midway between the two extremes is dropping a cookie. It may break into several pieces. Different types of cookies with the same force will break in diverse ways with different amounts of deformity. Similarly, various bones will break in different ways with the same force. However, the same part of a bone with the same force will break in a predictable pattern. To see this, you can snap brittle bread sticks in varied ways to produce transverse, oblique or spiral fractures.

A bone bruise at the knee is another low-energy injury, which may occur from running into something with your knee. Like a stress fracture, it has no displacement and is not seen on an x-ray. Stumbling while walking and twisting the foot is a low-energy injury and may cause a nondisplaced foot fracture. A fall onto the tailbone has a higher energy of injury and may cause a stable mildly displaced spinal compression fracture from the vertical forces on the spine. A fall from a single-story roof can create an unstable, displaced and angulated ankle fracture. High-energy forces with an automobile accident may cause the bone of the back to lose its shape with an unstable spinal burst fracture. This fracture can cause a paralysis of the legs from displacement of fracture fragments that damage the spinal cord (paraplegia).

Sports with high speed can produce elevated levels of injury when a mishap occurs. Each sport tends to have different injuries. We see motocross participants with serious displaced fractures while basketball players tend to have lower energy injuries. Higher levels of injury from automobile accidents may cause fractures of larger bones with multiple pieces, open fractures and multiple injuries (multiple trauma). Among the highest levels of bone injury energy are train wrecks and airplane crashes. They can produce crush injuries, complex open fractures and amputations.

Accidents with higher speed and greater mass create greater forces of deceleration. They tend to cause injuries over larger areas of the body. The energy level of injury and distribution area of the force determine the severity of injuries. When the area of the injury is more concentrated, the damage to a bone is greater with a greater number of small pieces. An elderly patient may fall and just break a wrist, but the forces can create so many small pieces in one area that we call it bone dust. It is an unstable fracture. In the same injury, if the energy is spread over the entire arm and shoulder, there may be no broken bones. Or, if there is a broken wrist, there will be fewer, larger pieces of bone, and it may be stable. In an automobile accident, the energy may be dissipated very effectively with functioning air bags. That patient may have widespread mild injuries but no broken bones.

Most bones will heal in 6 weeks if we immobilize them in a splint or a cast. The bone injury energy level and other attributes such as the size of the bone help us figure out how long a bone will take to heal. The healing response of each bone in the body is different. Each area of a bone is also different in how well it heals because of its blood supply anatomy and unique muscle forces. How we immobilize the bone will affect healing. A patient's activities of daily living that are too advanced may limit bone healing because of larger amounts of swelling and excessive stress on the bone.

An angled fracture in the hand at the base of the little finger or boxer's fracture takes only 3 weeks to heal solidly (distal fifth metacarpal fracture). It heals so quickly that if we need to improve the angle of the fracture, we should do it within 3 days of the injury (closed reduction under a local anesthetic). After it heals and the stiffness is gone, some angulation of that fracture does not impair function. However, a nondisplaced and non-angulated fracture of the same bone at the other end near the wrist will take 8 weeks to heal (proximal fifth metacarpal fracture).

We use surgery for some displaced fractures and all open fractures. What it takes to get every bone to heal in an acceptable position with good alignment is a little different. An orthopedic surgeon needs to repair displaced or angulated wrist fractures by manual manipulation (closed reduction). We do it with the help of a local anesthetic, intravenous sedation or general anesthetic. Some wrist fractures will need pins or a plate and screws in surgery to make and keep the correction. For an acceptable result, a displaced ankle fracture needs surgery with hardware, usually a plate and screws. We treat adult mid-thigh bone fractures best with a stainless steel or titanium metal rod. We push it down the bone marrow canal with locking screws across one or both ends of the rod (femoral shaft intramedullary rod dynamic or static fracture fixation). Hip fractures usually need a large compression screw and plate combination. For some hip fractures, we place multiple long screws through small incisions with x-ray control in the operating room.

Like the wide spectrum of injury levels, pain severity levels vary greatly in response to injury or disease. However, the same injury in different patients can have different amounts of pain. What the patient chooses to do or not do will directly affect the level of pain. Classic descriptions of pain are minimal, mild, moderate, moderately severe and severe. Occasionally, we substitute the term "slight" for mild. Sometimes we substitute the term "excruciating" for severe, along with many other descriptive terms for the same thing. The pain can be intermittent or constant. If constant, the pain intensity will vary with time. Pain may be increasing or decreasing in severity. It can be coming and going.

We can further clarify these terms for pain by describing the level of function or the lack of function. These insights are helpful, but different pain tolerances between patients limit their usefulness. Using the patient's words in describing the pain is more helpful. A patient's description of their pain, how often it is there, what affects it, their level of function and how they feel about it is a good start. An exact definition of what moderate pain consists of is not important. Patients may use many adjectives to describe pain. These words can give perspective to a doctor's exam. They help us know what is happening and what to do for the pain. Probing questions by a doctor, will often elucidate more characteristics of the pain than spontaneously described by the patient.

Because pain is a warning sign, we should never ignore a moderate pain, especially if it persists.

An ache may be increased pressure in a joint or a muscle. Aching might throb and can come and go. A pressure sensation may be more constant. Elevating the muscle or moving the joints early enough may be enough to resolve the pain. The longer a person waits to pay attention to pain, the more entrenched some of the problems become. Prolonged pressure can be from prolonged positions or tight muscles. Tingling is irritation of one or more nerves from prolonged pressure, which may cut off their blood supply. For stabbing pain or if the pain feels "like a nerve," it may be muscle spasticity in a small area of a muscle. In larger areas, muscle spasm may cause severe pain. A painful muscle cramp or "Charlie horse" is an involuntary spasm of an entire muscle.

Burning will occur in an area of a muscle that is subjected to prolonged pressure from swelling, tightness or stagnation of the veins (venous congestion). Blood flow congestion creates many problems because of stagnation of waste products from cell metabolism. When prolonged, it can irritate and then damage muscle in addition to all other soft tissues and bone. Eventually, it creates widespread subtle holes in bone (patchy disuse osteoporosis). If you have exercised "until it burns," it is the muscle that is burning. After stopping the exercise, the burning resolves in a few minutes with rest, movement and stretching.

It would be alarming if, after trying all the usual things, the burning did not go away in 20 minutes. Especially after an hour, most of us might become anxious. Then, our fear may increase, and we might think, "What if this never goes away?" Suppose the burning pain is still there a day or two later, despite your best efforts. Using ice will decrease blood flow and make the problems worse. Feeling constant burning symptoms is sobering. Many patients with chronic pain have constant burning pain for weeks or months at a time. Understandably, they get a little cranky, irritable and desperate. They cannot figure out what they should and should not be doing to decrease or resolve the burning pain.

At the other end of the pain level spectrum is the absence of pain for a period of minutes, hours, days or weeks. For patients with persisting pain, a helpful follow-up question is, "Have you had any periods of time without pain?" Another is, "What is your longest time without pain in the last 7 days?" Many patients struggle to answer these questions because they have not paid enough attention to the pain. Asking these questions will give them a chance to start figuring out the answers. Many say, "I am not sure if I have had any time without pain." Time without pain could be a few seconds or a few minutes. What they are doing when not having pain and what they just finished doing are important. By noticing and describing these periods without pain, the patient gives the physician a lot of help. By paying attention to pain, they can more often gradually have longer periods without pain. The principle is easy, but the application is difficult.

Things a patient can learn to do to lengthen out times without pain are critical for improvement and resolution of pain. They may be simple things such as being grateful for and appreciating the time without pain. Another, is recognizing trivial things that they can do without pain. Then, it becomes easier for the patient to identify things they are doing that bring the pain back. As a result, when they feel good, it is easier for patients to avoid doing too much. They can also avoid moving too far, too fast or too suddenly.

In 2001, the Joint Commission on Accreditation of Healthcare Organizations (JCAHO) that accredits United States hospitals mandated "pain management standards." When applied, the standards required hospital nursing staffs to monitor levels of pain by using a pain scale from 0 to 10. Zero is no pain and 10 is the most excruciating pain imaginable. For licensure, state governments require hospitals to receive an accreditation from the JCAHO based on complying with their requirements.

The intended result of the pain numbering standards by JCAHO was better communication with the patient. The unspoken objective was to gain power in health care. The unintended consequences are that the eyes, ears and judgment of nurses and doctors are less important. Nurses and doctors must focus on the numbers and may tend to listen to the patient less. They may also tend to look at the patient less because they have a number to deal with. To look past the obligatory numbers, it takes a diligent professional to hear and observe the patient while figuring out what needs to be done.

The required question a nurse or nursing assistant asks is, "What is your level of pain now on a scale from 0 to 10?" They record a number. If it is over a certain number, they must do something. That gives a manipulative patient a lot of power, especially those who are desperate to obtain opiate drugs. It gives the nurse and doctor, who have the patient's best interest at heart, less power. Unfortunately, the pain scale only helps when the pain is staying at the same level, which it rarely does. A patient may rate their pain at its worst, its best or its average without the nurse knowing.

A single number is meaningless, and two or three numbers is only slightly better. The pain number scale is too superficial. It does not address many painful experiences that come and go. Pain may vary day to day as well as minute to minute. The variation of pain is instructive, especially what makes it better and what makes it worse. Pain management standards were a response to bogus cries from some individuals of the, "widespread undertreatment of pain." In addressing that, the 2001 JCAHO pain standards may have inadvertently added to the opiate abuse problem. Since 2001, they mandated that all hospital patients be assessed for pain. In 2009, The Joint Commission felt compelled to subtly change the wording of their pain management standards to mandate that hospitals assess and manage a patient's pain. Among several revisions in January 2018, they mandate one treatment without drugs. They also want hospitals to facilitate referrals of opioid addicted patients to treatment programs.[100]

---

[100] "Joint Commission on Accreditation of Healthcare Organizations" was shortened in 2007 to The Joint Commission. David W. Baker, M.D., MPH, May 5, 2017, "The Joint Commission's Pain Standards: Origins and Evolution," Topics, Pain Management, https://www.jointcommission.org/topics/pain_management.aspx, accessed on May 9, 2018.

Pain standards have done nothing to slow the abuse of opioid prescription medications. With medical malpractice liability hanging over physicians, patients can often get whatever they want in the name of pain management. Making a verbal or written contract with a patient for the use of opiate medications and education have been touted as helpful. But they are of little help with a manipulative patient who knows what they want. Clinical "practice guidelines" and books for evidence-based medicine are of no help in a busy office or hospital practice. They give fodder to attorneys looking for variations. In orthopedics, nearly every patient we see has some variations. We find so many that books cannot list them all. Even the very large four-volume classic orthopedic surgery references do not cover all the problems we see.

Many patients describe their pain as constant because the pain is always there when they are upright. When lying down, however, they may experience no pain. Some patients only want to ignore their pain or cover it up. Many patients have given up trying to understand their pain or deal with it. A benign diagnosis gives hope. A malignant diagnosis of cancer helps understanding, thus giving hope as well. The pain level numbering requirement becomes a distraction from effective communication and, therefore, an accurate diagnosis. More important than pain scales are listening to and observing the patient, which give the health care professional many data points. The adage, "A picture is worth a thousand words," is true, but an evaluation by nurses or doctors are worth tens of thousands of words. Observations by family members may also be important. Diligent doctors consider all aspects when making decisions regarding a patient.

In determining a course of action or treatment, using a single number for a pain level at one point in time is useless. A single number for an average pain level for the past day or week is not any better. Treating a number is like treating an x-ray without paying attention to the patient. For example, one of my daughters was in labor with her fifth child. A nurse attending her asked for a pain number on a scale of 0 to 10. She had already endured labor pains with the births of her other four children. Even with my daughter's experience, she told me, "I didn't know what to tell them!" My daughter continued, "It was like they didn't know it would go away and would be worse with the next contraction."

Using one or two numbers for a pain level is like being lost in a forest on a moonless night without a compass. A lack of direction is scary. It becomes more frightening with fewer resources. In a forest during the daytime, you may have the sun to help give direction. Without the sun, you may have moss on the north side of some trees. With a compass, the direction is clear though there may still be cliffs, streams and other obstacles to negotiate. With a compass, experience and a map, a challenging path becomes easier to finish safely. A conscientious doctor has many resources to help a patient safely navigate away from pain.

Even if the patient rates the pain for the best and the worst pain, it does not communicate a picture. When a nurse communicates a number from the 0 to 10 pain scale, a good doctor will not ignore the information. They will use it in conjunction with better, more useful information. Doctors must ask patients, or nurses who call them, questions to elicit the nature, frequency, duration, cause and intensity of pain. Understanding well by listening and spending time with the patient are necessary for better treatment.

Attorneys, lawsuits and governments will never solve the problems they have created in health care over the past few decades. In Medicare, Veterans Affairs health care and in the rest of the medical industry, they need to get out of the way. A change in leadership can change health care benefits quickly. Benefits should allow more time, not less, with the doctor determined by the patient and the doctor. The medical profession does not need more regulation, practice standards or other fads. They should be paid fairly for what they do and the time they spend with patients. We need good, honest, elected representatives who will stay that way. We also need good, honest, diligent doctors who will stay that way in spite of abnormal economic, legal and illegal forces.

Chapter 32

Phantom Pain and More

Phantom sensations and phantom pain are common in amputees. They remind patients of the body part they have lost, such as an amputated foot or leg. After the amputation stump skin has healed, persisting phantom pain is an abnormal pain syndrome. It usually improves gradually over a period of months or years. The pain can be disturbing, uncomfortable and sometimes severe. Phantom pain can be chronic pain and can have associated disability. It has components of reflex sympathetic dystrophy with pain that is out of proportion to what we would normally expect for an amputation. There can also be nerve injuries associated with phantom pain. There may be stiffness, muscle spasm or muscle atrophy.

In 2008, Trevor Smith, a 21-year-old patient came to my office for a new appointment after having a below the knee amputation at a university teaching hospital in California. The amputation 4 months before was for an unsalvageable lower leg after multiple severe injuries from a motor vehicle accident. After surgery, the skin had healed well. They taught him how to use his leg prosthesis, which extended above the knee. He was walking on it, but he was not doing well despite the well-fitted prosthesis and physical therapy.

Trevor was having excruciating pain and severe itching in his stump, knee and thigh. The patient also told me that he had recurrent "bubbles" under the skin in the back of his knee that occasionally drained a water-like fluid. He said he tried to be more active on his prosthetic leg. He was doing what his surgeon and physical therapist told him to do. The patient and his family felt that things were getting worse and came to me looking for better answers.

When I entered the exam room, his leg prosthesis was already off. The inner liner, a removable micro-foam layer under the prosthesis, was still on his stump. The liner went from the end of his stump, 6 inches below the knee, up to the mid-thigh. When I asked him to take it off, he said that he was uncomfortable taking it off because the air bothered it. After I insisted, he hesitated but then took the liner off. Under the liner, his skin was wrinkled and an odd white color. Prolonged moisture had damaged his skin, which is skin maceration.

I could feel a soft 2-inch diameter fluid filled pocket under the skin at the back of his knee (soft-tissue effusion). It was not tender, and he did not have skin blisters. There was no open wound or drainage. There was no Baker's cyst. The stump was a normal length and shape. With his prosthetic liner off, the patient tended to rub his knee and upper thigh. He did it more often and repetitiously than when the liner was on. But he refused to touch his leg stump below the knee. He was hesitant to move the knee of his amputated leg. When I reached to touch the end of his stump, he reflexively jerked his whole leg away. He had a facial expression of fear.

When I asked Trevor to put the foam liner back on, he did it quickly and easily. He then again repetitively rubbed his knee, front and back. He said it itched. With the liner on, I asked the patient to touch the amputated stump below the knee, but he would not do it. He did not hesitate to move the knee fully in the liner. He had no trouble putting his prosthetic leg back on over the liner. Though he had a moderate limp, he was able to walk on his prosthesis. On x-ray, there was nothing remarkable. Nevertheless, he was going in the wrong direction, 180 degrees opposite from the direction he should have been going. Despite his young age, his soft tissues and muscles were breaking down.

Trevor was in a downward vicious cycle with no healing. By his history, the downward spiral was there for the last 2 months. He was otherwise healthy. He should have been healing, maturing and toughening the stump of his amputated leg. He was trying but getting nowhere. He was having soft-tissue complications, and soon the bone would atrophy as well. These were consequences of the choices the patient was making. His therapist and doctor encouraged him to use his stump and prosthesis. That should have been with the caveat of not getting into trouble.

The patient was overusing his amputated stump more than it was ready for. At the same time, he was underusing it in ways that were basic, simple and effective. The overuse and underuse combination in a patient is classic disuse. With more time in the wrong direction, the leg stump would become even less usable. I explained to the patient and his family what he should do and what he should not do. I told him to use crutches and keep his leg prosthesis off until I would tell him to start again. He was to taper off use of the prosthetic liner gradually and progressively, so he could allow the skin to air out and heal. He was not to flex his knee more than 45 degrees with the liner on. The liner was putting pressure on the soft tissues at the back of the knee, causing recurrent soft-tissue damage and fluid collections.

I gave him quadriceps and hamstring exercises, emphasizing the quadriceps. I also gave him instructions for holding his amputated stump with his hands. That included the end of his stump when he had the liner on. The patient was to avoid any repetitious rubbing, with or without the liner. He could hold all areas of his leg with his hands to help the itching. He was not to use his fingertips or fingernails. Instead, for holding, he was to use both hands together with all fingers without any rubbing motions.

When Trevor returned in 2 weeks, for the first time in months, he was doing better. I allowed him to resume limited rubbing motions if it was random, generalized and with both hands. He was to keep it short, less than 1 minute at a time. He was to use the prosthetic liner less than 30 minutes at a time. That would allow the skin to heal faster and keep the pressure off the back of the knee. Improving slowly in the right direction was thrilling for him. He had, however, no confidence that he could keep going in the right direction.

After more follow-up visits, the itching was gone. The soft-tissue fluid accumulations and the pain were gone. Trevor could hold the end of his stump with the prosthetic liner off. He was also able to properly hold and rub his leg without traumatizing it. I had not yet allowed him to use his prosthetic leg. So, he was still on crutches. I held him back from using the leg prosthesis to allow his stump soft tissues to mature and toughen in other critical ways. After 3 months, he was using his prosthesis for 60-minute intervals and had no recurrent itching, pain, swelling or fluid accumulations.

After 6 months, he was using the prosthesis for 2 hours at a time and was walking without crutches or a limp. His limits changed as all the structures in his stump and knee matured. The patient continued to go in the right direction. Full use of a leg prosthesis is realistic if a patient keeps heading in the right direction without damaging the soft tissues. That will happen if they stay within the training limits of skin, muscles and other soft tissues. Those limits are a moving target as they improve. We all have different limits. To stay within our physical limits when recovering, common sense plays a significant role. Overdoing use or activity is very easy and tempting to do.

At the worst part of Trevor's course, he was having phantom pain, nerve pain, muscle pain, muscle spasm, soft-tissue pain, skin pain and severe itching. The poor condition of his amputated limb was unusual with his age and otherwise good health. It took patience, time and both of us working together to get him over his terrifying experience. It also took spending a lot of uncompensated time with him at each visit. I did it willingly because of what I was learning with him. In retrospect, what the patient needed seems obvious.

His prior physicians took an easy path. They told Trevor to toughen the lower extremity and to use it more, and things will "work out." With that approach, some patients will eventually self-regulate and may gradually improve. However, the advice was 180 degrees different from what he needed. Whether the patient has an HMO or not, this pattern is all too common with many physicians who deal with HMOs. They are often in a hurry and do not take the time to listen to patients or explain things as they should. HMO groups also force their doctors to delegate patients to "physician extenders" who are not medical doctors.

Several physicians have told me that they always treat their HMO patients as well as their private patients. That sounds good and even admirable. However, economic realities are always present. What they do not say is that they make visits with their private patients quicker. Therefore, the visits are the same hurried, mediocre visits with all their patients. Similar economic forces also push doctor visits with PPO, Medicare and other insurance coverage in the same direction. The patient and therapist can also be in a hurry. The lack of attention to detail and what happened to Trevor are from, what I call, HMO mentality. Patients often do not know what to do and what not to do when they leave the doctor's office.

Many physicians do not take the time to explain things as well as they should. In time, their ability to explain things lessens. HMO insurance coverage has a dumbing down effect on the treatment offered by physicians. Innovative treatment is quashed with policy, "practice guidelines," time constraints and lists of "approved drugs" (formularies). High-tech toys such as electronic medical records (EMR) become a public relations marketing tool for some practice groups instead of real innovation. Electronic records can often be voluminous, distracting, disorganized and cumbersome to use, read and understand. The best innovation for standards of practice or the development of EMR comes without health plan or government mandates.

Most of the many electronic medical records I have reviewed over many years have many tiny details to allow a billing code for higher reimbursement. However, the detail of what the patient said in the history or what the doctor found on the physical exam is poor and often missing. Also, if a medical assistant takes the history, another assistant does an exam and the doctor does not bother to edit or add to them, credibility is lacking. Care in a university setting sounds wonderful, but as Trevor Smith found, any setting can miss the mark. Lack of detail in an exam can be tragic. The lack of detail in records can also create many problems.

We notice that public relations for HMO health plans are often more important than health care itself. VIPs and squeaky wheels are cared for more promptly. In other words, they "get the grease." Neglect of quiet patients may be inadvertent, but it may not be benign neglect. Conditions that are unusual or complex are common in orthopedic surgery.

The Miracle of Pain

They are disasters waiting to happen. Unless it is an emergency, an unusual medical or surgical problem often takes a back seat. Some people and some physicians say that HMOs are "not that bad." In some ways, they have gotten better.

In the 1970s and 1980s, they did not pay enough to attract the best physicians. They had a problem recruiting physicians. What changed? There are two major changes. First, HMO allied companies have made a lot of money and are paying their physicians better than they did. Second, physicians are finding it much easier to go to ready-made HMO practices. They go along with the economic flow. Heavy pressures on solo or small private practices from an intrusion of government and big insurers have been increasing over several decades. As a result, fewer young, bright physicians are willing to take the business risks necessary to start or buy into a practice without HMO contracts.

HMOs, PPOs, Workers' Compensation, Medicare, Medicaid, military medicine and Veterans Affairs health care are only a part of the government medicine machine. Big insurance companies and government contractors are taking over many aspects of care illegally. State and federal officials look the other way and use the excuse that it is "to protect the patient." Where has trust in physicians gone? Where are government insurance plans leading us? With a single payor or few payors, there is no competition. "Elites" in government and some in academia want us to trust them. They want us to let them or their large insurance allies sort out who is a good doctor and who is not. They discourage us from thinking that we, as patients and physicians, are smart enough or diligent enough to protect ourselves.

Word of mouth referrals and critiques from a credible person still offer significant, reliable protection. It is more reliable than credentialing by insurance companies or ratings by websites or magazines. Physicians without hidden motives still provide timely referrals to excellent local doctors. Despite the erosion of trust in doctors, many good doctors still give excellent care and compassionate service. Their patients trust them for the most part after doing their online homework.

Experiences with something unusual like reflex sympathetic dystrophy (RSD) of the hand, wrist and fingers are chilling. The problems are compounded when treated under Workers' Compensation, HMO or other managed care coverage. The worsening pain and stiffness from full-blown RSD is intimidating for any doctor to treat and is hard to watch. Often, an orthopedic surgeon sees it initially. Some will punt and send the patient elsewhere because RSD is difficult and time consuming to treat. Patients with RSD tend to be frustrated, and they are frustrating to the doctor. To many patients, it sounds good when the doctor says, "I want to send you to a pain specialist." It sounds good because the patient has already sensed that the doctor has lost interest in trying to help them.

Likewise, there has been similar punting for poor spine surgery results. The fallout of that approach in the 1990s built up the pain management specialty. The impulse to punt after spine surgery by orthopedic surgeons and neurosurgeons should not happen. Surgical training programs in the 1970s and 1980s fairly uniformly taught that if you operate on a patient, you "marry" them. In other words, you do not abandon them. The patient can always abandon the doctor, but the surgeon should never abandon the patient. That approach has waned with the influence of government sponsored HMOs since the 1970s and government allowed PPOs since the 1980s. Punting leaves fewer headaches for the surgeon to follow up on. It unleashes incentives to do a high volume of surgeries though indications for the surgeries may be marginal.

A very common cause of hand RSD is a wrist fracture. The incidence is about 5 percent of wrist fractures. The onset is often after the fracture has healed, 1 to 2 weeks after the cast is off. Normally after a cast is taken off, we ask patients to move the wrist joint to get rid of stiffness. If they, instead, try to move it by using it to get things done, the results can be frightening. Swelling, stiffness, a dusky discoloration and pain can increase quickly, and RSD occurs when a patient is going in the wrong direction. It is a recovery phase problem after an injury, surgery or other stimulus.

For many injuries, we normally start to lengthen out the time between office visits after 1 to 2 months. That is the most common time for RSD to occur. At the earliest suggestion of RSD, bringing the patient back earlier for an office visit is helpful. However, the sooner RSD occurs after an injury or surgery, the denser and more resistant the symptoms tend to be. Patients who start getting RSD symptoms more than 3 months after the injury usually develop milder symptoms. A hand crush injury is less common than a wrist fracture. However, the crush injury has a much higher rate of RSD, approaching 70 percent. Small hand injuries with complications such as a nerve injury have an RSD incidence rate of 5 percent, similar to a wrist fracture. Minor injuries to the hand tend to have a low incidence rate of less than 1 percent.

Elizabeth Parker, a right-handed hospital manager, had a paper cut of her right middle finger at work in 2006. I saw her in the emergency room for the first time a few days after the injury. At that time, she had skin and soft-tissue death at the site of the paper cut (necrosis). She also had an infection of the entire middle finger in the soft tissues (cellulitis). It could have also involved the closed channels of the flexor tendons (infectious tenosynovitis). I hospitalized her and ordered intravenous antibiotics for her. I also called an infectious disease consultant who saw her later in the day for optimal antibiotic coverage.

The signs of infection cleared in a day or two with the intravenous antibiotics. However, skin and soft-tissue death on the thumb side of her middle finger increased at the paper cut, near the middle knuckle (proximal interphalangeal joint). In the operating room, I explored the wound and cut away the dead fatty tissue and dead skin (debridement). The finger sensory nerve was intact but was dangling across the open wound. The bed of the wound had no blood supply or healing tissues. A skin graft or a skin and soft-tissue flap graft would not have survived. Tendons and tendon linings were normal.

As dressing changes continued, slowly over a few days, healing of the soft tissues appeared (granulation tissue). When the wound base began to appear healthy, I gave her the option of a skin graft or a flap graft. The patient declined. The new healing soft tissues encased the nerve. I offered to free the nerve or remove it, but she again declined. After a few weeks at home, the skin healed fully, but the patient began wondering if she wanted to keep the finger. It was becoming increasingly stiff and painful. Stiffness was accumulating in the other fingers and thumb of the same hand. There was also stiffness in the wrist. Her Workers' Compensation insurance adjuster authorized limited hand and wrist therapy with an occupational therapist. The patient noticed some improvement.

Elizabeth kept trying to use her hand, but it was getting her into trouble. Stopping her from using it was difficult. She also tried going back to modified work, but it caused more pain, swelling and stiffness. She had to stop. Her fingers, hand and wrist had an abnormal, clawed appearance. This posture of the hand included flexion of the index, middle, ring and little fingers at the middle and end joints. There was also mild hyperextension at the base of the same fingers.

When trying to flex the fingers, she started by actively flexing the wrist and then the fingers (palmar flexion). That strained the finger flexor muscles and fed into a painful vicious cycle. She kept trying active motion and tended to avoid using easier passive motions even when encouraged. After showing her many times, she slowly began using passive motions. She also tended to use irritating isolated finger motions, but she was slowly willing to learn better ways.

By 2 years after the injury, Elizabeth's basic hand function and motion had improved towards normal. She told me that she was glad that she did not have an amputation. However, she had limited strength and endurance for using the hand and middle finger. The skin was healed, but she had a soft-tissue deformity of her middle finger. It was ⅜ inch wide, ¾ inch long and ⅛ inch deep on the palm and thumb sides of the finger. There was shrinkage of the soft tissues at the tip of the finger (atrophy). She could use the tip of her finger for limited tasks, but she had to watch her finger as she used it, so she did not bump or traumatize it. Sensation of the finger was abnormal on both sides, more on the thumb side.

The Miracle of Pain

In the beginning within a short amount of time, her paper cut spiraled out of control. It developed infection, pain, soft-tissue death, nerve damage and reflex sympathetic dystrophy of the fingers, hand and wrist. Her experiences show the early and late effects of infection and RSD on top of the effects of the injury. Within 2 months of the injury, the patient was wondering about amputation. Her other fingers and the rest of her dominant arm could have easily been worse with a middle finger amputation because RSD tends to spread. In addition, she would be missing a finger. Elizabeth learned to appreciate her limited use of her right middle finger and hand. That attitude helped her to improve by more faithfully staying within her limits.

In patients with a healed wrist fracture who develop RSD, the pain, stiffness and swelling tend to spread easily from the wrist to the hand and fingers. Before finger stiffness accumulates, the right movements will minimize stiffness, pain, swelling and the discoloration from stagnation of blood flow in the veins. They should use passive motion for gentle flexion of the wrist with extension of the fingers and then relaxation, using 3 to 4 repetitions (wrist palmarflexion). They should follow that with gentle passive extension of the wrist and flexion of the fingers, again with a few repetitions (wrist dorsiflexion). If without pain, this will allow better muscle relaxation. Then eventually, making a fist becomes possible.

This pattern is the opposite of what those with hand and wrist reflex sympathetic dystrophy tend to do. The error is trying to flex the fingers by flexing the wrist. Then, to extend the fingers, they try extending the wrist. Those motions are counterproductive and quickly cause muscle strains, tendinitis, stiffness and swelling. Another error is trying to use the hand to get things done. We can see a normal looking hand and wrist in as little as 7 to 10 days develop an alarming amount of pain, swelling, stiffness, discoloration, muscle cramps, muscle spasm and muscle irritability.

The farther down the vicious cycle path the patient goes, the journey back is harder. If a patient is willing to learn and change, they can always improve. They need to learn motions that help the pain and do not hurt. They need to avoid doing things because doing things causes muscle tension and strain. Muscle tension means that the muscle is tighter than normal muscle tone. It always causes problems. Prolonged positions of the hand below the heart will add to the same problems. Isolated, active flexion motions of one finger, which RSD patients tend to do repeatedly, can cause muscle strains and tendinitis. After a delay of an hour or so, painful abnormalities then easily multiply. These movements in a normal hand may feel awkward. In a hand with RSD, they are painful and more quickly counterproductive.

We should flex our fingers together passively when trying to resolve pain, stiffness or swelling. Using the other hand to gently help is often the best way to start. The same should be said for extension. After combined passive motion is reestablished, some limited, isolated passive or active movements of the fingers are okay if they feel good. An example could be extending the index finger or little finger for pointing. Each of those movements are possible because of two specific forearm muscles which are for that purpose (extensor indicis proprius and extensor digiti minimi). Spreading or separating the fingers is less important but is okay passively when the patient does not overdo it and when the motion feels good.

Passive motions tend to create fewer problems. An example of passive motion of the little finger is the Boy Scout sign. We make the sign with the right thumb holding down the right little finger in a flexed position passively while extending the other three fingers actively (Picture 19). Because the thumb is helping the little finger, the motion is passive for the little finger. When the left hand helps instead, the passive motion is even easier. Passive motions use help from another body part, gravity or any surface to push. I am not sure what the resistance to doing passive motions is. It may be that they are too easy to overdo and thereby cause pain. To get good at not overdoing them, we must remind ourselves to do passive motions easier, more slowly and more carefully, but we should do them often.

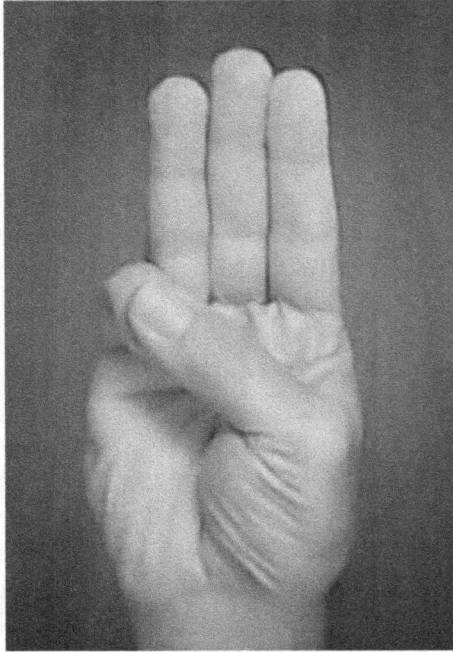

Picture 19, Scout sign

Small motions, elevation and time are other tools that will solve pain if the muscles relax. That allows movement without reinjury. Injury, amputation and phantom pain are bad enough, but reflex sympathetic dystrophy added on top of them can be much worse. Learning what to do and learning to severely limit activity along the way can help to resolve some very frightening vicious cycles.

Chapter 33

"Give Up All My Vices?"

Habits, good or bad, become patterns of behavior that directly affect our ability to avoid pain as well as recover from pain. Bad habits such as eating too much, taking excessive risks or frequently going to bed late are destructive. They are a form of self-abuse. The consequences of them include obesity, risky behavior injuries and being tired during the day. Controlling what and how much we eat, assessing and controlling risk and going to bed early are good habits. They can improve our health and our minds.

Keeping our minds active and strong is like exercising muscles. Using our brain for reading good literature and memorizing songs, poems or scripture verses builds them. Good habits are a challenge to cultivate, yet they are worth every effort. Hope for good things in the future is a motivating force needed to develop a good habit. Because overuse of a good habit may turn it into a bad habit, we must prioritize, balancing good activities and habits. When trying to overcome a bad habit, it helps to think of a good habit to replace it. We then have something to look forward to.

Without the desire to change, bad habits and vices can become worse and more engrained. Those who become involved with bad habits frequently describe them as "chains." There is a loss of choice. We have no choice but to accept the consequences of the bad habit until we change. The longer we go without changing, the harder change is. Then, we will find more adverse effects. Bad habits create dependency, addiction, weakness and captivity. Bad habits are voluntary enslavement. We call them "bad" for good reasons. Bad habits are easy to develop, and there are many. Replacing a bad habit with another bad habit is not helpful.

For obesity, of course, controlling the amount of food we eat, measured in kilocalories (Kcal) is a good idea. If a person focuses on food all day long, including what to eat and what not to eat, food becomes a habit or a fixation. Eating is a necessity, but we can find better things in life to spend our time on. For those who have a desire to lose weight, we should lose an average of 1 pound per week. Decreasing food intake by decreasing portion size of all parts of the meal is the key. This slow weight loss is safer and more effective in forming better eating habits than losing weight quickly. Though slow, the above two tools result in a weight loss of 50 pounds per year. Use the same weight scale each day. Pick a reasonable weight goal for your height. It does not matter how long it takes if we are going in the right direction.

Using a balanced diet with 7 food groups is important. The 7 food groups in the order of amounts our body needs are water, grains, vegetables, fruit, dairy, protein/meat and oil. Each of the 7 food groups are a necessity. Desserts are not a food group and are not a necessity! Do not worry about water weight changes. They will vary as much as 3 to 5 pounds from day to day. Stay well hydrated with water, so the urine is clear once or twice a day. Water can diminish appetite and cravings before meals. It can do the same at the end of meals. Water sounds too simple, but it works.

Having an increased activity level more often is vital. Sitting on a couch or at a computer is okay, but we need to balance that with other physical activity. It can simply be reading a book, checking on the yard, exploring the neighborhood or talking to a neighbor. Immense sources for learning new things are available to us through reading. An active mind that learns, creates or figures things out is using more kilocalories than a brain passively engaged with a TV show or movie entertainment. The kilocalories we use for reading while sitting are 50 percent greater than watching TV. Desk work, compared to watching TV, burns over 100 percent more kilocalories.[101] Active games are better for exercise and for the ability to properly focus compared to repetitive card or video games. At first, learning something new can be difficult. It puts us on a path to form good habits and learn new things that will easily replace overeating or other bad habits.

---

[101] Harvard Health Publications, Harvard Medical School, "Calories burned in 30-minute activities," Table from the July 2004 issue of the Harvard Heart Letter, www.health.harvard.edu/diet-and-weight-loss/calories-burned-in-30-minutes-of-leisure-and-routine-activities, accessed May 9, 2018.

Landing a skateboard trick gives a skateboarder an addicting adrenaline rush. Limited success with risky behavior can contribute to more risky behavior. Those thriving on it never know when an accident will occur. Increasingly, they become willing to accept the risk. Doing something that has a 10 percent risk and doing it 10 times creates a 100 percent probability of the risk occurring, assuming no improvement. Worse, risky behavior allows injuries and permanent physical limitations to accumulate. Before doing something with risk, we often do not think of all the consequences.

On a snow campout in February 2003, our Boy Scout troop planned to go to higher elevations for better snow after breakfast. One of our scouts, Sam Reed decided not to wait. After I asked him not to do it, he slid down a nearby snowy hill. Because he cut his shin on the campground table metal leg, we could not go to higher and better snow. While he propped his cleansed, bandaged leg up in the car, the other scouts played in the snow at our campsite for an hour. Then we took Sam to the emergency room for stitches, which was well within the 6-hour golden period for closing a wound. Taking risks not only affects us but often those around us.

Common risky behaviors include smoking, fast driving, gambling, hiking alone in the mountains and dealing with dishonest people. Impaired driving with alcohol, marijuana or drugs is also very risky. In the emergency room at Riverside Community Hospital, I saw many patients with multiple trauma from automobile accidents. It is a Trauma II hospital in the center of five nearby freeways. While taking orthopedic trauma call there for 30 years, until December 2009, I noticed a high percentage of patients with alcohol on their breath. The stench of alcohol on a patient's breath is etched in my brain. Also, trauma patients or their families often offered their observations that the other driver, who hit the patient, was drunk or had alcohol in the car. Impaired driving from alcohol is a greatly dismissed and an under-reported tragedy. It injures and kills many individuals who are not drinking alcohol.

In the last 15 years of my orthopedic practice, I noticed an alarming trend. About 90 percent of the orthopedic multiple trauma patients in the emergency room were from motor vehicle accidents with alcohol present. Several of my emergency room physician colleagues agreed with that percentage. This experience is much higher than the 40 percent of critical injuries that are alcohol-involved motor vehicle accidents during the same time, estimated by the National Highway Traffic Safety Administration (NHTSA).[102] According to them, one third of all Americans will be involved in an alcohol-impaired crash during their lifetime.[103]

The 2016 data published in October 2017 by the National Highway Traffic Safety Administration, continues to focus on the 10,497 fatalities involving 9,885 drivers with a blood alcohol concentration (BAC) of at least 0.08 grams per deciliter (g/dl). What they did not emphasize were the additional 2,044 drivers in 2016 who were involved with motor vehicle fatalities with less alcohol.[104] Tragically, the number of injuries is much larger. Over an estimated half million injuries and fatalities occur in the United States per year in the presence of alcohol with levels of 0.01g/dl or greater.[105]

Although the presence of alcohol does not establish fault, alcohol is a prominent factor in the numerous ongoing road and highway tragedies. Injuries, disability and death related to alcohol are much more common than they should be. Driving after drinking alcohol is an abuse of the privilege to drive. The curse of injuries and property damage, for both innocent and alcohol-involved persons, remains striking and

[102] National Highway Traffic Safety Administration, Lawrence J. Blincoe, Angela G. Seay, MSc, Eduard Zaloshnja, Ph.D., Ted R. Miller, Ph.D., Eduardo O. Romano, Ph.D., et al., "The economic impact of motor vehicle crashes, 2000," May 2002, DOT HS 809 446, MAIS 5 on page 36, tables 8 and 10, crashstats.nhtsa.dot.gov/#/, accessed May 10, 2018.
[103] National Highway Traffic Safety Administration, "Risky Driving, Drunk Driving Overview," www.nhtsa.gov/risky-driving/drunk-driving, accessed April 7, 2017—website screenshot available, "Overview" changed since then.
[104] National Highway Traffic Safety Administration, "Traffic Safety Facts, 2016 Data, Alcohol-Impaired Driving," October 2017, DOT HS 812 450, page 6, crashstats.nhtsa.dot.gov/#/, accessed May 9, 2018.
[105] National Highway Traffic Safety Administration, Robert B. Voas, John C. Lacey, "Alcohol and Highway Safety 2006: A Review of the State of Knowledge," March 2011, DOT HS 811 374, pages 9, 12 and 35, www.nhtsa.gov/sites/nhtsa.dot.gov/files/811374.pdf, accessed May 9, 2018.

underappreciated. Research measurements for driving skills have gradually improved in sensitivity. In the year 2000, a published technical literature review showed, "strong evidence that impairment of some driving-related skills begins with any departure from zero BAC. By 0.05 g/dl, the majority of studies have reported impairment by alcohol. By BACs of 0.08 g/dl, 94 percent of the studies reviewed reported impairment."[106]

Vices create problems that impact all of us. We can deal with them more effectively. That would include more individual responsibility and swift punishment for crimes that are committed. Those who shield offenders from personal consequences are enabling their behavior. Problems with healing are known to increase with drinking, smoking, obesity, risky behavior and high levels of activity. Problems include a delayed recovery, including delayed fracture healing, loss of fracture position in casts or after surgery, vein clots and infection. Bad habit patterns or vices slowing a recovery from pain, injury or surgery also affect those around us.

Patients occasionally ask, "Does that mean I have to give up all my vices?" It depends on what they want. Do they want the best chance of healing and want a chance to get back to normal? If yes, each vice or bad habit we choose to give up is an opportunity for improvement and wonderful benefits. That will not happen until we have decided to do better and to make changes that we know are right. Change may be difficult, but it will be worth it. We will be less likely to suffer from chronic pain and injuries that do not heal.

Do you have trouble waking up? Are you tired in the morning, or are you sleepy in the afternoon? Are you "a late person?" I want to challenge those who are trying to recover from injuries or surgery to give going to bed early a try. Early means going to bed with lights out by 10:30 PM. You will be more refreshed in the morning and have a better energy level

[106] National Highway Traffic Safety Administration, Herbert Moskowitz, Ph.D., Dary Fiorentino, "A Review of the Literature on the Effects of Low Doses of Alcohol on Driving-Related Skills," April 2000, 4.1 Major Findings, www.nhtsa.gov/people/injury/research/pub/hs809028/Discussion.htm#Major, accessed May 9, 2018.

even if you do not fall asleep right away. You may have to toss and turn frequently. You may have to get up for a few minutes at a time, but do not stay up. The effect of going to bed early is energizing and is much more natural and effective than pills will ever be for normal sleep. If you have any doubts, take my challenge by trying it every day for a week. Remember, most young children get up by 6:00 in the morning. They are excited to play, learn and have a quick breakfast. We may not have their energy level, but we can do better than we have been doing with our bad habits. Try getting up by 6 AM without any caffeine, and see what you can accomplish in the quiet of the morning.

Some medical leaders continue to push for a group mentality instead of individual responsibility. Large studies of populations may play a role in learning what is needed, but they create gaps in individualized thinking and treatment. We have given little attention to a greater need for patient participation in choices and options after a full discussion with the patient by the doctor. We hear little concern from medical leaders about the need for individual responsibility in many health issues. That includes individual responsibility for the consequences of obesity, brain injury, depression, diabetes mellitus and automobile accidents with multiple trauma. Most football players know that their head is at risk.

Life is a wonderful teacher. Being here on earth gives each of us a responsibility to learn. Each person is a son or daughter of two parents who brought them into this life. If we are a son, daughter, mother, father, brother or sister, each role carries a responsibility. Other roles add to our responsibilities. For both patients and physicians, our choices during this mortal existence also have consequences that follow us in time. The example we set affects us and others around us. Many seem to want to forget our individual responsibilities. Those who binge on Halloween candy or those who abuse drugs will have more consequences than they realize at the time. Those who engage in risky behavior will have more consequences that catch up to them than they will admit. They are too busy rationalizing their behavior to admit that anything is wrong.

Some of life's problems come for unknown reasons. Challenges also come our way because of the faults of others. Can we forgive them? We must, or their behavior affects our behavior and healing. Giving forgiveness to others heals our wounds, but anger keeps our wounds festering. All problems are not because someone else crashes into us or because our parents or genetics do it to us. If our individual choices are part the problem, why do we want to ignore that? If our choices are the entire problem, why would we ignore that? Will doctors, governments or our families protect us from ourselves if we refuse to make better choices? Doctors or governments may promise a lot, but their track records are poor without us doing our part. Our part is taking as much responsibility as we are able. Then, using our conscience, we can make the best choices possible. We should learn from our choices and accept responsibility for those choices.

Most patients do not want to hurt themselves. A patient hurting themselves intentionally is a form of abuse and can be part of their bad habits. Malingering is faking pain. Disuse is different than both abuse and malingering. Disuse is when a patient does too many of the wrong things and not enough of the right things to help their body heal. This can be true even for something as simple as an ankle sprain. Disuse occurs frequently in the same day or even in the same hour without us realizing it. Most patients are not aware of it happening.

Disuse is not intentional. It occurs from pride about what we think we know and also from what we do not know. Disuse is going in the wrong direction, sometimes 180 degrees in the wrong direction. It begins when a patient does something to cause setbacks. Even little setbacks can do it. If we have occasional setbacks, disuse continues. It can happen after an injury, after a surgery or with a disease. Disuse is sometimes merely from going back to activity too soon. It can be from putting weight on a leg sooner than is prudent.

With the use of crutches, a patient can protect an ankle sprain. But they may not understand that the length of time up on the crutches is the reason that the swelling is not going away. Sitting at a computer can be worse because of the lack of movement. Appropriate elevation and protection for a reasonable time after the ankle sprain helps swelling. Then, in the correct directions, working on range of motion helps. At first, we can do up and down motions. However, movement in the direction of the sprain done too early will reinjure the ligament and delay the recovery (ankle inversion or eversion). Too early means within 2 weeks for a minor sprain (grade I). It means 4 weeks for a moderate ligament injury without instability (grade II). And it is 6 weeks for a complete ankle ligament tear (grade III injury).

Ignoring pain or swelling adds to the manifestations of disuse. Amounts of swelling or pain that are out of proportion to what we expect for the degree of injury are signs of disuse. If swelling or pain lasts longer than we would expect for an injury, it is another sign of disuse. Increasing swelling or pain more than 2 or 3 days after an injury is another sign. Another manifestation of disuse is numbness or tingling in an entire arm or leg, especially if not present initially after an injury or a surgery. It may come and go and does not follow the pattern of a specific nerve. It happens from nerve irritability with tight muscles or persisting swelling affecting an area.

Signs of disuse can occur early or late after an injury, surgery or other triggering condition. Another sign of disuse is stiffness lasting longer than we would normally expect. Another sign is subtle, generalized, dusky discoloration of an entire arm or leg. This occurs because of large areas of stagnation in the veins (venous congestion). If unchecked, over time this can lead to large areas of increased pigmentation, especially common in front of the shins (stasis dermatitis with brawny discoloration). Within 3 months, disuse also leads to shrinkage or atrophy of muscle and weakening of bones with scattered visible holes in the bone on an x-ray (disuse osteoporosis).

Some features of disuse are also components of reflex sympathetic dystrophy (RSD). Those characteristics put disuse patterns and reflex sympathetic dystrophy in the same ballpark. Disuse is a beginning phase of going in the wrong direction. RSD is a faster and more dangerous, downward vicious cycle.

It adds more pain and other severe problems during the body's attempts to heal. With some exceptions, these severe problems are the consequences of our choices during recovery from injury or surgery. Exceptions may include previous nerve or vein damage and muscle stiffness from old injuries. Disuse may or may not evolve into reflex sympathetic dystrophy. The pain severity spectrum extends from mild pain with early disuse to severe pain with full-blown reflex sympathetic dystrophy. After several months there can be mild to severe atrophy from chronic disuse or reflex sympathetic dystrophy.

Keys for resolving disuse are recognition, turning around and going in the right direction. Helping the patient to see the right direction and learn what to expect with better choices are always important. Elevation at or above the heart level and movement of joints that do not need immobilization are important to help the swelling and pain. Then, for most areas, keeping the time in upright positions limited is critical to resolve swelling and help healing. The exceptions are the shoulders, neck and head, which are naturally elevated in upright positions.

If it does not add stiffness, light strengthening may start after basic healing when the swelling is gone. The sequence is light resistance, progressing to light use, then heavier resistance strengthening and interval training for endurance. Each step in the recovery process should be slow enough to minimize risk and avoid reinjury. It takes less of an injury to cause a reinjury. Minimal repeated reinjury can create a disuse pattern at any stage along the recovery path. Disuse slows or stops recovery if not recognized and changed. We should always be alert for and recognize other explanations for disuse symptoms, such as bleeding complications, clots and cancer, and we must deal with them first.

All of our vices, habits and choices have consequences, whether we are aware of them or not. Learning better ways can be fun. It is an adventure that opens many exceptional opportunities to heal and recover fully!

Chapter 34

"I Have Good Days and Bad Days"

I love to ask patients during follow-up visits, "How are you doing?" A common answer for a patient struggling with persisting pain is, "I have good days and bad days." Often that answer comes at a time when patients are not sure where they are going. Their answer may show some complacency, a degree of hopelessness or some frustration. Then I ask them, "How many good days have you had in a week?" Many do not know. Most others must think about it because they have not paid enough attention to the pain to put a number on it for a time period. Even if the number of days varies, there is an average, and we should record it. If patients quantify it, we have a better idea of where they are in their recovery.

Patients with good and bad days usually offer no explanation for the bad days. They seem to want to forget them. Often, the patient is in a rut with persisting acute pain or with chronic pain that is going nowhere. It is like they are on a boat without a rudder, tossed on waves of the sea. They have no ability to get where they want to go. The observation by a patient that they have good and bad days acknowledges a change in the pain from day to day. They compensate for the probability that bad days will keep coming back by doing more on their good days. They feel that they have little control over the pain. Usually they do not see the reasons or factors contributing to the bad days.

The good and bad days, however, create an opportunity for me to ask them more questions. I want to make them think about what they are doing. If we can help patients pay attention to their pain, they will eventually understand it better. Pain never stays the same. Ups and downs are normal for pain and for life. Except for truth, nothing in this world stays the same, especially pain. As we learn a basic truth about our pain, our choices expand by learning how to use what we have discovered and how often to use it. Our understanding of principles about pain adjusts over time as we apply them.

Patients who continue to have good and bad days should recognize that the choices they make when they have a good day usually contribute to their bad days. They tend to minimize the significance of their choices by saying, "I hardly did anything." That means that they do not understand what is contributing to the pain. What are the influences on choices that contribute to having bad days? On good days, patients are easily tempted to do too much. They feel guilty for not doing things. Others often encourage them to exercise or be active, so they, "do not become weak." Patients do not want to be labeled as "a wimp."

Doing things on good days is also tempting because patients know that when it gets bad again they, "cannot get anything done." Having them verbalize what they did and did not do is difficult because they often do not remember very well. Verbalizing what they did helps them remember and learn from their choices. Regarding what caused the good days, unless patients are paying attention, they have no idea. They may think that they had some good luck that day. We should reassure patients that things they had to do on their bad days contributed to their good days. The things they did right may be because they could not do anything else or because they had to behave.

Doing small things right can be spontaneous and without knowing it. Learning can occur with patients noticing little things they did that were right. That knowledge allows them to remember to use those little things. Then, they can use them more often. Learning can continue by helping patients sort out their choices that were significant and those that were not. Helping them understand requires asking both specific and open-ended questions. Their answers allow opportunities for important follow-up questions to understand better and to help them think of other things they have forgotten.

Occasionally, a patient only wants me to tell them what to do and what not to do without learning anything else. I can give examples to them, but covering every situation is impossible. They should learn from what they feel and use principles. The tasks of learning and using principles are harder than being told what to do. If the patient or the doctor learns little during the visit, then little if any learning happens before the next visit, and the patient suffers. The doctor learning from the patient is as important as the patient learning from the doctor. Changes in pain are good. If the pain level were constant, no matter what the patient did, there would be no hope of learning what to do and what not to do. Even if pain never goes away, it always changes intensity.

When the pain level goes up and down enough, there will usually be a time without pain. It might be gone for only a few seconds or minutes at a time. The amount of time that pain is absent may change, allowing us to learn at different levels. Resolving pain at a higher recovery level with longer periods without pain requires more learning. A good question to ask is, "What is your longest period of time without pain in the past week?" The answer helps us know where the patient is. We can ask the same question for any warning sign, such as swelling, numbness or popping.

Nothing stays the same in our amazing, but imperfect, mortal bodies. When a patient says, "The pain is still the same," they rarely offer details. We need to ask questions. If they say that the pain is constant and never changes, patients are either not paying attention to the pain or malingering. Some rationalize the use of alcohol or drugs to avoid feeling pain and are okay with being mindless. Some people are proud of their ability to ignore pain and tend to continue in the same direction in spite of pain.

Those approaches come at a huge cost. Not paying attention to pain is not very smart and has led to the axiom, "no pain, no brain." Patients and others around them give the other adage, "no pain, no gain," as a reason for putting up with pain and pushing through it. That is a distortion of its original meaning. When we understand both sayings correctly, they are right. They denote a need to learn from pain and to not keep making the same mistakes. Succinctly, the sayings encourage us to use our brain and to not be afraid to learn.

Something needs to remind us of a principle more than once before we learn, remember and apply it. Repetition is how most of us learn and get good at something. In diverse situations, the application of truth may be a challenge to learn.

I had to learn not to be frustrated with patients who asked the same question multiple times. They merely asked a question. It did not matter whether patients were challenging my judgment or not. I simply had to tell myself, "Just answer the question." If I did that, they learned, and I learned. We were both uplifted. If we keep making the same mistakes, we have not taken the time and made the effort to learn, remember and apply what we have received from good sources.

If we can learn from big ups and downs in pain levels, we can also learn from small ups and downs. Not only are good and bad days important to learn from, good and bad hours and minutes are important to learn from as well. Pain intensity changes minute to minute and hour to hour, not just day to day. To be able to learn from little ups and downs, patients have to put in the time and effort to learn from what they feel. That takes focusing on it as well as trial and error. After patients have learned from their experiences, the application of what they have learned is the hardest part. It takes remembering, patience, endurance and diligence, all of which are not easy.

If we make a mistake every few days that causes pain, how far are we going to get with that? If we are not improving or worsening, to turn it around, we must be willing to learn why. When we are learning what not to do and doing most of what we should be doing, the healing process can speed up as we avoid mistakes to a more normal rate. Even if we feel only slow improvement, we know that we are going in the right direction, and it is reassuring. With a chronic back sprain, patients going in the right direction will notice a difference within 3 weeks and a big difference within 3 months. Many other musculoskeletal conditions respond in similar periods.

Many patients with chronic pain have expressed to me the wish to be able to, "heal like a child." I have pondered that plea many times. Over the years, I have seen children recover from both little injuries and from life-threatening injuries. I have seen children die from illnesses or injuries. Children are brave, trusting and willing to learn. The wish of an older patient to heal like a child may indicate they fear that healing will take longer than they would like. Patients also fear that they will not heal. Admitting that we are not as young as we used to be is okay. Most of us do not want to go back and relive our childhood over again. Nevertheless, some child-like qualities are good to learn from and use.

Children have a natural curiosity and a willingness to learn from what they feel. They easily learn from surrounding sources. Especially under 8 years of age, children are honest, innocent and less polluted by misinformation from the adult world. Children do not like pain. On the other hand, many adult patients with chronic pain express pride that they, "have a high tolerance for pain." Some adults have told me that they thought they were getting better because it was hurting. A friend or even a therapist may have told them that, "it has to hurt before it is going to get better." That approach of rationalizing and ignoring pain is false. A child with a high pain tolerance heals more like an adult. Children with a high pain tolerance are uncommon. They tend to have slower healing rates and higher rates of complications.

We see a dramatic difference in most children compared to adults when we notice what children do with pain after an injury. If a child comes to my office with a broken leg, they know not to move it. They have already tried moving it, and it hurt. If the parents reach for the leg to help the child, the child cries in anticipation. Or, if I reach for the leg to examine it, the child screams like someone is torturing them. After the leg cast is on, the child gains confidence quickly because they feel relief of pain. Then I show them how they can move their exposed toes without pain. Most children then begin to do it spontaneously without any other encouragement before they leave the office. When they return home, a child has a natural tendency to hold back on activity until they have confidence the pain is gone. After that, holding them back from doing things can be difficult but is necessary.

Sometimes a parent gives pain medicine too readily. They try to help their child with a fracture remain without pain. Some have given doses regularly every 4 hours in anticipation of pain. Unfortunately, when anything close to that happens, the child cannot find their limits. The self-regulating pain mechanism lessens or is gone. Those children will often return with a destroyed cast and sometimes with a displaced fracture that was not initially displaced. It is from over activity. The parent may complain that they, "cannot stop them from running or jumping."

If that child is still receiving any pain medicine, stop it. That includes any over-the-counter pain medication, such as acetaminophen (Tylenol or other brand names). Then, as the child with a fracture feels pain again, they react accordingly. They quickly learn what to do and what not to do. They spontaneously limit their activity, including risky behavior. The child will maintain a good range of motion of the adjoining joints that we do not immobilize in a cast. They do not like pain. Encouragement by a parent in the right direction is a great help. They can teach the child the consequences of their good and bad choices.

After a leg or arm fracture heals, we take the cast off. We encourage the child to get the stiffness out by moving all the joints. To do that, we show them that it does not hurt if they warm-up to it and use movement in small amounts. It is important to show the child that the fracture does not hurt anymore by touching and pressing on the fracture site (palpation). As I answer the parent's questions, I look back and watch the child. Often, without the parent noticing, the child spontaneously tests the movements I had just encouraged. Children like the little motions because they feel good. At this critical time in fracture healing, children are not afraid.

We must caution both the parent and the child to hold back on activity and use. If a well-meaning parent instead encourages the child to use the leg or arm in spite of the instructions, the child usually figures it out and still holds back from using it. They do what feels good, but they test it. Most young children easily find their limits short of what it takes to cause pain. Initially, the child will limit use spontaneously. However, as the area continues to stay pain free, holding the child back from using the leg or arm is hard but again necessary. The child needs guidance by the doctor and encouragement by a parent in the right direction.

For a child's forearm fracture, the cast comes off 6 to 8 weeks after the injury. By then the x-rays usually show that the bone has healed enough. If so, we see a knot of new bone and no residual fracture line. But the bone strength is still only 90 percent. That amount of healing is enough for range of motion but not for activity. We cannot keep a cast on too long without causing significant stiffness of immobilized joints, especially the elbow. Follow-up x-rays are a huge help for judging the adequacy of the new bone healing.

Less than 100 percent bone strength means that with enough force the bone will break again at a weak spot (a stress riser). The force can be less than the original injury. A refracture can be defined as a reappearance of at least part of the original fracture line on an x-ray. It is not true that a bone is stronger after a fracture has healed, even if the new bone makes the bone look bigger. As a bone heals, it slowly approaches 100 percent strength with gradual use and maturation. The time needed for bone healing depends on the size of the bone and the quality of bone healing.

After the cast comes off, any activity where the child may fall should be avoided. For a healed forearm fracture, I need to tell the child and parent, "No horseplay with a brother or sister and no use of a scooter, skateboard or anything where they may fall for at least 1 month." The parents should help limit risky behavior. If the parents are not willing to help the child with that or if the child does not listen, they have an increased risk of refracture.

Most children will initially protect an arm or leg fracture sufficiently as it heals in a cast and then matures out of the cast. They must be held back from most activity as the strength returns in the bone and surrounding muscles. After an arm cast is off for 2 weeks and when the range of motion is good, the muscles surrounding the fracture are ready for gradual strengthening and use. At that time, the bone and muscles are still not ready for sports, high-level activity or risky activity.

In another month, the surrounding muscles can return to normal strength and the joints to normal flexibility. Those characteristics protect the bone from reinjury as bone strength also returns to normal. When muscle strength and joint flexibility are the same as the other side or at a higher level, the risk of reinjury will be greatly lessened. Questions about when a child is ready to return to gymnastics, soccer or other sports after a fracture are critically important. Repeat physical exams and repeat x-rays by an experienced orthopedic surgeon will help answer those questions.

What are the principles we can learn from children, so those of us with acute or chronic pain can heal injuries better and with fewer setbacks?

1. We should have a natural curiosity and willingness to learn new, simple things.
2. Do not be afraid to move if it does not hurt. You have to try it to know. Then, do it easy but often.
3. Do not ignore pain. Learn from it.
4. Trust good sources, and let a trusted medical doctor who will listen guide you through the maze.
5. If you use pain medication, stop it as soon as possible, especially before resuming activity.
6. Resolve stiffness with warm-ups and stretching before trying to do things and before strengthening.
7. Test limited use slowly as strength returns.

A youthful age is a help but is not the biggest element in healing. The size and location of the bone and the degree of injury are usually big factors. However, choices we make day to day and minute to minute are the most important controlling influences that can help or hurt healing. During healing, a lot of ups and downs in pain will slow the healing at any age. As we learn, we can look forward to more good days and have fewer bad days! If we expect no bad days at some point, we must continue to learn a better way, stop making mistakes and go more consistently in the right direction.

Now What?

The areas of pain I have focused on are mostly the back, neck, arms and legs. Unintentionally, some of the principles may apply to other areas of the body and sources of pain I have not mentioned. For example, stomach pain after eating jalapeños, chili pepper or other spicy food is always a warning sign that we should learn from. How often do we need to feel pain before we learn from it? Some patients have told me that they have a cast iron stomach and have no problems with hot sauce or other spicy foods. I have seen a lot of stomachs during my career and have never seen a cast iron stomach. Many of those who say they have "no problems" compensate with more food, milk, bread or medication (antacids, proton pump inhibitors and histamine-2 receptor antagonists). Others choose to ignore pain. All of them are accepting the risk level of the habits they have chosen.

Our bodies were not created to be able to withstand abuse for an unlimited amount of time. Yet, the amount of abuse we expect our bodies to take is astonishing. That we can learn from our experiences, if we are willing, is extraordinary. It is even better when we learn from the experiences of others, so we can avoid some of the problems they have had. As we learn and set a good example, others will learn from what we are doing. Although not popular, there is nothing wrong with saying, "I do not want any hot sauce." I have also said, "I like my stomach the way it is." Or we can say, "No thanks, I do not want to wear out my stomach." We are not missing any essential nutrients by avoiding spicy food.

If we keep abusing our stomach, back, knee or any other body part, the likelihood of wearing it out is high. If we try to delay it by using medications, the body gets accustomed to most of them and they become less effective. Also, the medications can only do so much, and they may have side effects of their own. Many cultures have some who are proud of their ability to "tolerate" spicy food or alcohol. They see it as a sign of bravado. However, many patients are hospitalized with bleeding ulcers from the use of alcohol or arthritis medications (NSAIDs). Too often, upper gastrointestinal bleeding can be lethal. If spicy or acidic foods give us stomach pain or heartburn, why would we not pay attention to that? Some cultural habits of risk taking are okay to get rid of. Why wait until we work ourselves into a corner that can be difficult to get out of?

The reasons for many medical conditions are not as clear and may not be a result of our choices. An example is frozen shoulder (adhesive capsulitis of the glenohumeral joint). Others are autoimmune diseases, many congenital deformities, many cancers and many injuries. However, the treatment we choose and our other hour-to-hour choices of what to do and what not do about them can determine how well things turn out. Knowledge of what frozen shoulder is and what to do and not do can help. Frozen shoulder is a stiffness and strain vicious cycle that becomes painful and disabling. Muscle spasm may come with it. Pain and a limited shoulder range of motion are moderate to severe.

Frozen shoulder often develops for no known reason. Or it starts within a few months of a shoulder injury, bursitis, fracture, surgery, heart attack, stroke or other stimulus. The pain can be difficult for patients, doctors and therapists to deal with. Within a few weeks of the onset, a mechanical block of joint movement develops from scar tissue that attaches to the surrounding structures (adhesions). We must stretch out the scar tissues with motion. A physical or occupational therapist is especially helpful when they give enough time to the patient. If improvement stalls, at the right stage of this condition an experienced orthopedic surgeon can do an outpatient shoulder manipulation without incisions. It helps the patient improve quickly. We do it during general anesthesia with relaxation of muscles given by an anesthesiologist.

We may prevent frozen shoulder with easy stretching if we avoid the vicious cycles of pain, strain and spasm. To keep from developing a frozen shoulder is much easier than recovering from it. It occurs often in middle-aged women and less often in middle-aged men. The key to solve it is early recognition of shoulder pain and stiffness. More advanced manifestations may include muscle pain and stiffness in surrounding areas of the shoulder girdle, neck and back. Some patients develop components of reflex sympathetic dystrophy of the arm and hand and are more difficult to deal with. Their symptoms may include swelling, burning pain, hypersensitivity to touch and a dusky arm and hand (shoulder-hand syndrome). Easy shoulder stretches can help the stiffness and pain of frozen shoulder. They employ the help of gravity, the help of the other hand or help from a table or wall. In the 1990s, I fine-tuned the motions because helping frozen shoulder patients by sending them to physical therapy became harder. Increasing overhead and declining insurance reimbursements were pushing physical and occupational therapists to decrease the time they spent with problematic patients.

After realizing the clear benefits of continuous passive motion (CPM) for the knee in the 1980s, we tried to apply the same principles to the shoulder. For all the available shoulder CPM devices, the patient was in a sitting position, and they had uncomfortable, fixed angles for the arm and elbow. The machines were expensive to rent, bulky and awkward. Patients often had increased pain with them. CPM machines were not as successful for the shoulder as they were for the knee. Knee CPM machines were used on a bed. They decreased scar tissue after joint fractures. They also decreased the need for knee manipulations after total knee replacement surgeries.

In 1995, I wanted to create a better shoulder CPM machine, and I drew out some plans. A medical equipment manufacturer gave me a price of $4,075 to build the prototype. While I was working on the patent application, however, I thought of a few more stretching variations. If they did not cause pain, patients could use them without the expense of a machine. As patients began using the exercise variations, I found more modifications. I put building the prototype and applying for the patent on hold.

The shoulder movement variations became an excellent tool and changed my desire to build a machine and hold a patent. Proper use of shoulder movement exercises is critical and includes doing them often, doing them consistently and avoiding pain with the exercises. Does that sound familiar? These principles are the same for all exercises, but a frozen shoulder is extremely sensitive. Shoulder stiffness and pain is easy to make worse. If an exercise causes pain, with or without therapy, the pain-spasm vicious cycle takes over and all progress stops. It becomes not only a physical block but also a mental block. Muscle pain inhibition from the brain is real and is a protective mechanism in response to pain.

Shoulder stretches with variations and modifications are dangling, using a table, hanging on and lying down:

1) In an upright position, dangle the arm by simply allowing the weight of it to stretch the shoulder muscles with gravity. With the hand hanging down straight, on the lap or somewhere in between, we can vary the amount of weight. We can have more variations by leaning the upper body slightly in different directions. We should keep repetitions less than 15 seconds each to keep them from hurting. If it feels good, come back to it often, but do not stay there.

2) In an upright position, lean towards a table. Slide the hand on the table away from the body with the opposite hand. Use a table with different heights or surfaces for variations. Use neutral arm rotation variations that are comfortable. More modifications are leaning forward and, at the same time, backing away from the table. These motions allow raising the shoulder without gravity at comfortable angles. Keep them short and without pain.

3) While standing, scoot the hand up a wall using the fingers with the palm on the wall. When the hand reaches a solid support on the wall, hang on to it and bend the knees to allow the arm to go up further. The support can be at various levels. The body can be at different angles to allow the most comfortable position. Help the arm back down.

4) In a horizontal position, help the hand up over the head in line with the body by pulling the wrist with

the opposite hand, allowing comfortable elbow and arm rotation. For variation, slide the hand or elbow on the back of a couch or a supportive surface.

Further stretching modifications are also important for individual adaptation. Each exercise repetition should be done with a short amount of range of motion, so the pain-spasm cycle is not initiated. This gives the patient and the muscles confidence that the repetitions will not hurt. More than 80 to 90 percent of the repetitions should not hurt, and as soon as possible, none of them should hurt. They should not do more than 4 to 5 repetitions at one time. Most of the repetitions should be done at 50 percent of the amount of motion it takes to cause pain.

If there is no pain, the last 1 to 2 repetitions can go further than 50 percent because the muscles have had a chance to warm up. On the last repetition, if the patient reaches the point where they would have felt pain but now feel none, they have accomplished something. Warming up well is crucial, but then not overdoing it is also important. These two principles break the vicious cycle of pain, spasm and stiffness. Patients should do warm-up repetitions often. Small cool-down repetitions afterwards can also be helpful.

Dangling the arm is one of the simplest stretches, but it is the most important to help break the pain-spasm cycle. Not overdoing the dangling weight or length of time is important. But again, come back to it often. If we do it to the point of pain, the pain-spasm cycle restarts and stiffness continues. After frequent dangling without pain for several days, add position and body angle variations.

Later, by moving the body, add small swinging motions of the arm. Dangling is more important than swinging because it allows muscle relaxation more consistently. Do not work on shoulder rotation because that will come easily later after the shoulder raising motion is full. By using shoulder stretching modifications and variations correctly, most frozen shoulder patients recovered within 2 to 3 months. Some were regaining near full motion and achieving no pain within 3 to 4 weeks without physical therapy.

Even with an underlying tear of the rotator cuff tendon, frozen shoulder rarely needs a surgical incision. Once stiffness from frozen shoulder is gone, the shoulder pain is gone. When they feel no pain and function is full, the patient with a rotator cuff tear is usually not interested in rotator cuff surgery and rightfully so. If they have recurrent pain, those patients with a rotator cuff tear may need surgery. With the pain and stiffness from frozen shoulder gone, patients will do better with surgery. The surgery can remove bone spurs and repair the rotator cuff tear. Those who have not resolved stiffness before surgery will struggle more with their recovery after surgery.

For frozen shoulder, some orthopedic surgeons have used arthroscopic surgery. In my experience, frozen shoulder does not need arthroscopic or any invasive surgery. By the year 2000, my stretching variations almost eliminated the need to do shoulder manipulations under anesthesia. Patients were regaining their shoulder motion and resolving their pain. With nonoperative care, orthopedic surgeons can solve many problems if we will try. We should only consider surgery when it is the best choice. With an attitude of learning and innovation, we can do many new, good things, both with and without surgery. A priority for all of us should be avoiding ineffective and unnecessary procedures.

The best reason for starting physical therapy is a patient not making progress on an easy home program within a few weeks. To be successful with frozen shoulder, a therapist must be willing to spend a little extra time during the first few visits even if not reimbursed for it. We should stop physical therapy if the patient is not making progress with it or if it stays painful. Patients can do the stretching exercise variations I have described without a machine. They can do them with or without physical therapy. Depending on the cause of the frozen shoulder, a patient who spends time with the stretches often and does them without pain will have a shorter recovery. Patience is always required.

Those of us, who have had pain for lengthy periods of time, dream of being pain free. Remembering what it is like to be without pain gets harder after several weeks. Because life goes on, the path to improve gets murky, especially after 2 to 3 months. Whether it is gastrointestinal ulcers, frozen shoulder, cancer or a fracture that is struggling to heal, how do we become pain free? The healing of pain is not fate, luck or coincidence. Besides using common sense, how do we obtain the best knowledge needed for a specific painful condition? Ask good sources, including a reputable medical doctor. You should be comfortable with them. They should have the proper medical or surgical training in the area that concerns you.

Another good source is God, our Creator. Ask Him, in the name of Jesus Christ, to help guide you and the doctor in the right ways. Do not be shy or afraid to pray to Him since all good things come from God. He knows our pains and knows that those pains will help us learn if we endure them well for the length of time that we must. Follow His counsel when you feel His comforting influence or hear His words in your mind that are right. When you find an answer, acknowledge His hand and give thanks to Him. The admonition to pray is not for religious persons only. All men and women in all nations and cultures everywhere have been invited by Him to pray. We should pray humbly and honestly seek Him. After seeing a vision, the apostle Peter learned a new concept he had not known. He described it by saying, "God is no respecter of persons: But in every nation he that feareth him, and worketh righteousness, is accepted with him."[107] Fearing God means to respect and trust Him, regardless of the setbacks we face.

The knowledge we need to be pain free is an ongoing battle that will continue to unfold as we look for and find answers. If many good answers are given to us quickly, often we cannot remember and use them all. We need things repeated, and we will need practice. Forgetting, resuming old habits and then losing the knowledge that we find is easy to do. Practice and diligent use are not easy. The work it takes to remember what we learn is worth the effort. Share large improvements with others. Do not underestimate the value of

[107] The Holy Bible, New Testament, Acts 10:34–35, written by Luke who quotes the apostle Peter, www.lds.org/scriptures/nt/acts/10?lang=eng, accessed May 9, 2018.

small improvements and the small things we learn. Be thankful for them. Others will not understand or want to hear about our small improvements. They will notice when our behavior changes for the better. They may notice our courage. When we form better habits and are consistent, they may learn from us and follow our good example.

Robert Louis Stevenson (1850–1894) described the courage it takes to make better choices, "Everyday courage has few witnesses. But yours is no less noble because no drum beats for you and no crowds shout your name."

Remember:

1) After all that you can do, learn to have patience in dealing with painful experiences.

2) A sudden loss of pain is always possible. Most often it is a gradual journey that teaches us along the way. Always have hope for a brighter, better tomorrow.

3) Be grateful for the challenges of pain, from which we can learn. We could not have learned the same things in an easier way. One of the purposes of life is to expand our capacities and knowledge.

4) Basic things that we learn from pain will help us lessen normal ups and downs of pain. Remember them, and use them often.

5) Learning to decrease pain takes practice. Do little things that are right consistently and faithfully.

6) Making mistakes and having recurrent pain along the way temporarily is normal. It is okay as long as we learn from it and do not keep making the same mistakes.

7) Get good at good habits, so they can replace bad habits.

8) Do not be afraid to lie down to resolve pain. Do not feel guilty when slowing down to resolve pain. Life goes on and gets busy quickly.

Our mortal body is a marvelous creation. If you are curious, experiment with good things you find. As I have, you will learn new things. Real science is honest and inquisitive.

Anyone can use it. True science is consistent with the reality of God. The beauty and order in the heavens, the earth and our souls imply that an eternal, loving, just and living God is behind it all, encouraging us onward and upward. That does not mean that our mortal life is fair. The adversary, Satan or Lucifer, is real and wants to pull us the wrong way. He teaches that God does not exist and that there is no devil. Satan teaches that we should not pray. He is the father of all lies and all evil in our mortal world. Because of misinformation in our world, many patients suffer because they lack the guidance of simple truths that God has already brought to light.

Seek for help with good advice from honest, competent, reliable sources, especially an honest medical doctor. There is no need to experiment with bad advice, marginal treatment or substandard approaches. They can be dangerous distractions. A better way to treat pain is not difficult though it takes a little more time. The knowledge and insights that are available to us are gifts to be used wisely. Many patients who have had pain have expressed gratitude for things they have learned and are using to lessen and resolve pain.

All of us have many painful experiences and challenges to learn from. I do not have all the answers for pain. When someone I know is in pain and asks for help, I love to listen and learn from them. If I can, I love to help them. I enjoy hearing about their results and what they have learned. Never lose hope. In a courageous heart, we can cultivate many good desires. In doing so, we can help ourselves and then those around us.

The Miracle of Pain

❧ Index ❧

Index

The Miracle of Pain

Notes

www.ingramcontent.com/pod-product-compliance
Lightning Source LLC
Chambersburg PA
CBHW021027210326
41598CB00016B/929